Health Fitness Management

Health Fitness Management

A Comprehensive Resource for Managing and Operating Programs and Facilities

SECOND EDITION

Mike Bates, MBA

University of Windsor

Refine Fitness Studio

EDITOR

Human Kinetics

Library of Congress Cataloging-in-Publication Data

Health fitness management : a comprehensive resource for managing and operating programs and facilities / Mike Bates, editor. -- 2nd ed.

p. cm.

Includes bibliographical references and index.

ISBN-13: 978-0-7360-6205-3 (hard cover)

ISBN-10: 0-7360-6205-X (hard cover)

1. Physical fitness centers--United States--Management. 2. Physical fitness--Study and teaching--United States. I. Bates, Mike, 1972-

GV428.5.H43 2007

613.7'068--dc22   2007029345

ISBN-10: 0-7360-6205-X

ISBN-13: 978-0-7360-6205-3

The Web addresses cited in this text were current as of August 2007, unless otherwise noted.

Acquisitions Editor: Michael S. Bahrke, PhD; **Developmental Editor:** Maggie Schwarzentraub; **Assistant Editors:** Jillian Evans and Kyle G. Fritz; **Copyeditor:** Alisha Jeddeloh; **Proofreader:** Erin Cler; **Indexer:** Bobbi J. Swanson; **Permission Manager:** Dalene Reeder; **Graphic Designer:** Nancy Rasmus; **Graphic Artists:** Patrick Sandberg, Tara Welsch, and Angela K. Snyder; **Cover Designer:** Keith Blomberg; **Photographer (cover):** © Banana Stock/Robertstock; **Photographer (interior):** © Human Kinetics, unless otherwise noted; **Photo Asset Manager:** Laura Fitch; **Visual Production Assistant:** Jason Allen; **Art Manager:** Kelly Hendren; **Associate Art Manager:** Alan L. Wilborn; **Illustrator:** Argosy; **Printer:** Edwards Brothers

Printed in the United States of America   10 9 8 7 6 5 4 3

The paper in this book is certified under a sustainable forestry program.

Human Kinetics
Web site: www.HumanKinetics.com

United States: Human Kinetics
P.O. Box 5076
Champaign, IL 61825-5076
800-747-4457
e-mail: humank@hkusa.com

Canada: Human Kinetics
475 Devonshire Road, Unit 100
Windsor, ON N8Y 2L5
800-465-7301 (in Canada only)
e-mail: info@hkcanada.com

Europe: Human Kinetics
107 Bradford Road
Stanningley
Leeds LS28 6AT, United Kingdom
+44 (0)113 255 5665
e-mail: hk@hkeurope.com

Australia: Human Kinetics
57A Price Avenue
Lower Mitcham, South Australia 5062
08 8372 0999
e-mail: info@hkaustralia.com

New Zealand: Human Kinetics
Division of Sports Distributors NZ Ltd.
P.O. Box 300 226 Albany
North Shore City, Auckland
0064 9 448 1207
e-mail: info@humankinetics.co.nz

This book is dedicated to all of the contributors.
This project would never have started or finished if it weren't for your involvement and expertise.

contents

contributors

Anthony Abbott, EdD
President, Fitness Institute International, Inc.

Brenda Abdilla
Management Momentum

Mike Bates, MBA
University of Windsor, Refine Fitness Studio

Karen Woodard Chavez
Premium Performance Training

Sandy Coffman
President and owner, Programming for Profit

Casey Conrad, JD
President, Communication Consultants
President, Healthy Inspirations

Terry Eckmann, PhD
Minot State University

Mike Greenwood, PhD
Professor, Baylor University

Dave Hardy, MBA
President, Club Fit Corp.

Kevin Hood, MEd
Operations director, Cherry Hills Country Club

Cheryl Jones
Vice president of programs and services, Town Sports International

Scott Lewandowski, MS
Regional fitness director, Fitness Formula Clubs

D. Jane Riddell, MA
COO, GoodLife Fitness Clubs

Bud Rockhill, MBA
President, Westwood College Online

John Wolohan, JD
Professor, Ithaca College

If you are looking for a fast-paced, constantly changing profession where you will have the opportunity to make a difference in the lives of thousands of people, then this book is for you. If you love interacting with people and motivating them to be the best they can be, then this book is for you. If you want to be a part of one of the fastest-growing and most challenging industries in the world, then this book is for you. If you are interested in a 9-to-5 desk job, you should probably stop reading right now because this book is definitely not for you.

This second edition of the popular reference and textbook, *Health Fitness Management*, is written for everyone who has an interest in managing a health and fitness facility. The contributors to this text are some of the most experienced and knowledgeable people in the fitness industry. Whether you are a student being exposed to this topic for the first time or a seasoned veteran, we are confident you will find this text helpful. Several new chapters, a more practical emphasis, enhanced learning tools, as well as new instructor resources, make *Health Fitness Management, Second Edition*, the best text on the topic.

The manager of the health and fitness club is the single most important person in determining the long-term success of the club. While some people may debate this, those of us who have worked in the industry know it is true. This is the person who gets the call at 5:00 a.m. when a staff person has overslept and the club has not opened on time. This is the person who is often left dealing with the most difficult and challenging customers. The club manager is the one who assembles the team of sales, service, programming, and maintenance staff. He or she is also the one who pays the price when things go wrong with the staff.

On the other hand, the manager is the one who gives people an opportunity to succeed in an extremely satisfying industry. This is the person who coaches staff along until they are able to overcome some of their greatest fears and challenges. The manager's job is an extremely rewarding one that comes with a significant amount of responsibility and enjoyment.

This book is divided into three parts. The first part on human resources is going to give you all the information you need to get started in the areas of organizational development, hiring, evaluation, and compensation. This part is potentially the most important part of the book. As a manager, your job is to hire, train, and retain the best people you can find. This part will help you understand all of these areas.

Part II covers member recruitment, retention, and profitability. In order for your club to be successful, you need to be able to attract new members and keep current members. And, in order to make a profit, you'll need to sell products and services to those members.

Part III covers operational and facility management—information that you'll need to know in order to run a successful club. As a manager, you need to know how to read financial statements and how to implement systems that ensure your club is clean and the equipment is up to date and in good working condition. You also need to have a solid understanding of the risks that are associated with running a fitness club, both for your staff and the general public. It takes only one accident for you to regret not understanding this side of the business. This final part ends with a chapter on how to properly evaluate a fitness business.

Within each chapter you'll find various tools that enhance the overall learning experience. Each chapter begins with a list of learning objectives to help you focus on what you should be learning while you're reading. After the objectives, you'll read an anecdote from the author that illustrates the main topic of the chapter. Most of these stories are based on the authors' actual experiences and are a great way to get students involved in a class discussion. Additional real-world experiences are integrated throughout the chapters so that you'll know how to apply the material. Because most of the authors have used this information in an actual fitness facility, you know it has the potential to work in the real world. We have also highlighted "the bottom line" throughout each chapter. These are key points that summarize and emphasize the most important topics in the text. Key terms—words and phrases that readers should be familiar with—are also highlighted within the text.

For instructors who are using this as a class text, this second edition comes with a test package and instructor guide. The test package features multiple choice questions that are based on material from each chapter. The instructor guide includes summaries of each chapter and various teaching tools that will help the instructor prepare for lectures and class discussions. The instructor guide also has various assignments for students using this text. These assignments are practical in nature and will allow students to apply the information presented in the text.

If you think you are ready for a career in the fitness industry, I applaud you for your interest. The true test will be how you use the information in this book to make your club or center the best it can be for you, your staff, your members, and the public.

[acknowledgments]

If you had told me when I was an undergraduate student in kinesiology at the University of Windsor or when I was managing my first fitness club that I would be editing and coauthoring a book on managing health and fitness facilities, I would have said you were crazy. Life does not always let us know where it is going to take us, but if we are open to new ideas and willing to share our experiences, it can be a great ride.

There are many people who need to be thanked for their contributions to this book. I would like to start with the authors of the first edition of *Health Fitness Management,* Robert Patton, Tracy York, Mitchel Winick, and the late William Grantham. The success of the first edition of this book paved the way for a new edition. Although the majority of the information in the book is new, we were able to keep a significant amount of some chapters, which is a testament to the original authors' work.

In my opinion, there has never been a book with more experts and combined years of industry experience than this one. Our list of contributors is a who's who within the fitness industry. They are all considered experts in their fields, and it has been a pleasure working with each and every one of them. This book would not have been completed without these contributors making the time to write their chapters. Thank you to each and every one of you. In the end, it was all worthwhile and I truly appreciate you taking the time from your busy schedules to contribute to this book.

I have been with Human Kinetics as managing director of Human Kinetics Canada for 8 years.

Throughout this time I have been challenged and rewarded beyond my expectations. I would like to personally thank Brian Holding and Rainer Martens for trusting that I could make this project happen on top of all of my other duties. I have worked closely with Mike Bahrke on many projects and appreciate the expertise he gave me along the way. Our developmental editor, Maggie Schwarzentraub, was an absolute gift from above. Her insights and overall approach allowed us to take a bunch of random thoughts and turn them into what is now a reference for anyone in the field. To everyone at HK Canada who keeps the ship running when I am out of town or taking on new projects: I would not have been able to take on this project if I didn't have your support and expertise.

Some of the others I would like to thank are Howard Ravis from Club Industry, Katie Rollauer from IHRSA, David Patchell-Evans, Michele Colwell, and everyone else at GoodLife Fitness Clubs, everyone at Can-Fit-Pro, the Faculty of Human Kinetics at the University of Windsor, Ted Farron, and all of the other great teachers and coaches I have had over the years.

Last but definitely not least, I'd like to thank my family. My wife, Laura, and my son, Jackson, put up with me and my crazy schedule and desire to take on too many projects, this probably being one of them. I love you both very much and appreciate everything you do for me. To my parents and my sister, who gave me the foundation to become who I am today: I continue to learn from you. Thank you for everything you have done for me.

An Overview of the Health and Fitness Industry

Managers of successful fitness centers no longer can get by on their passion and knowledge of fitness. They must have a thorough understanding of marketing, operations, and financial concerns that affect their club. In the early days of the industry, this was not critical to the success formula, because there was little competition. This has changed, as you will read in the following paragraphs. The industry is now highly competitive and there is no room for managers who do not understand the business side of fitness. This text will give you the knowledge base you need to be successful as a health and fitness manager.

Since the first edition of this book came out in 1998, the health and fitness industry has undergone some major changes. In 2005 the global industry grew to over 105 million members, with more than 92,000 clubs worldwide. Within the United States, the largest health club industry worldwide, there were more than 41.3 million members in more than 29,000 clubs; in 1985, there were only 9,222 commercial fitness clubs. This is a remarkable growth rate. Here are some other key industry data:

- In the past 10 years, fitness clubs have increased the total industry revenue by 105%.
- This revenue increase has been fueled by the increase in the number of facilities (118%) and members (71%).
- Clubs have increased revenue per member by 20%.
- In 2005, 57% of fitness club members were female and 43% were male.
- As of 2005, the 18- to 34-year-old market made up 36% of club membership base, and the 35- to 54-year-old market made up 33%.
- The under-18 group made up 12% and the over-55 group made up 19%.

- Since 1995, the number of members over the age of 55 increased by 305%.
- The average fitness club member had a household income of $82,900.
- People with household incomes over $75,000 account for 50% of the membership base.
- Despite the large percentage of members coming from these income levels, the fastest growing portion of the industry is the $50,000 to $74,999 income level.

One striking statistic from International Health, Racquet, and Sportsclub Association (IHRSA) is that, for the first time in about 10 years, the total number of health club members stayed relatively the same between the years 2005 and 2006. There are many potential reasons for this; the inability to reach the inactive, sedentary marketplace (by far the largest percentage of the population) and the increased competition are just two examples.

Despite this marked plateau in growth, the leading corporations are growing at a much quicker pace than the overall average. This growth has come in the form of acquisitions, expansions, new clubs, and initial public offerings. There is no doubt the industry is here to stay. As with any maturing industry, ours is beginning to see clubs differentiate themselves or get swallowed up by the large chains. Independent clubs have been forced to redefine themselves as they realize they cannot compete with the resources of larger fitness corporations with budgets in the tens and hundreds of millions.

Regardless of the size of the fitness center, a solid management team can make the difference between a club that is just getting by and one that is a benchmark for the industry. This text will help you create that team.

Human Resources

Human resources are often the most overlooked aspect of running a fitness club. Throughout this book, we talk about the importance of member retention—keeping the members you have from year to year. Equally as important is staff retention. Keeping staff members motivated and challenged will have a positive impact on member retention levels. Members like to see the same people when they come in to your facility. The relationships that members form with staff will make them want to keep coming back. If the facility is constantly losing staff, the result will be the eventual loss of members. Successful clubs realized a long time ago that spending the time on developing their human resources will pay off in the long run.

Chapter 1 discusses the importance of the leader within the fitness club. As with any business, a strong leader is necessary to build a great team. Jane Riddell tells you about the major mistakes managers made and what it takes to become a great manager.

In chapter 2, Scott Lewandowski explains how various fitness businesses are organized. You will see that there are many potential ways to design your organizational structure. It is critical that everyone on the team knows the role that they play and how their role contributes to the company's goals.

Kevin Hood addresses the topic of recruiting and hiring the best staff in chapter 3. A section on the importance of building job descriptions and designing appropriate interview questions is also included. Each of these areas is a critical component of all successful businesses.

In chapter 4, Brenda Abdilla shows you that the most successful clubs differentiate themselves by offering training programs that build great employees. One common denominator among successful fitness businesses is their investment in people and their consistent training and development programs.

In chapter 5, Bud Rockhill explains how to properly evaluate your staff and give them feedback so that they and the organization are working at the highest level possible. Giving employee feedback and conducting formal evaluations can be very complicated. Bud lays out the framework for designing a performance appraisal system, including the always sensitive topic of terminating employees. While this last topic is never fun, it is important to the business and the employee that managers understand how to do this properly.

Part I concludes with chapter 6, in which Mike Bates discusses how to design a compensation program that motivates and rewards the best employees. Various industry approaches to compensation are discussed. Once you have an understanding of each approach you should be comfortable discussing the advantages and disadvantages of each.

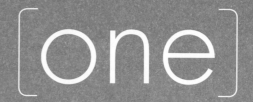

Recognizing the Importance of Leaders and Managers

D. Jane Riddell

LEARNING OBJECTIVES

After studying this chapter, the reader will be able to

- understand basic management and leadership theory,
- identify the roles of the manager and the leader,
- recognize the critical skills required to be a successful manager,
- identify behaviors that limit the ability to be a successful manager, and
- develop a strategy for managing talent.

Tales From the Trenches

Susan was the manager of a brand new fitness club in a very competitive market. The club was in a great location (the busiest mall in the city) and contained a huge cardiorespiratory training area, several lines of selectorized strength training equipment, a large free-weight area, a studio for group exercise, a running track, and a swimming pool. Susan had worked in a smaller club for 2 years before being promoted to manager of the new facility and had performed well, showing an affinity for sales. She and her team of three salespeople surpassed their presales targets despite delays in construction that resulted in the club opening 2 months late.

Because the club opened before it was fully completed, Susan had to deal with the inevitable construction problems on top of training new associates and ensuring that members were properly oriented to the club. She worked an inhuman schedule, often arriving before the club opened and staying until close and working at least one day on the weekend. She complained of being tired, and she became increasingly irritable with both associates and members. She refused to delegate even mundane tasks and spent little time training her staff since she was doing almost everything herself. Her justification was that it took less time for her to do things than to teach someone else and she knew they would be done properly. If she had a problem with an associate's work, instead of talking to the employee, she chose to leave strongly worded notes and make pointed remarks to other associates. When confronted about her behavior, her response was that she didn't have time to deal with the person directly.

Despite these shortcomings, the club continued to do well. Over time, however, the cracks in Susan's performance started to widen. She had trouble keeping associates and was constantly hiring new people. And most alarmingly, member attrition was far too high for a new club. Susan's supervisor met with her to outline the changes that needed to happen in order for her to keep her job. She needed to hire and train an assistant manager and to allow her department heads to take on some real responsibility. She had to invest time in building relationships with her associates, and she needed to take a course on dealing with conflict and confrontation. She had to treat members with respect and make time for them to discuss their concerns with her. Susan was shocked that she was being given an ultimatum since the club was continuing to beat its sales targets and was far ahead of budgeted financial goals. She either wouldn't or couldn't change her behavior, and as a result she was asked to leave shortly thereafter.

Enter Michele, who had worked under Susan for 2 years and had managed to stick it out because she loved working with members. Shortly after Michele assumed the role of manager, it was discovered that the locker rooms had been built in a part of the mall that contained asbestos. The plan called for immediate removal of the asbestos, which would require the locker rooms to be sealed off completely for a minimum of 8 weeks. Members would be able to use small washroom facilities in another part of the club but would not be able to shower. The only positive aspect of the mess was that the asbestos removal would occur over July and August, the quietest months for club usage.

When the removal began, Michele called an emergency associate meeting, outlined the situation, and asked for their assistance in formulating an action plan. It was decided at the meeting that members should receive a written communication indicating what the course of action would be, how it would affect them, and what the club was prepared to do to help the members get through it with a minimum amount of inconvenience. Michele lobbied the owner to suspend the members' dues for the 2 months and he agreed. With the backing of her associate team and the owner, Michele felt she was prepared to meet the challenge. She invited members to meet with her, and she also made time to meet with her associates and provide additional training in dealing with angry and upset members. Still, club usage dropped off dramatically.

Michele built a good relationship with the foreman who was coordinating the asbestos removal and he kept her informed about the progress they were making, which she promptly passed along to her associate team. As September edged ever nearer, the tension grew. It became apparent that the job would not be finished until closer to mid-September. She informed the associates and posted the news for the members and waited for the screaming to start. Surprisingly, most members took the news well, and many commended Michele for the way she was dealing with the problem. The locker rooms reopened 20 weeks after they had been shut down. Only 32 members cancelled their memberships as a result of the asbestos problem, and in the month after the construction was finished, the club had its best sales ever.

Michele's ability to successfully manage the crisis was attributed to her ability to build good relationships with her associates and members and her ability to plan and prioritize. She understood that in order for the club to come through the crisis successfully, she needed to have the associates on her side. And she understood that the more she communicated with the stakeholders (the members, associates, and construction foreman) and relayed information in a timely fashion, the less likely people were to be upset even if it wasn't what they wanted to hear. Michele went on to become one of the most successful managers in the history of the company. Under her guidance, the club achieved sound financial results and had one of the best member retention rates in the company. Her associate retention also remained high, and she mentored several associates who went on to become successful managers in their own right.

Two different managers, both new to their positions and both faced with circumstances that were out of the ordinary. One achieved extraordinary results and the other failed. What was the difference? By the end of the chapter, you will be armed with the knowledge you will need to replicate Michele's success and avoid the pitfalls that led to Susan's downfall.

Exploring Management and Leadership Theory

Over the years, there has been intense interest in the question of what makes managers and leaders effective, as well as whether or not there are differences between the roles of managers and leaders. The following overview of the theory of management and leadership will allow you to draw your own conclusions about the answers to these important questions and understand current thinking regarding these subjects.

Management Theory

There are three classifications of management theory.

1. *Scientific management approach.* This theory defines the relationship between incentive and performance and advocates rewarding people based on their output rather than hours worked. An example would be to reward salespeople via commission and bonuses (commonly termed *incentive pay*) rather than placing them on an annual salary or hourly rate. Although this approach was developed almost a century ago by Frederick Taylor (1911), it is still effectively used today by many club operators.

2. *Human relations management approach.* This theory evolved in the late 1920s and early 1930s from studies on more than 20,000 workers that demonstrated that if employees felt valued, they became more productive. Mayo (1933) hypothesized that when employees felt important, they had higher levels of job satisfaction, which in turn led to higher levels of productivity. The theory has been supported and augmented by several other researchers since Mayo, most notably Maslow (1954), Herzberg (1966), and McGregor (1960).

3. *Process (or administrative) approach to management.* Originally developed 70 years ago by Gulick and Urwick (1937) and since refined by Hersey, Blanchard, and Johnson (2001) as well as Koontz, O'Donnell, and Weihrich (1984), this approach has a broader perspective on the manner in which managers take actions and make decisions. Five processes revolve around the central construct of taking actions and making decisions: planning, organizing, directing, staffing, and controlling or evaluating (see figure 1.1). Decisions made in one of the five processes always affect the other four; in other words, all five processes are interrelated. At the risk of stating the obvious, planning is most often the process that is used first. However, an effective manager will most likely perform more than one process simultaneously.

According to Mintzberg (1973, 1990), the typical manager assumes 10 distinct roles (i.e., sets of expected behaviors associated with a managerial position). These roles can be classified into three categories: interpersonal, informational, and decisional.

- Interpersonal
  1. Figurehead—acting in symbolic and ceremonial ways
  2. Leader—influencing and coordinating the work of followers to achieve the goals of the organization
  3. Liaison—developing and cultivating relationships with individuals and groups outside the organization

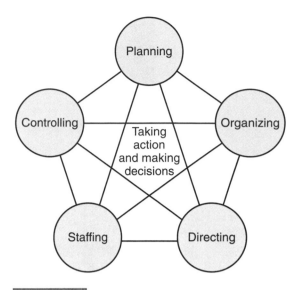

Figure 1.1 The process approach to management.

- Informational
  4. Monitor—scanning the environment for information about trends and events that can affect the organization
  5. Disseminator—transmitting information to stakeholders in the organization
  6. Spokesperson—transmitting information to individuals or groups outside the organization
- Decisional
  7. Entrepreneur—searching for opportunities to improve the organization
  8. Disturbance handler—responding to unexpected situations that may disrupt normal operations
  9. Resource allocator—determining how to best allocate resources to achieve the goals of the organization
  10. Negotiator—conferring with individuals or groups outside the organization to obtain concessions or gain agreement on important issues

Leadership Theory

Leadership theory may be divided into three approaches. Understanding leadership theory will allow you to gain greater insight into how leadership has been viewed from a historical perspec-

tive. More importantly, this understanding will also allow you to make decisions about your own personal leadership style, which will help you maximize your effectiveness.

Trait Leadership Theory

This theory is based on the premise that leaders can be identified by physical, intellectual, or personality attributes and is perhaps best summed up by the statement, "Leaders are born, not made." Although discredited for some time, this school of thought generated renewed interest more recently when Kirkpatrick and Locke (1991) demonstrated that core traits such as drive, desire to lead, honesty and integrity, self-confidence, cognitive ability, and knowledge of the business are assumed to be good predictors of the potential to lead, although they do not guarantee successful leadership.

Behavioral Leadership Theory

This theory hypothesizes that if critical behaviors of leaders can be identified, then a blueprint for successful leadership can be created and duplicated (Likert 1961). This analysis focuses on what leaders actually do, whereas trait theory focuses on their attributes and characteristics.

Behavioral theory divides leaders into either job centered (concerned with attaining either personal or organizational goals) or employee centered (concerned with building good relationships with peers and followers). These two categories are not mutually exclusive; indeed, leaders and managers are most effective when they are focused on getting the job done and building relationships.

Situational Leadership Theory

Situational leadership theorists observed that a variety of leadership styles could be used simultaneously in response to changing situations. Several models of situational leadership theory have been applied to leadership; four of the most well known are briefly outlined here.

- *Fiedler's contingency model.* Fiedler (1967) theorized that the effectiveness of a leader depends upon the leader's personal style and the amount of control the leader has over the situation. In this model, the leader is either primarily task oriented or relationship oriented. Fiedler believed that the environment can be manipulated to match the leaders' personal style (which he believed could not be easily changed) by either assigning followers who are compatible with leaders' personal style or seeking out situations that match the leaders' style, thereby allowing for a higher probability of success.

- *Path–goal model.* This model suggests that followers are motivated by their estimates of the probability that their behaviors will result in a valued outcome and by the level of personal satisfaction they will experience based on their work. Evans (1970) proposed that the primary role of the leader is path clarification, whereby the leader describes the behaviors that will lead to the reward. According to House and Mitchell (1997), leaders who are aware of both the personal characteristics of their followers and the environment can modify their behavior to maximize motivation under the given circumstances.

- *Situational leadership model.* This is a three-dimensional model developed by Hersey and Blanchard (1969). The leaders' behavior depends upon the mix of task (directive) and relationship (supportive) styles. There are four behaviors, which comprise different degrees of task and relationship styles. For example, if task is high and relationship is low, then leaders' behavior will tend to be more controlling and they will tell people what to do. If the task is low and relationship is high, leaders will be more participative. The third dimension of this model is how ready the follower is to perform the task. Aptly termed *readiness,* once the leader is able to identify how prepared the follower is to perform the task (the readiness level), the model can be used to select the most appropriate style and communication pattern for that follower.

- *Full range of leadership model.* This model encompasses three leadership styles—transactional, laissez-faire, and transformational. Transactional leadership is a negotiated and agreed-upon deal between leaders and followers outlining rewards and punishments for levels of performance by the followers (Bass 1985). Laissez-faire leadership is, as one would expect, the "do nothing" approach to leading people. This is the least effective of all leadership styles. Transformational leadership, on the other hand, focuses on the four *Is*—idealized influence, inspirational motivation, intellectual stimulation, and individualized consideration (Avolio, Waldman, and Yammarino 1991). These leaders are considerate, trustworthy, encouraging, and risk taking. Research suggests that the most effective leaders engage in all three styles to different degrees—transformational leadership most often, transactional leadership occasionally, and laissez-faire leadership seldom if at all (Bass and Avolio 1994).

Acknowledging the Difference Between Managing and Leading

It will not come as a surprise to learn that every successful organization needs a leader. A leader's role is to formulate the vision for the organization, provide clarity for what the future will look like, and inspire group members to align themselves with the vision. Essentially, the leader sets the course for the group. Recently, more than 200 Canada geese were found dead in a frozen Manitoba wheat field. Initially, it was thought that they had been poisoned; however, autopsies on the birds revealed that the birds had all suffered a traumatic death, with their breastbones shattered and necks broken. It was concluded that the leader had become disoriented during a dark, moonless night and had flown at full speed into the frozen ground and the rest of the flock had obediently followed. There are two morals to this story. The first is that you need to choose your leader wisely. The second is that, if you are going to lead people, you had better do a good job because if you don't, the consequences can be dire.

Leaders, by definition, must have followers. In order to get people to believe in your leadership capability and to therefore follow you, you need to develop good relationships with your key people. They need to trust you and believe that you genuinely care about them. The best leaders are those who take the time to learn about their associates, to understand what motivates them, what they are proud of, what their goals are, and who or what is important to them. The most effective leaders are fully engaged in the performance of their people, continually coaching and providing timely, constructive feedback. Leaders provide vision, create clarity, foster hope by telling people that they believe in them, and, of course, deliver results.

All of this, with the exception of providing vision, sounds suspiciously like what we expect managers to do. So is there a difference between managing and leading? The literature in this area is controversial. On one hand, you have Peter Drucker, one of the most respected management gurus of the modern era, telling us that leadership and management are identical (Drucker 1998). And then we have Marcus Buckingham (2005), who is equally respected, telling us that the core activities of the leader and the manager are totally different.

The manager looks inward—into the processes, the systems, and most importantly, the people. The leader, on the other hand, looks outward—to industry trends, external factors such as competitive influences, and best practices from other companies and industries. Thus, managers and leaders perform distinct but complementary roles within the organization.

Is it possible to be both a great leader and a great manager? In fact, the best managers must also be good leaders. In Robert Slater's book, *Jack Welch and the GE Way*, Jack Welch tells us that leaders speed things up and managers slow things down (Slater 1999). This, as Martha Stewart would say, is a very good thing. Leaders are all about vision and forward thinking, and the sooner they can get the organization to the goal, the better. From the leader's perspective, if it could happen tomorrow that would be okay, but today would be better and yesterday would have been ideal. They are not interested in the *how*—most great leaders regard details as necessary evils. Managers, on the other hand, are intensely interested in the *how* because they are charged with the responsibility of making the goal happen. They have to marshal the people and the resources to accomplish the task and formulate the action plan.

If we use the analogy of the ready, aim, fire sequence, the leader is essentially concerned with fire, whereas the manager is all about ready, aim. However, great managers must have the ability to organize people around achieving the common vision or goal. They must be able to inspire their group to work hard, smart, and together, and this is where leadership comes into the manager's world. It is impossible for a manager to achieve significant success without good leadership skills. The reality is that in a small organization, you and probably others on your team will need to don the leadership hat from time to time. Great organizations grow leaders at all levels. Organizations like Southwest Airlines and Starbucks empower their associates to make decisions to preserve their well-deserved reputation for outstanding customer service. The good news is that most research shows us that anyone can become a great leader—it is not a genetic gift.

Characteristics of Great Leaders

The following section outlines a few of the most important characteristics that great leaders share. It focuses on culture as a critical component for the success of the leader and the organization.

Great Leaders Create the Group Culture

In an intensely competitive industry such as ours, arguably the only **sustainable competitive advantage** you have is culture. In other words,

when everyone in the industry has access to the same knowledge and technology, the only way to achieve a long-term edge on the competition is through the culture developed within the company. Great leaders carefully craft the culture of the organization and then promote and protect it at every turn. It may be worthwhile mentioning that if you don't consciously create the culture, one will be created for you—and it may not be one that you find desirable.

What is that elusive quality we call *culture*? It is the combination of values and beliefs that guide behavior. It is reflected in how associates treat members, each other, and themselves. If your culture is strong, you will attract like-minded people to your company. They will feel comfortable operating within the values and beliefs espoused by the group. When their behavior is consistent with the culture of the company, it will be rewarded, recognized, and reinforced by their leaders, managers, and peers. Similarly, those who cannot internalize the culture of the company will leave, either voluntarily or with a gentle push. When your culture is strong, members will experience consistent treatment from your associates, whether or not a manager is present.

THE BOTTOM LINE

If you want a quick report card on how you are doing as a manager, take a look at what happens when you are in the club versus when you are not. If your associates conduct themselves with the same high level of dedication and commitment regardless of whether you are present, then you will know that you are in the top 10% of managers in the industry. Congratulations!

How can you create culture?

- Clearly define your values and communicate them tirelessly.

- Champion and reward positive behaviors and discourage and eliminate negative behaviors.

- Have all key people in the organization walk the talk—all the time, not just when it is convenient.

- Create **cultural heroes,** those associates who, through actions consistent with the values of the company, create an amazing experience for a member. These heroes are then held up to the rest of the organization as shining examples of what appropriate behavior looks like, and they are rewarded accordingly.

Great Leaders Inspire Trust

Great leaders don't necessarily have to be charismatic, larger-than-life figures. Some of the best leaders are those who quietly toil behind the scenes, building great teams that are capable of extraordinary performance. Regardless of their personal characteristics, all great leaders are able to rally people to them, because people feel that they are trustworthy. They believe that such leaders will deliver on their promises because they have a proven history of doing so. If you truly want to become a great leader, make sure you can fulfill your commitments. Before verbalizing a promise, you need to understand what you must do in order to keep it. Great leaders underpromise and overdeliver. You will quickly build a reputation for being trustworthy if you always deliver on your promises.

Finally, when great leaders don't have the answers, they don't fabricate them. When Mayor Rudy Giuliani was asked questions to which he didn't know the answers in the terrible days after September 11, 2001, he replied honestly and with great compassion. In so doing, he won the trust of the nation.

Great Leaders Communicate the Goals of the Organization

Great leaders understand that people are drawn toward the vision of success. If the vision is unclear or is continually changing, people start to question what they are doing and why they are doing it, and they begin to disengage. It is the leader's responsibility to ensure that the vision of the goal is clearly communicated to every member of the organization. Dave Patchell-Evans, the founder and CEO of GoodLife Fitness Clubs, never wavered from his vision of what success would look like for his company. Everyone in the company knew that success would be 100 clubs by the year 2005. Having achieved that milestone, he communicated his new vision in an equally clear and compelling manner: "One hundred more in four," or 100 more clubs in the next 4 years.

Characteristics of Great Managers

The following section discusses a few of the critical traits that great managers must possess. You can be a good manager if you possess only some of these qualities, but great managers possess all of them.

Great Managers Have a Nose for Talent

Great managers have a sixth sense about people. They are continually on the lookout for promising candidates outside of the organization and are continually assessing the talent they currently possess. We are in a war for talent in North America—the workforce is shrinking, as is the birth rate, and the traditional sources of skilled workers are drying up. This has been predicted for years, but in the words of Peter Drucker (1998), "The future has already happened," and most health club managers are struggling to adjust. How can you avoid the frightening prospect of having no talented candidates to fill the inevitable vacancies you will experience?

One obvious strategy is to keep the people you currently have, as we'll discuss later. Another is to constantly be scouting for people who have the right attitude and would be a good fit with your company culture and values. Prime scouting areas include the hotel, restaurant, and retail industries. These places are where you are most likely to find employees who are genuinely interested in people and who have the service mentality required to be successful in the health and fitness industry. Whenever you experience exceptional service, make sure you compliment the employees and present them with a low-key recruiting pitch. Recruitment is the highest form of flattery, and it is identical to selling. You may not lure prospective associates to your club immediately, but you will plant the seed so that if they consider switching careers at some point, they will think of you.

Great Managers Continually Assess Talent

Great managers need to constantly be evaluating and assessing their current talent. How can you ensure that you are consistently, fairly, and accurately assessing the merits of your people?

In our company, we use the following method of evaluating people, which is similar to one outlined by Jack Welch in the book *Jack Welch and the GE Way* (Slater 1999). We place people into one of four quadrants (see figure 1.2).

We have found this method provides clarity for decisions that may otherwise be difficult to make. And more importantly, it allows us to make decisions that are based on consistent, unchanging criteria. The easiest decisions are arrived at for those associates in quadrant 1—the people who consistently deliver on commitments and results and also act in accordance with the company values. One trait that sets great managers apart from average managers is their understanding that top

Quadrant 1	Quadrant 2
• Delivers results • Lives the core values Reward, recognize, and promote	• Delivers results • Does not live core values Terminate
Quadrant 3	Quadrant 4
• Does not deliver results • Lives the core values Evaluate, train, or reassign	• Does not deliver results • Does not live core values Terminate

Figure 1.2 Four quadrants for ranking associates.

performers require coaching and feedback just as much as lesser performers. Quadrant 1 associates are the people who need consistent recognition and rewards. The key word here is *consistently*. Always recognize your top people, publicly if possible. These are also the people you need to take care of, so reward them fairly. And, of course, these are the people who are deserving of promotion. They are your future leaders and represent the backbone of your succession plan.

The other group whose future is relatively easy to determine are the quadrant 4 dwellers—those who don't produce and don't act in accordance with the company values. These are people who somehow got into your organization and make you scratch your head and wonder about your selection process. Those in quadrant 4 should be introduced to the harsh reality of the employment market and have their futures freed up—in other words, they should be terminated, and the sooner, the better. The first rule of good leadership and good management is to honestly evaluate your employees and get rid of the bad apples. No amount of coaching, caring, or feedback will change them, and you will be wasting valuable time and resources on them at the expense of developing people with high potential. If you find yourself spending the majority of your coaching time fixing bad hiring decisions, then it's time to reevaluate how you hire people.

The more difficult decisions are those regarding associates who end up in quadrant 2 (good producers but poor values) and quadrant 3 (poor producers but good values). You will be sorely tempted to keep those good producers in quadrant 2. It takes a very special manager not to agonize over the decision to terminate a good producer for exhibiting behavior that is contrary to the core values of the company.

The **core values** are the foundation of the culture of the company, and they must be passionately protected. However difficult it may be, the cost of keeping associates who continually bend the rules or act without integrity is much higher in the long run than terminating them. What is the message that you send to your remaining employees by not letting that person go? In effect, you are telling them that you really don't care about the core values and all that truly matters is to win (i.e., make money) at any cost. They will believe the company (and you) to be unprincipled, uncaring, and soulless, and you will drive away associates who believe in the core values of the company.

The following true story illustrates how potentially destructive delaying the decision to rid your organization of these people can be. Paul was an associate who rose quickly through our organization. He started as a membership coordinator selling memberships and he excelled at it. He was rapidly promoted to general manager of a small club and then a large facility. From a financial perspective, both clubs performed exceptionally well under his guidance. However, it eventually became apparent that despite the solid financial performance of his clubs, there was an unusually high rate of associate turnover. Exit interviews with former associates revealed that Paul was managing through fear and intimidation. He was prone to berating employees in public and throwing temper tantrums. When confronted, Paul refused to accept responsibility for his actions and attempted to place blame on others. He was given the option of anger management training, which he declined, so the decision was made to terminate him.

Within a week, two other high-performing general managers told us that they were considering leaving the company because they saw how inconsistent Paul's behavior was with our core values and they thought the company was turning a blind eye to his actions because he was putting up great numbers. They had no interest in working for a company that they could not trust and that they perceived as being hypocritical. And these were the two people who had the courage to speak up about how they felt—who knows how many other associates were struggling with the same decision? The manager who replaced Paul did not possess his drive or business acumen but was a solid performer with consistent alignment with our core values. Within 6 months, the club had regained the ground it lost, and it continues to be one of the best-performing facilities today. The moral of the story is, quickly get rid of the people who do not fit into your culture or your values. If they don't fit, they can cause your business irreparable damage.

Let's take a look at the quadrant 3 dwellers. They are great people who love your company and take the core values to heart, but they just don't produce. What should you do? Start with training, and if that doesn't make a difference, try them in another position. You really don't want to lose these people unless there is absolutely nowhere else in the organization for them to go.

Perform this ranking exercise at least once per year—more often if you are adding new people to your organization at a rapid rate. It allows you to see at a glance the strengths and weaknesses of your most valuable assets and to take the appropriate action quickly.

Great Managers Understand That Everyone Is Different

Great managers understand that they cannot treat everyone in exactly the same manner. Marcus Buckingham (2005) likens this to chess versus checkers. In the game of checkers, each piece moves in exactly the same way. In chess, however, each piece moves in a different way and performs different roles. So, too, different people are motivated by different triggers and respond differently to feedback and coaching. For example, some people love to be praised. They thrive on public recognition; it's what makes them get up in the morning and come to work with a smile on their face. Others are uncomfortable in the spotlight and prefer to receive their rewards privately. Another example is that you can be very direct when giving feedback to some people whereas you will need to soften your approach for others. Great managers intuitively understand this and are constantly working on

building great relationships with their team members so that they can better understand how to help all members achieve their potential.

How do great managers seem to build those relationships so easily? Some managers have that elusive sixth sense about people. They tend to be keenly observant, ask lots of probing questions, and are excellent listeners. They are genuinely interested and care deeply about the success and happiness of their charges. For those of us who are not as gifted, here are a few practical ways to find out what makes your associates tick and how you are performing in their eyes as their manager and leader. Figure 1.3 illustrates a goal-setting process that you can use to acquire the basic information you will need to develop meaningful relationships with your associates.

We use this goal-setting worksheet to provide structure for meaningful, caring conversations with associates about their past accomplishments and their aspirations for the future. These conversations provide the foundation for a great relationship. Once you understand what is important to your associates, you will be able to provide meaningful coaching and support as you assist them in moving toward their goals.

In our company, we also use the 12 questions as a major form of feedback for our managers and leaders. The 12 questions are from the 1999 book, *First Break All the Rules*, by Marcus Buckingham and Curt Coffman. In this book, they describe the rationale behind each question. The first two questions—"Do you know what is expected of you?" and "Do you have the resources required to do your job?"—are the most relevant to our discussion and elicit the most important information from your perspective as a manager. If people don't know what you expect of them or don't have the tools to do their jobs properly, then they don't have even a faint hope of being successful. Buckingham and Coffman use the analogy of climbing a mountain. You cannot move up to the summit without spending the requisite amount of time acclimatizing at base camp; otherwise, you will die. Until your associates can strongly agree with both questions, any attempt you may make to motivate or empower them will ultimately end in failure. This is your foundation and until it is solidly in place, you dare not move on.

Answers to the remaining 10 questions will provide feedback on you as a leader or manager, how well the individuals fit into the company culture, and what they believe their future in the organization looks like—all great information. We ask for the evaluation to be completed quarterly. Building

Life and Work Goals for 2007

Name: _____   Date: _____

Mission
My mission is to make a positive difference for each person I come into contact with every day.

Core Values That Guide Me
Care, trust, integrity

Significant Life and Work Accomplishments
Completed two marathons.

Married for 16 years to the same person.

Promoted to general manager (GM) in 2005.

Graduated with an MA in exercise physiology.

Professional Development Goals
Win GM of the Year.

Join Toastmasters.

Present at Can-Fit-Pro.

Work Goals
Achieve all financial targets for my club.

Improve member retention by 3%.

Recruit and hire an excellent member-care manager.

Personal, Family, Marriage, and Health Goals
Take a family vacation in Italy.

Learn to speak Italian.

Run two half-marathons.

How to Make My Goals Happen
Work Goals

Set up a monthly meeting with my divisional manager to review statements and correct variances. Beef up personal training revenue by 20%.

To improve member retention, handle all cancellations myself whenever possible. Focus on training front desk for world-class meet and greet. Once per month, meet with member focus group to invite feedback.

To recruit member-care manager, recruit from local restaurants and retail and post internally to see if there are any members who would be great. Once hired, set up a rigorous training program. Develop an incentive program based on reducing member cancellations.

Professional Development Goals

Work out an action plan with my divisional manager to win GM of the Year. Get clearly defined expectations and performance standards.

Contact Can-Fit-Pro and find out how presenters are selected. Join Toastmasters in November to improve presentation skills. Ask my divisional manager to allow me to present at GM meetings.

Personal, Family, Marriage, and Health Goals

Book and pay for the holiday—that way we can't cancel!

Buy Italian language CDs and commit to listening three times per week for 1 hour.

Join the half-marathon running group in January.

Figure 1.3 Goal-setting worksheet filled out by an associate. Managers can learn about their associates' motivations by asking them to fill out similar worksheets.

a history of responses from all associates will enable you to monitor their (and your) progress and will indicate potential sources of trouble or success if a score changes dramatically from one evaluation period to the next. For example, if an associate who previously answered the second question with a 5 (strongly agree) dropped the response to a 2 (tend to disagree) on the next evaluation, you would need to initiate a meaningful conversation with that person to ascertain what changed and how it might be rectified. We find this a valuable method for scoring the effectiveness of our managers and how engaged people are. It is short, easily understood, and quickly interpreted.

Another useful tool for determining how to best manage people is to use the StrengthsFinder profile (www.strengthsfinder.com). You will need to buy one of either *Now, Discover Your Strengths* by Marcus Buckingham and Donald Clifton (2001) or *Strengthsfinder 2.0* by Tom Rath (2007) in order to access either one of the online questionnaires. The information you receive will be well worth it. You will be able to define the top five strengths for each person who fills out the questionnaire. Even more importantly, you will gain invaluable insight into how to effectively manage each associate. This information will give you tips as to which situations and projects will allow different people to thrive and which ones will cause them to become frustrated and disengaged.

Great Managers Encourage Feedback

A climate where feedback is encouraged is an invaluable tool. If people feel safe giving you honest feedback about what works for them and what doesn't, you are well on your way to becoming a great manager. It sounds easy, doesn't it? Tell people what you really think about their behavior on a consistent and timely basis. What is so hard about that? Unfortunately, most of us struggle with honest communication. You can create a feedback-positive climate in your organization by building relationships based on trust and caring. The adage "They don't care how much you know until they know how much you care" is highly applicable to managing. People will forgive you for many mistakes if you create an environment where they understand that you sincerely care about them and their success and you are prepared to invest in them.

A word of caution is warranted, though—there is a huge difference between caring and caretaking. Don't fall into the caretaking trap. The caretaking trap sounds something like this:

"Justin hasn't hit his sales goals in 6 months and he was told that if he didn't perform this month, he would be out. I know I should just go ahead and fire him, but he and his wife are expecting their first baby next month."

"I can't tell Kim what I really think of her performance because she is so sensitive. I know if I'm totally honest with her, she will get really upset."

If you are unable to be honest with associates because you think that they will be unable to handle the truth, then you have fallen into the caretaking trap. On the other hand, the highest form of caring is to give honest, timely feedback to people in a manner that allows their dignity and self-respect to remain intact. It may be challenging initially, but like anything else, it gets easier with practice, and eventually you will be able to develop meaningful relationships because they are based on mutual trust and respect. Caring is the most important implement in your managerial tool kit. Use it often and wisely.

Great Managers Provide Clear Expectations

Great managers are very clear about what they expect from their associates. Once again, this characteristic seems so basic that it isn't even worthwhile stating. After all, how would you know if you were doing a good job if you didn't know exactly what your job was? However, you would be amazed to discover how few people in supervisory roles are able to state clear expectations for their direct reports. If you are in doubt about how good a job you are doing in this area, use the 12 questions (from *First Break All the Rules,* by Marcus Buckingham and Curt Coffman), and pay specific attention to responses to the first question.

When defining expectations for associates, be aware that a job profile is really just the beginning. You need to have meaningful discussions with people about what it looks like to perform well. For instance, a job profile for people who work the front desk may state, "The phone must be answered in a professional and courteous manner." Your definition of professional and courteous may be quite different from theirs. Thus, it is important to provide training in this skill and observe associates' performance so that you can provide caring, honest feedback that will clearly show what it looks and sounds like to answer the phone in a courteous and professional manner. As noted previously, the greatest gift you can give or receive is honest, timely feedback delivered in a manner that both provides clarity as to future expectations and enhances the receiver's self-esteem.

Consider this example. You walk into your club earlier than usual one morning to find the person at the front desk reading the paper and paying no attention whatsoever to the members who are checking in. You have several choices:

- Rant and rave like a deranged maniac, scaring the associate and everyone else in earshot.

- Ignore the behavior (more about the effectiveness of this strategy later).

- Ask the associate to come to your office when the next person shows up to work the front desk.

Hopefully you chose the last option. Your mandate for giving feedback should always be to reward in public and reprimand in private. How might you deliver appropriate feedback that will leave no doubt as to your future expectations but will also leave people feeling good about themselves? Great managers seek "first to understand," in the words of Stephen Covey (1989). It is all too easy to jump to the wrong conclusion about the motivation for someone's behavior only to make an idiot out of yourself and damage the relationship. Take a deep breath and find out first why the associate felt compelled to read the paper at a time when it was clearly not appropriate. For instance, you may be shocked to find she considers this to be appropriate behavior because no one had ever told her it wasn't. Or you may find out that she was responding to a query from a member to find the time and location of a particular movie for him. If, however, you know that she understands that the behavior is inappropriate and simply made a bad decision, you need to take the appropriate action. In order not to damage her self-esteem, make sure you isolate how you feel about her behavior from how you feel about her as a person.

For example, you might open the conversation with a question such as, "Sarah, when I came into the club this morning I observed that you were reading the paper. I am curious to know why you were doing that." This is an open-ended, nonjudgmental question (hopefully your body language and voice tone are neutral and nonthreatening). Now, let's assume that this particular associate knew and understood that she had made an inappropriate choice and she admits it to you. An effective response from you might be, "I trust you to conduct yourself in a professional manner at all times when you are in the club, Sarah, whether or not I am here. To our members you are a walking, talking personification of our core values. I know I can count on you to make decisions about your behavior that are in the best interests of our members. Although I am disappointed in your behavior this morning, you need to understand that I think you are a fine individual, and I am proud to have you working here. And I know that this is the last time you and I will have to have a conversation about this."

Struggling as a Manager: Ten Pitfalls to Avoid

Over the past 26 years, more than 500 people have come through our organization and developed into club managers. Many of them have succeeded and, unfortunately, many more have struggled and failed. Here are 10 of the most common behaviors that will cause you to struggle and ways to avoid them.

1. *Hiring those who have similar strengths to yours and failing to hire those who are stronger.* Good managers are able to honestly assess their own strengths and weaknesses and to surround themselves with people who are strong in the skills and abilities that they lack. Good managers build teams who are capable of greatness, and the best teams have people who are different but who complement each other and clearly understand their roles so that the total is greater than the sum of the parts. Poor managers, on the other hand, will hire people who have similar skill sets to theirs; they are not comfortable with those who are different from them, and they are especially not comfortable with those who are stronger. If you have great organizational skills but do not naturally have a sales mentality, you need to go out and find people who do have that sales ability—you don't need another organizational whiz. Poor managers are also guilty of consistently hiring those who are weaker than they are because they are threatened by those who are stronger. A club or an organization that is in decline will exhibit the following downward spiral: Those at the top—the managers, or the 10s—will hire 9s, who will hire 8s, and so on. The best will hire the best because they understand that by doing so they will be pushed to a higher level of performance.

2. *Undertraining.* Great managers understand that the best investment of their time is to train people early in their tenure with the club and train them well. They know that if they can teach people to master a task properly, they reduce the time they will have to spend correcting the performance or,

worse, performing the task themselves. If this is so simple, then why do so few managers grasp the concept? When pressed, most managers who have failed to train their associates say that it is too time consuming to train people, it is easier to do the task themselves, or they just plain don't like training. New managers especially are guilty of not training or delegating enough, and as a result they end up burning out because they are doing everything themselves. In addition, associates are not given the opportunity to learn and take on more responsibility, so the good ones leave. Information from the exit interviews we have conducted corroborates this: The number one reason associates leave is that they do not have the tools to be successful. Managers thus become caught in a vicious cycle. They must continually hire new people to replace the people who left because they were not trained, so the managers have even less time for training, and so the cycle continues.

3. *Failing to invest the time and energy necessary to hire the right people.* If you are going to be successful in any business, but particularly in this business where you deal with people from the time the lights come on in the morning until you lock the doors at night, you had better have great people. In other words, using the simple but insightful analogy created by Jim Collins in *Good to Great* (2001), you had better have the right people in the right seats on your bus. The hiring decision is a critical responsibility, yet most managers hurry through the selection process just to find a body. You need so much more than that if you are to be successful. As tempting as it may be, don't rush to hire. You will save time, energy, and money by finding the right fit for your club. Be very clear about your requirements and don't compromise. And a word to the wise—check the candidate's references thoroughly. The best predictor of future performance is past performance.

4. *Avoiding confrontation.* Here are eight words that characterize poor managers: "If I ignore it, it will go away." Ignoring poor performance or tension among your stakeholders (associates or members) will not result in it going away. It will get worse and your blind eye will drive your team to question your ability to lead them. Before addressing the problem, you need to gather the facts and understand that in any conflict, there are at least two sides to the story. Addressing conflict and confrontation is a skill that can be learned like any other, and with practice you will get very good at it. Even if you don't handle it quite right, it is far better than pretending it doesn't exist. When people see you taking a leadership role in addressing conflict and treating those involved with respect, you will, in turn, earn their respect.

5. *Ignoring the good performers.* We have already discussed this previously, but it bears repeating. The best workers need your time and attention as much as the weak performers and perhaps even more so. Ignore your stars at your peril. If they feel unappreciated, you risk sending the message to the rest of your team that it is not really important when people excel, so why should they bother? Very few people are totally intrinsically motivated. Most of us are shallow enough to require some external recognition in order to stay inspired. Look for opportunities to recognize good performance at every turn. You don't need to make a big splash; a simple, sincere thank-you is a good start. Seek out ways to catch people doing things right and let them know you appreciate their efforts. This sounds easier than it is; in practice, your time will inevitably be drawn to fixing problems and fighting fires, so you will need to continually remind yourself to focus on the positive.

6. *Managing time inefficiently.* This is perhaps the challenge that new managers wrestle with more than any other. It takes great skill to create a schedule with enough flexibility to allow for the inevitable unanticipated events that will require your attention, and it takes even greater discipline to stick to it. There are many books written and many courses offered on the best way to manage your time. Steven Covey, author of *The Seven Habits of Highly Effective People* (1989), among other books, is one of the best authorities in this area. The reality is that virtually any system will work providing you have the discipline to execute it. Managing your time well means that you are able to prioritize tasks and responsibilities and place the most important tasks on your schedule where you know they will get done with minimal interruption.

As a club manager, many people require your time and attention. If there is a secret to successfully managing your time, it is that you need to manage your interruptions. Train your team to respect your schedule. Create specific times during the day when they have access to you for asking questions. Also, apply the 80:20 rule, also known as **Pareto's Law,** when you are analyzing your work. Focus on the 20% of your tasks that yield 80% of the results, and then place those tasks on your schedule at times when you are most productive. Whenever possible, delegate tasks that do not meet the 80:20 criteria. This will help you focus on the most important items and will allow your people to assume more responsibility. No matter how well you plan and how disciplined you are, you will have days where nothing goes according to schedule, but as long as the majority of your days do not fall into that category, you will be winning the time management battle.

7. *Forgetting that members come first.* New managers are often so overwhelmed with the responsibilities of their positions that they forget who is most important—a classic case of not being able to see the forest for the trees. In our industry, members always come first. This needs to be much more than rhetoric. It needs to be an attitude and a philosophy that are so thoroughly woven into the operation of your club that they cannot be taken for granted or forgotten. Members put food on your table, clothes on your back, and a roof over your head. As such, they need to be treated like gold. And happy, satisfied members will become ambassadors for your club, which will ultimately bring you more members. Poor managers somehow forget this or overlook it. They don't make time to stay in touch with members. As the manager, you need to walk the talk in this area more than in any other.

A member of a club once complained that the manager was harder to find than Osama Bin Laden, and this complaint was corroborated by the low member retention in that club—not exactly a ringing endorsement of the members-first philosophy. The manager was transferred to a different position that was a better fit for her (she was enormously gifted in organization and administration and truly believed in the core values of the company) and replaced with a manager who went out of her way to create meaningful interactions with members. She set up time in her daily schedule to walk the workout floor during busy times and inquire about concerns that members had with the club. It would be too simplistic to say that member retention improved due to this one act. But improve it did, and this certainly was a contributing factor. Perhaps more importantly, this manager was able to convert the rhetoric of "members come first" into action on several levels. Her team saw how much she valued the members and took their cue from her as to how they should act with members, and it paid off.

8. *Micromanaging.* To the untrained eye, there is a fine line between coaching and telling, but to the trained eye and to those on the receiving end, there is a world of difference. The difference is that a good coach will act as a guide but will allow associates to find their own way, within reason. If you find yourself consistently telling people how they should act or fixing problems for them, then you have crossed the line into the realm of **micromanaging.** The net effect of micromanaging is that people never have to think for themselves—you are always doing it for them. They will become incapable of find-

ing workable solutions to problems because they have you to do it for them. Aren't they lucky? Not really, and neither are you. Micromanaging means that associates will not grow and develop; you will have to spend an inordinate amount of time at the club since when you aren't there, things fall apart; and people will never feel that you trust them. Ambitious people will leave and the people who are content to have you do their thinking for them will stay—and you will never experience the level of success that you are capable of.

9. *Being complacent with the status quo and failing to invest in your own growth and development.* As managers acquire the skill that comes with experience and taste success, there is a real possibility that they may become complacent with what they have achieved. If ever there were a pitfall in club management, this is it. The moment you are content with standing still, you start to lose ground. This industry demands that you stay current in sales, marketing, performance management, human resource principles and legislation, exercise physiology, programming, customer service, and financial management. You must continually work to improve yourself and your associates.

10. *Not fostering an atmosphere of fun.* All work and no play will make your club a very dull place to work. People spend such a significant portion of their time working that if they aren't enjoying what they are doing then they are not living their life to its full potential, and that's a shame. We do important work that makes an incredible difference in peoples' lives, and we need to enjoy ourselves while we do it. One of the ways enjoyment becomes apparent is that your people have fun while they work. This doesn't mean playing practical jokes or using slapstick humor, although there is a time and a place for that. It means laughing together and laughing at yourselves. Lighten up and see the humor in what you are doing. It will allow you to keep everything in perspective and to maintain your sanity, and it will make your club a desirable place to work and to be a member. People love to laugh. Read *Fish: A Remarkable Way to Boost Morale and Improve Results* by Stephen Lundin (2000), and watch the *Fish* video. Work with your team to brainstorm ways to have more fun at work. If a fish market can be that much fun, just imagine what can happen at your club!

These 10 pitfalls will derail your success if you let them. The first step to mastering them is awareness. What you do with the information is now up to you.

Becoming a Better Manager

Fitness First, the largest fitness and health club company in the world with more than 400 locations in Europe, Asia, and Australia, has a policy that their club managers invest 10% of their after-tax income on their learning and development (T. Kew, personal communication). The International Health, Racquet, and Sportsclub Association (IHRSA) offers great learning opportunities via conferences and seminars around the world, as do the Canadian Association of Fitness Professionals, also known as Can-Fit-Pro (www.canfitpro.com), and Club Industry, which has an annual conference and trade show (www.clubindustryshow.com).

It is highly recommended that you attend conferences and network with others in your profession. Find out what is working for them, and just as importantly, learn from their bad experiences. You don't have to reinvent the wheel; you just need to know how to use it. Develop relationships with successful club operators and visit their clubs to learn firsthand why they are doing well. You will also need to look outside the industry to keep your education well rounded. Find out what is working for other companies in other industries. Learn from best business practices elsewhere. The Gallup Organization is an excellent source of information (www.gallup.com), as are *Fortune* magazine and the *Harvard Business Review*, to name but a few. Become a lifelong learner—it will keep you energized and focused.

Succeeding as a Manager: A Strategy to Manage Talent

If you could choose only one component that would have the most impact on your success as a club manager, what do you think it would be? If you guessed people, you are right. You need a talent management strategy to ensure your success. You may find it useful to use the ACE (alignment, capability, and engagement) model described in figure 1.4 to visualize your talent management strategy.

If your associates are aligned with the values, beliefs, and goals of the organization (alignment), if they are capable of good performance and are properly trained and equipped to do their jobs (capability), and if they are fully engaged around their work and giving 100% of what they are capable of (engagement), then they are operating in the sweet spot of performance. This is comparable to what athletes refer to as the *zone*, that state where they are working at peak performance and loving what they are doing. People who are successful and love their jobs seldom leave.

Keeping good people is essential to the success of your club. You first need to measure associate retention just as you would measure member retention. What gets measured gets managed. Calculate how much it costs to replace one associate, and you will understand how important it is to keep good people. In order to calculate accurately, include the costs of recruitment, lost productivity by the manager while hiring and training the new associate, lost productivity by not having the position filled, lost productivity during the associate's learning curve (the time it takes to get to full productivity), and training the new associate.

THE BOTTOM LINE

In our company, we estimate that the cost of replacing one membership coordinator (sales associate) is approximately $17,500. When you use this type of analysis to gauge the cost of poor associate retention on your bottom line, it will quickly become apparent how much time and energy you need to invest in keeping good people.

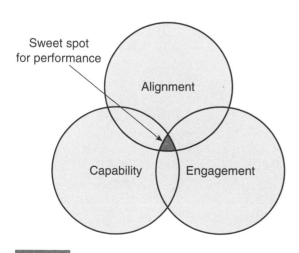

Figure 1.4 The ACE model.

You also need to closely monitor associate retention (or attrition). In this instance, not all positions are equal. The *A* positions—those who have the most direct and significant impact on the financial performance of your club—are those that should be of primary concern to you. This is the strategic part of your role and requires application of the 80:20 rule. You need to focus most of your time, attention, and resources on these positions because these are the people who are fundamental to your financial success. We consider these positions to be the club managers, membership coordinators, and front-desk associates. Whatever your *A* positions are, you need to be continually working to improve retention in them. Realistically, you will never reduce your turnover to zero. But if you have a mental picture of writing a check from your bank account for $17,500 each time a membership coordinator leaves the company, it will help you to stay focused on this critical goal.

Managers who have the lowest associate turnover in our company (and not coincidentally, consistently deliver the best financial results) have these three traits in common:

1. They are extremely skilled in developing great relationships.
2. They give people the coaching and training they require to quickly become successful in their jobs and achieve their full potential.
3. They recognize and reward good performance and confront poor performance immediately and in a caring manner.

If you are able to develop these traits in yourself and consistently treat people in accordance with them, then you will find yourself in the enviable position of having experienced, productive, and engaged people working with you. When that piece of your success strategy is in place, your success and the success of your club will be guaranteed.

KEY TERMS

core values

cultural heroes

micromanaging

Pareto's Law

sustainable competitive advantage

REFERENCES AND RECOMMENDED READINGS

Avolio, B.J., D.A. Waldman, and F.J. Yammarino. 1991. Leading in the 1990s: The four Is of transformational leadership. *Journal of European Industrial Training* 15:9-16.

Bass, B.M. 1985. *Leadership and performance beyond expectations.* New York: Free Press.

Bass, B.M., and B.J. Avolio. 1994. *Improving organizational effectiveness through transformational leadership.* Thousand Oaks, CA: Sage.

Buckingham, M. 2005. *The one thing you need to know.* New York: Free Press.

Buckingham, M., and D. Clifton. 2001. *Now, discover your strengths.* New York: Free Press.

Buckingham, M., and C. Coffman. 1999. *First break all the rules.* New York: Simon & Schuster.

Collins, J. 2001. *Good to great.* New York: Harper Business.

Covey, S.R. 1989. *The seven habits of highly effective people.* New York: Simon & Schuster.

Drucker, P. 1998. *On the profession of management.* Boston: Harvard Business School.

Evans, M.G. 1970. The effects of supervisory behavior on the path-goal relationship. *Organizational Behavior and Human Performance* 5:277-298.

Fiedler, F.E. 1967. *A theory of leadership effectiveness.* New York: McGraw-Hill.

Giuliani, R. 2002. *Leadership.* New York: Talk Miramax Books.

Gulick, L., and L. Urwick. 1937. *Papers on the science of administration.* New York: Institute of Public Administration.

Hersey, P., K.H. Blanchard, and D.E. Johnson. 2001. *Management of organizational behavior: Leading human resources.* 8th ed. Upper Saddle River, NJ: Prentice Hall.

Hersey, P., and P. Blanchard. 1969. The life cycle theory of leadership. *Training and Development Journal* 23(5):26-34.

Herzberg, R. 1966. *Work and the nature of man.* Cleveland, OH: World.

House, R.J., and T.R. Mitchell. 1997. Path-goal theory of leadership. In *Leadership: Understanding the dynamics of power and influence in organizations*, ed. R.P. Vecchio, 259-273. Notre Dame, IN: University of Notre Dame Press.

International Health, Racquet, and Sportsclub Association (IHRSA). 263 Summer Street, Boston, MA, USA, 02210. www.ihrsa.org.

Kirkpatrick, S.A., and E.A. Locke. 1991. Leadership: Do traits matter? *Academy of Management Executive* 5(2):48-60.

Koontz, H., C. O'Donnell, and H. Weihrich. 1984. *Management*. 8th ed. New York: McGraw-Hill.

Likert, R. 1961. *New patterns of management.* New York: McGraw-Hill.

Lundin, S. 2000. *Fish: A remarkable way to boost morale and improve results.* New York: Hyperion.

Maslow, A.H. 1954. *Motivation and personality.* New York: Harper.

Mayo, E. 1933. *The human problems of an industrial civilization.* New York: Macmillan.

McGregor, D. 1960. *The human side of enterprise.* New York: McGraw-Hill.

Mintzberg, H. 1973. *The nature of managerial work.* New York: Harper and Row.

———. 1990. The manager's job: Folklore and fact. *Harvard Business Review* 68(2):163-176.

———. 2004. *Managers not MBAs.* San Francisco: Berrett-Koehler.

Rath, T. 2007. *Strengthsfinder 2.0.* New York: Gallup.

Slater, R. 1999. *Jack Welch and the GE way.* New York: McGraw-Hill.

Taylor, F.W. 1911. *The principles of scientific management.* New York: Harper.

Tichy, N.M., and N. Cardwell. 2002. *The cycle of leadership.* New York: HarperCollins.

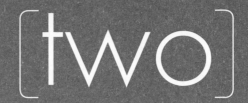
Understanding Organizational Design

Scott Lewandowski

After studying this chapter, the reader will be able to

- recognize key employees and their responsibilities;

- understand the importance of job descriptions in facility operations;

- discuss the differences among for-profit, not-for-profit, and corporate-based fitness facilities; and

- identify behaviors of successful leaders in the fitness industry.

The culture of health and fitness clubs is fast paced. You must expect the unexpected, be prepared to maintain your composure, and execute superior service. Along with operations issues that can change the flow of anyone's day, many employees, especially the frontline staff, work part-time. Unless part-time employees have a significant number of hours, their commitment to your club may not be a priority.

It is the manager's responsibility to provide a healthy, challenging, and rewarding work environment that encourages a greater commitment from and builds confidence in both part-time and full-time employees. A clear and concise organizational chart listing all job positions is essential for employees to understand everyone's role in reaching the goals of the club. Well-structured job descriptions are critical for employees to know their responsibilities and expectations. Finally, management must provide some training for staff in other departments besides their hired position to create a sense of confidence in case they have to handle a crisis like the one described in Tales From the Trenches.

THE BOTTOM LINE

Job satisfaction is directly related to maximally using your employees' skills, and employee retention is directly related to member retention. Create volunteer executive retention teams that focus on welcoming new members, retaining old members, retaining staff, providing social activities besides exercise, and getting members to participate in group exercise.

Organizational design is important in the daily operations of a facility. By hiring qualified personnel with a clear understanding of their responsibilities, employees perform their best and understand how their position contributes to the facilities' goals. Concise job descriptions define the roles of the employee, determining how the position will contribute to customer service, revenue of the individual department, and retention of employees and members. It must also be noted that although staff members may have job descriptions, it is not unusual for them to assume multiple job functions. The focus of this chapter will be to describe how various health and fitness organizations are set up and discuss the key positions of these organizations. Four types of organizations will be examined in this chapter, including for-profit commercial organizations, not-for-profit organizations, hospital-based organizations, and corporate-based organizations. (Key components of job descriptions are discussed in chapter 3.)

Though these four types of health and fitness organizations have some differences in organizational design in order to achieve their business goals, they do share common themes, positions, and processes. These organizations strive to promote an environment that is welcoming, friendly, and fun.

A common theme among all of these organizations is superior **customer service** to improve member satisfaction, increase member referrals, and retain members. Each organization has a front desk where members and guests are greeted by name with a smile. Members are encouraged to provide feedback in the form of comment cards located throughout the clubs. Member appreciation parties are offered to foster staff–member relationships and member–member relationships. Staff must be educated on every program and service offered at the club so that they can answer the numerous questions asked during their shifts.

Selling fitness is another common theme among these organizations. Marketing staff and sales staff look for new members, generate leads, sell memberships, and continue to foster those relationships for member referrals. Each organization has personal trainers who offer individualized workouts and niche programming to assist members in reaching their goals. They also include elaborate group exercise schedules that offer complimentary classes in different formats.

THE BOTTOM LINE

All employees in a health and fitness facility sell fitness. They may not be selling memberships or performing personal training, but they are selling the benefits of your facility in helping members reach their goals. Keep this in mind when interviewing—a common mistake in hiring is an employee who dislikes selling.

Comprehensive processes for staff and member integration have been implemented to improve success and retention. Initial and ongoing staff training improves the likelihood of job satisfaction, and IHRSA studies have shown a direct correlation between staff retention and member retention (International Health, Racquet, and Sportsclub Association [IHRSA] 2004). The integration process includes a specified number of complimentary sessions or discounted club services to help members become acclimated to their new facility and to direct them on their fitness journey at the club. The more connected the member is to the facility, the greater the chances are of member retention.

These organizations are fast paced and staff members must be proficient in multitasking. A scheduled task could change within minutes of a member's question, concern, or specific need. An entire day's work can change with a staff absence, club emergency, unexpected appointment from neighborhood businesses or vendors, or e-mail or voice mail.

To ensure their future existence, these organizations continue to develop new fee-based programming to increase **nondues revenue.** Members participating in more than just the club membership are more likely to remain members because they are more financially invested.

Although these organizations share common themes, positions, and a few processes, their organizational design and job descriptions for similar positions are arranged differently in order to meet facility goals. The organizational design and job descriptions may focus on profit, community service, hospital involvement, or corporate wellness. We will compare a few different organizational designs. See Essential Web Sites on page 24 for sources of additional information on organization and other topics of interest to the health and fitness industry.

For-Profit Commercial Organizations

For-profit commercial facilities larger than 20,000 square feet (1,858 square meters) with more than 50 employees are very fast paced (see figure 2.1). Expectations at the beginning of the workday are seldom completed. These organizations focus on membership, retention, and revenue. Earnings before interest, taxes, depreciation, and amortization (EBITDA), as well as revenue growth sales, membership retention, net membership growth, revenue per member, revenue per indoor square foot, and nondues revenue, are tracked monthly and compared against the current budget, last year's budget, and industry standards.

For-profit commercial facilities smaller than 10,000 square feet (929 square meters) maintain the same financial and retention goals as larger facilities (see figure 2.2). The main difference is in staffing and marketing. These facilities staff up to 7 employees, but normally not more than this. Most of these employees have titles like *member counselor* and *wellness coach.* They sell memberships, set up exercise programs, and clean up the facility. They have to be demographically sound because unless they are part of a franchise, they don't have much capital for large direct-mail promotions. Instead, they spend their time and money offering screening at community events and corporate health fairs.

Employees in larger facilities have more clearly defined roles and responsibilities. Key positions in a large commercial facility include the general manager, membership director, membership consultants (sales representatives), fitness director, and personal trainers. Following are sample job descriptions for each position.

General Manager

The primary role of the **general manager** is ensuring that the annual budget is met, developing a marketing plan with the membership director for continued membership growth, keeping a high profile in the club, and working with department managers to achieve desired results. The general manager has the most difficult job when it comes to organization. When there is a problem, it is the general manager who is called upon. The general manager must be available to assist departments when needed and have a strong presence throughout the club, especially during peak times. It is the general manager who can truly say there are not enough hours in a day.

Primary Responsibilities and Goals

- Adhere to the core values and core purpose as established by ownership.

- Improve the overall service level of the club. This is measured via a semiannual quantitative customer satisfaction survey.

- Increase the demand, usage, and net revenue capabilities of the club during off-peak hours. To date this has primarily been accomplished by ownership ability to establish **subtenant** relationships in addition to off-peak membership sales. (A subtenant, such as a juice bar or a pro shop, rents space from the fitness club and operates its business within the walls of the club.)

- Implement the strategic plan for the club.

- Hold quarterly all-staff meetings for the purpose of reinforcing the annual goals; team building; informing staff of new programs, services, and amenities; gathering staff ideas; and training.

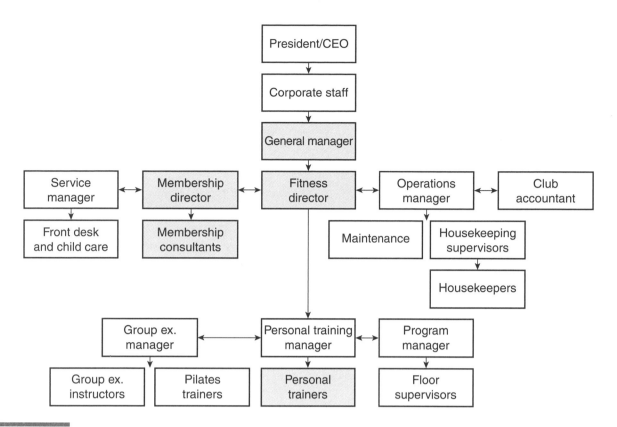

Figure 2.1 Organization chart of a for-profit organization (larger than 20,000 ft² [1,858 m²] and more than 50 employees). Shaded areas indicate positions described in the text.

Reprinted by permission.

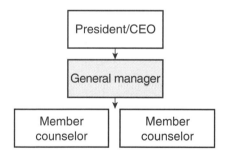

Figure 2.2 Organization chart for a small for-profit organization. These organizations typically are smaller than 10,000 square feet (929 square meters) and have fewer than 10 employees.

- Hold regular meetings (weekly) with the management team.
- Nurture the subtenant relationships.
- Establish specific goals for each department manager and tie them directly to the managers' budget performance and compensation.
- Establish the annual club budget (to be approved by ownership).

- Meet budget profits by implementing the approved budget and making adjustments to the budget plan if profit goal is not being met by midyear.
- Participate in the manager on duty (MOD) program on a regular basis.
- Produce a monthly variance report that documents financial variations from the budgeted versus actual income statement.
- Work diligently on the marketing efforts of the club, with a special emphasis required for the membership director and the staff.
- Actively participate in the development of the marketing plan yearly. Work closely with sales department to help sell memberships.
- Keep a high profile in the club, getting acquainted with as many members as possible.
- Work with the operations manager and director of human resources (corporate staff) to provide regular, thorough training of all employees.

- Conduct performance reviews first at 90 days and then every 6 months for all department managers.
- Approve hiring of all new employees, as well as all changes of employment status.
- Submit assigned operating and retention reports.

Job Summary

The general manager position is full-time. The position reports to the regional operations director (corporate staff).

Membership Director

With 70% to 80% of total revenue coming from dues, the primary role of the **membership director** is setting sales goals with membership consultants to maintain a constant stream of new members. One responsibility is prospecting outside the club through various mailings, participating in networking functions, and building relationships with local businesses. Many of these prospects are offered guest memberships to try out the facility. Another responsibility is prospecting within the club with current members. New members are offered guest memberships for family and friends to enforce a support system for the new member and to recruit new members. A member **referral program** rewards members who assist in recruiting a new member.

The purpose of this position is to lead, motivate, and organize a team of sales professionals in achieving or exceeding monthly and individual sales numbers and quotas, monthly dues, annual dues, guest fees, seasonal memberships, and **I-fees** (enrollment fees charged when the member first joins).

Qualifications

- Demonstrate good communication skills.
- Demonstrate good leadership qualities.
- Demonstrate strong sales ability.
- Display good organizational skills.
- Have a minimum of 2 to 5 years of sales or sales management experience.
- Maintain regular attendance and punctuality.

In addition, the ideal candidate will possess all of the following skills and attributes:

- Outgoing personality
- Sales and promotional aptitude
- Telephone sales skills
- Ability to effectively use one-on-one sales closing techniques
- Ability to effectively present and close corporate accounts

Responsibilities

- Meet quotas as set forth in the membership director salary, commission, and quota agreement.
- Fulfill all assignments as requested by general manager.
- Work within approved guidelines of pay structure and follow proper procedures for hiring, disciplining, and firing.
- Train, coach, and manage membership consultants.
- Have monthly one-on-one meetings with each membership consultant.
- Chair weekly team meetings.
- Compile, publish, and maintain sales standards, including incoming and outgoing calls, number of tours, referrals, referral attempts, commissions, payroll, closing percentages, bonus records, and so on.
- Ensure membership department meets monthly goals.
- Set up and maintain standards of cleanliness and orderliness for the membership staff and membership consultant offices.
- Maintain professional dress and appearance for self and staff.
- Set up and maintain standards of protocol with nonmembers for all staff.
- Set up systems to ensure consistent inventory of all membership and collateral materials.
- Ensure that membership staff promote and sell all club services and products.
- Stay up to date on sales and marketing information and disseminate this information to staff.
- Develop member referral programs with the regional membership director (corporate staff).
- Develop consultant recognition and reward programs.
- Lead by example, especially in the areas of appearance, punctuality, and professionalism.
- Be an active participant in club management meetings.

- Use training and quality-control techniques to ensure membership consultants' compliance with their job description.
- Create membership budget.
- Write monthly variance reports as requested by the general manager.

Position Requirements

- Proficient in scripted sales method, for which training will be provided.
- Proficient in asking for the sale, for which training will be provided.
- Must work during closeout, the last 3 days of each month.

Job Summary

The membership director is a full-time position and reports directly to the general manager.

Membership Consultants (Sales Representatives)

The purpose of the **membership consultant** position is to reach individual quotas of monthly dues, annual dues, guest fees, seasonal memberships, and I-fees and thus help ensure the membership team meets budgeted goals; to serve members on a daily basis; and to actively pursue inside and outside prospects.

Primary Responsibilities

- Reach monthly quotas.
- Process all contracts and paperwork in a timely and accurate manner.
- Prospect inside and outside leads on an ongoing basis.
- Serve all prospects and members by exceeding their expectations.

General Responsibilities

- Complete all assignments as given by the general manager or membership director.
- Adjust schedule as required.
- Meet sales skills standards (phone presentation, building rapport, greeting, needs, touring, trial closing, overcoming objections, and closing).
- Schedule and confirm appointments with prospects.
- Track membership activity using daily, weekly, and monthly tracking sheets. Keep specialty mailing files up to date (e.g., past tours, guest passes, cancelled memberships).
- Obtain referrals from current and new members.
- Send thank-you notes to all new members.
- Attend all required membership meetings and training sessions.
- Research competition by touring and calling other clubs on a regular basis.
- Represent the club in outside sales capacity, including corporate memberships, chamber of commerce lunches, and after-hours special events.
- Contribute ideas to and help implement internal and external marketing campaigns.
- Meet and exceed individual and team goals.
- Organize and file all membership-related paperwork.
- Always be available to work month-end closeouts.

Position Requirements

- Proficient in scripted sales method, for which training will be provided.
- Proficient in asking for the sale, for which training will be provided.
- Must work during closeout, the last 3 days of each month.

Physical Requirements

- Must be able to walk stairs repeatedly during shift.
- Extended time spent on the phone.
- Must be able to lift 15 to 20 pounds (7-9 kilograms).

Job Summary

The membership consultant position is part of the revenue-generating membership department. It is full-time and reports directly to the membership director.

THE BOTTOM LINE

If the membership department does not have a structured follow-up plan with new members, the chances of retaining those members decreases. This is especially true with members who decide not to participate in their integration appointments or sign up for a fee-based fitness program.

Fitness Director

The primary responsibility of the **fitness director** is retaining members by offering a variety of programs that help members attain their health and fitness goals. They are responsible for developing, evaluating, and growing programs to increase participation and revenue. Clubs offer a balance of free and fee-based programs that add value to the membership. Free programs include an integration program, a group exercise schedule, seminars, and motivational contests. Fee-based programs include personal training, Pilates training, weight management programs, sport-specific programming, leagues, and special events. To offer this variety in programming, the fitness directors actively recruit, train, and evaluate employees for continued success. Successful fitness departments produce 25% to 30% of the total revenue (IHRSA 2006).

Purpose

The purpose of this position is to originate, coordinate, promote, supervise, implement, and evaluate quality fitness programs that will assist all members in achieving their fitness goals, and to ensure that the fitness department is profitable and meets or exceeds the annual budget goals.

Qualifications

- Bachelor's degree in exercise physiology or exercise science required. Master's degree in exercise physiology preferred. One or two **third-party nationally accredited certifications** required, as well as current cardiopulmonary resuscitation (CPR) and automated external defibrillator (AED) certification.
- Three to 5 years of experience in a health and fitness facility, 2 years of experience at a fitness facility or in program management, and 1 to 2 years of supervisory experience required. Must be experienced in conducting submaximal fitness assessments. Must have experience in performance management and staff motivation.

Primary Responsibilities

- Provide a clean, safe, and healthy environment for members, guests, and coworkers.
- Help retain current members and attain new members through club promotion and customer service excellence.

General Responsibilities

- Acquire, maintain, and serve members by supporting their participation in programs and activities.
- Define performance standards and objectives for fitness staff.
- Develop, promote, grow, and evaluate fitness programs.
- Conduct all facets of fitness assessments.
- Maintain knowledge of all programs taking place within the club.

Specific Responsibilities

- Conduct staff training sessions on fitness and service on a regular basis.
- Conduct performance evaluations for fitness managers.
- Track completion of managers' evaluations of fitness staff performance.
- Track attendance, vacation, and sick days of fitness staff.
- Attend national industry trade shows and conferences.
- Instruct group exercise classes.
- Provide personal training for club members as necessary.
- Provide education and training on proper use of exercise equipment available to members.
- Recruit, hire, train, and supervise fitness department managers (personal training, group exercise, and program managers).
- Contribute articles to company quarterly newsletters.
- Actively participate in all phases of major club functions and special events.
- Participate in the MOD rotation.
- Submit annual fitness department budget as per instructions by the general manager.
- Help develop the fitness department operations manual.
- Oversee the maintenance, cleanliness, and upkeep of the facility and equipment.
- Inspect all fitness equipment to ensure the highest standards of maintenance and cleanliness.

Position Requirements

- Proficient in scripted sales method, for which training will be provided.

- Must be proficient in asking for the sale.
- Must work during closeout, the last 3 days of each month.

Physical Requirements

This position requires bending and standing. Must be able to move fitness equipment and lift weight plates and dumbbells.

Job Summary

The fitness director is part of the revenue-generating fitness department. It is full-time and reports to the general manager.

Personal Trainers

The entry-level position in the fitness department is the **personal trainer.** Personal trainers are responsible for integrating members into a facility and generating revenue by helping members reach their fitness goals. To maximize personal training sales and membership penetration, personal trainers should be hired as full-time employees. It is difficult for employees to build rapport with members, let alone a client base, if they spend little time interacting with members.

Members who spend additional money beyond their dues reinforce their commitment to the club. According to IHRSA's *Profiles of Success* (2006), there is a direct correlation between clubs that have a high percentage of nondues revenue and clubs that have high retention rates. The trainers must be held accountable to monthly individual and team goals.

The personal trainer position will include selling personal training sessions and packages and establishing, implementing, monitoring, and maintaining individual exercise recommendations for clients in a professional manner to ensure member satisfaction and retention.

Qualifications

- Bachelor's degree in exercise physiology or an allied health field or a third-party nationally accredited personal trainer certification and 1 year of experience required.
- Current CPR and AED certification required.

Position Requirements

- Proficient in scripted sales method, for which training will be provided.
- Proficient in asking for the sale, for which training will be provided.

- Responsible for $1,500 in personal training sales in the first month, $3,000 in personal training sales in the second month, and $5,000 in personal training sales in the third month and beyond.
- Work 36 to 40 hours in club and maintain 25 paid personal training sessions per week by the third month of employment.
- Complete 20 complimentary sessions per month.
- May be required to work during closeout, the last 3 days of each month, based on individual or department budgeted goals.
- Must be available to work certain fitness floor shifts to ensure proper service for and safety of all members and guests.

Position Responsibilities

- Member service:
  - Provide a clean, safe, and healthy environment for members, guests, and coworkers.
  - Help retain and attain new members through club promotion and customer service excellence.
  - Conduct a fitness consultation orientation for all new members within their first month of joining. All members must be given a workout card upon completion.
  - Assist members with specific fitness concerns on the fitness floor.
  - Conduct 8-week reassessments on all members.
  - Provide and monitor quality exercise recommendations for individual clients, ensuring the attainment of their specific fitness goals.
  - Wear appropriate attire at all times while training clients.
- Maintain and update a 2-week schedule for appointments.
- Client files maintenance:
  - Physical Activity Readiness Questionnaire (PAR-Q)
  - Medical health history
  - Needs analysis
  - Informed consent
  - Fitness evaluation
  - Copy of exercise program

Physical Requirements

Physical strength and manual dexterity are required.

Education and Training

- Maintain current involvement in professional organizations.
- Maintain current certification through continuing education and current CPR certification.
- Attend all required department and continuing education meetings.
- Provide a free personal training session to all new sales staff.

Equipment

- Spot members during exercise sessions.
- Restack all weights.
- Maintain supply of towels on the floor.
- Clean weight and cardiorespiratory equipment after client or personal use or when necessary.

Special Events and Community Service

- Volunteer for special events and programs and various community events.
- Participate in member appreciation parties.

Job Summary

The personal trainer is a full-time position. It reports directly to the personal training manager, fitness director, or general manager.

THE BOTTOM LINE

Qualified, energetic, and well-organized personal trainers are successful whether they are full-time or part-time employees. However, with full-time personal trainers scheduled for 40 hours per week, you can control their schedules, keep them on higher revenue goals, and hold them to a minimum number of paid sessions and integration appointments per month. You can accomplish some of these expectations with part-time personal trainers, but their schedules are limited and they are usually only present for their appointments, limiting their interaction with other members during slower times.

Not-for-Profit Community Facilities

Not-for-profit community facilities are unique in that they receive tax-exempt status for providing affordable health and wellness programs for their community. These organizations include YMCAs, Jewish Community Centers (JCCs), and hospital-based, faith-based, and park and recreation centers. A board of directors made up of local business members governs these facilities. The board members serve a 2- to 4-year term dependent upon the organization and, along with the president and CEO, develop the budget and plan major renovations and purchases. As not-for-profit organizations, revenue generated through memberships and programs pays the operating expenses, with the remaining revenue benefiting the community.

Not-for-profit organizations also campaign for donations to provide scholarships to offset membership and program costs for families in need. The goal of these organizations is not to turn a profit on their activities but to provide programming that meets the needs of today's youth, family, adults, and seniors regardless of their financial situation. These programs focus on health and fitness, child care and development, education, arts, and summer and overnight camps. Key positions of these facilities include the individual directors of the various programs as well as the director of fund-raising. Unlike many for-profit centers that focus on a niche market, not-for-profit facilities try to provide something for everyone. A sample not-for-profit community facility is shown in figure 2.3, and two of its key positions are described in the material that follows.

THE BOTTOM LINE

Fund-raising is an important source of revenue for nonprofit organizations. Along with the finance development team, the entire staff is constantly conducting fund-raising competitions and events. Staff members also set fund-raising goals for themselves.

Finance Development Executive

The **finance development executive** will assume the primary responsibilities of capital development and annual fund-raising along with developing and executing a communication plan for the com-

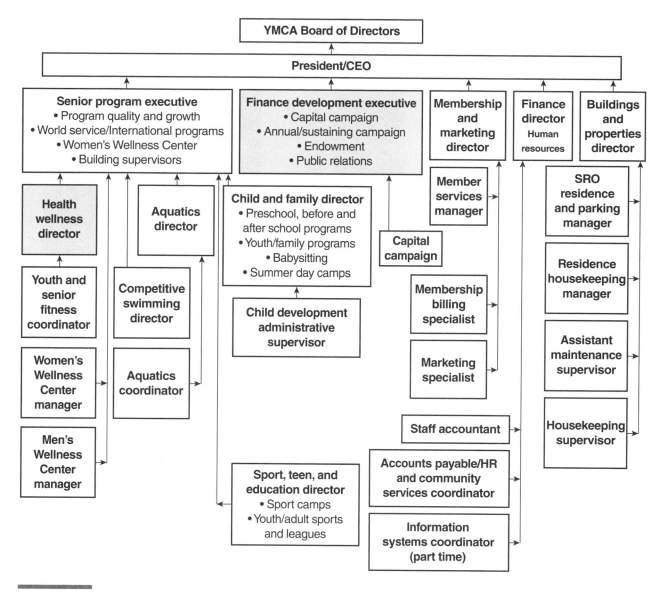

Figure 2.3 Organizational chart for a not-for-profit community facility. Shaded areas indicate positions that are described in the text.

Reprinted by permission.

munity, members, donors, and board members. The finance development executive will establish a recognition system for donors and volunteers who contribute to the annual fund-raising efforts; develop and implement a communication plan that interprets the club to the community, donors, members, and board members; work with the board of directors to maintain a high profile within the community; and consult with the senior program executive on the budget to meet fiscal objectives.

Preferred Qualifications

Successful financial development experience in a nonprofit or public setting with increasing levels

of responsibility required. Experience in a paid or volunteer position preferred. Previous fund-raising or capital campaign experience preferred. Must possess excellent written and verbal communication skills, be proficient in all Microsoft Office applications, and have experience in training others.

Health and Wellness Director

The **health and wellness director** is responsible for the organization, delivery, and quality of all health, fitness, and wellness programs for all age groups. Emphasis is on the quality of the programs, remaining up-to-date on fitness trends, increasing the number of participants served, and budget management.

Functions and Duties Specific to Health and Fitness

- General: Perform all duties required for successful fitness, health and wellness, and related programs for all ages.
- Staffing: Hire, manage, recruit, and supervise, and oversee job performance of fitness staff.
- Character development: Commit to developing character in all participants, especially young people.
- Communication: Keep fitness staff informed of new programs, program time changes, special fitness events, and other fitness-, health-, and wellness-related events. Market the department programs to the community.
- Staff meetings: Conduct informal or educational staff meetings at least once during each session to pass information from program director and department head meetings, creating positive information flow both ways.
- Facilities and equipment: Secure all internal facilities needed for program implementation, and seek areas outside the facility in the community as programs grow. Maintain, monitor, inventory, and purchase equipment. Collaborate with all other departments regarding needs and status of facility and equipment.
- Budget and reports: Develop and monitor programs to meet fiscal objectives of the budget with program executive and finance director.

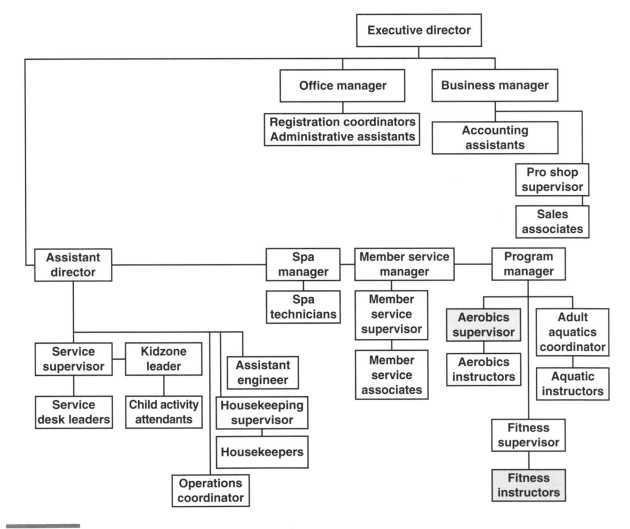

Figure 2.4 Organizational chart of a hospital-based fitness center. Shaded areas indicate positions that are described in the text.

Reprinted by permission.

- Fund-raising: Facilitate fund-raising to meet budget goal and collaborate with other directors regarding events and ideas.

Functions and Duties Specific to Director Status

- Program related:
  - Promote and incorporate core values and character development model in all programs and activities.
  - With marketing department, market and distribute program-specific information each session.
  - Compile program statistical reports as needed.
  - Develop and maintain collaborative relationships with other community organizations.
  - Assist in fund-raising activities and special events.
  - Respond to all member and community inquiries and complaints in a timely manner.
  - Assist with and attend program staff meetings (1-2 times per month), department head meetings (2 times per month), and other meetings as needed.
- Member services:
  - Keep front-desk staff informed of all programs, special events, and changes at all times.
  - Assist member services during busy registration times as needed.
- Relationship building:
  - Consider every interaction with members as an opportunity for creating a relationship.
  - Maintain an average of 10 to 12 contact hours per week with members (teaching, personal training, or other interactions).
- Teamwork:
  - Work in cooperation with all staff to ensure safety and quality member service as the main priority.
  - Work within all set deadlines, following all procedures as related to meeting communication and report expectations (i.e., purchase orders, new-employee documents, bulletin board messages, marketing requests, check requests, budgeting and operational goals, brochure information, and so on).

- Assist in maintaining building cleanliness and repairs through service requests.
- Other duties as assigned by supervisor.

Qualifications

To perform this job successfully, an individual must be able to perform each essential duty satisfactorily. The requirements listed are representative of the knowledge, skill, and ability required. Reasonable accommodations may be made to enable individuals with disabilities to perform the essential functions.

- Education: Bachelor's degree in exercise physiology, physical education, or related field required; master's preferred.
- Additional certification from a national organization.
- Knowledge: Must show sensitivity to needs of populations served; strong organizational, communication, and fiscal skills.
- Experience: Must have 1 to 2 years experience and ability to provide leadership in developing program designs, fitness testing, exercise prescriptions, personal training, and programs for special populations.
- Language skills: Must be able to read, analyze, and interpret general business periodicals, professional journals, technical procedures, or government regulations; ability to write reports, business correspondence, and procedure manuals; and ability to effectively present information and respond to questions from supervisors, members, customers, participants, and the general public.
- Mathematical skills: Must be able to calculate figures and amounts such as discounts, proportions, percentages, area, circumference, and volume; ability to apply concepts of basic algebra and geometry.
- Reasoning skills: Must be able to solve practical problems, deal with a variety of concrete variables in various situations, and interpret a variety of instructions furnished in written, oral, diagram, or schedule forms.

Physical Requirements

Physical demands described here are representative of what must be met by an employee to successfully perform the essential functions of this job. Reasonable accommodations may be made to enable individuals with disabilities to perform essential functions. While performing duties of this job, employees are regularly required to stand and walk for long periods. In teaching class, the employee must to be able to run, jump, or dance for a period of up to 75 minutes; have the upper- and lower-body range of motion required to demonstrate and perform all aerobic, toning, and strengthening exercises included in class; have the upper-body strength to lift 80 pounds (36 kilograms); and have the manual dexterity to lock and unlock doors and to move and operate stereo and exercise equipment. The employee must be able to talk and hear during prolonged conversations and often under noisy conditions. The employee is occasionally required to sit.

Work Environment

Environment characteristics described here are representative of those the employee encounters while performing essential functions of the job. Reasonable accommodations may be made to enable individuals with disabilities to perform essential functions. The noise level in the work environment is usually moderate but may be intermittently high.

Hospital-Based Fitness Centers

Hospital-based fitness centers are more often not for profit than for profit. Many of these centers have community members and physicians serving on a health system board or board of directors, setting standards of health care that integrate prevention, lifestyle changes, and rehabilitation of members and patients and that create a continuum of care for the community. Most patients will have temporary access to the fitness center.

Not only do these fitness centers offer cardiorespiratory equipment, strength equipment, group exercises, and programs typical of for-profit centers, they also offer programs such as cardiac rehabilitation, arthritic programming, osteoporosis programming, smoking cessation, aging seminars, and cancer wellness because of the involvement of physicians at the hospital. Most of the centers are located on a hospital campus, allowing for ease of blood cholesterol testing, bone density testing, and stress testing. The success of medical programming depends upon enthusiastic physicians who firmly believe that exercise can assist in the prevention and rehabilitation of many diseases. In some cases, a hospital may have a health promotions department that works closely with the program manager of the fitness center to run these wellness programs.

Employees at a hospital-based facility come in contact with a wide range of members. Some members will be apparently healthy but a majority will have some complication or injury they are recovering from at the hospital. Doctor involvement is not unusual in fitness programming. Most importantly, the employees need to be comfortable with reading health history forms and be aware of exercise limitations for various conditions such as cardiac rehabilitation, asthma, arthritis, and high blood pressure. This is important for any facility, but particularly a fitness club that is associated with a hospital.

A sample organizational chart of a hospital-based fitness center is shown in figure 2.4, and two key positions are described in the material that follows.

THE BOTTOM LINE

There has been much discussion about the opportunities of medical referrals for fitness centers. Hospital-based centers are more likely to be successful with medical referrals because in many circumstances the fitness center is owned by the hospital and some of the medical programming from the hospital occurs in the fitness center.

Aerobics Supervisor

The supervisor is responsible for coordinating and supervising the aerobic exercise programs. In doing so, he or she prepares work schedules, trains exercise instructors, monitors adherence to policies and procedures, and assists in resolving difficult problems or complaints. He or she also assists in developing the annual operating budget and administers it and implements policies and procedures to improve the aerobic exercise program.

Corporate Philosophy

It is the obligation of each employee to abide by and promote the mission and values of the corporation to ensure that excellent services are delivered with compassion.

Principal Duties and Responsibilities

The following duties and responsibilities are all essential job functions.

- Responsible for supervising the daily activities of personnel engaged in designing and leading various levels of aerobic exercise classes. In doing so, develops aerobic programs, establishes exercise class contents and schedules, maintains supplies and equipment, and so forth.

- Prepares periodic work schedules in order to ensure adequate coverage of aerobics classes. Monitors attendance at classes and recommends changes to the schedule in order to better meet the needs of members.

- Interviews, hires, orients, trains, and evaluates the performance of subordinate instructors, and when necessary, disciplines and discharges subordinate instructors. Works with supervisor to resolve difficult problems in employee relations.

- Prepares and administers annual operating budget for assigned area, ensures adherence to same, and notifies supervisor of significant variances.

- Maintains aerobics equipment and music system in proper working condition, orders routine supplies, and recommends purchase of capital equipment.

- Acts as a resource for assigned personnel in resolving complaints and problems. Evaluates suggestions for improving the aerobic exercise program and implements new routines and classes in order to enhance the program.

- Develops, recommends, and implements policies and procedures for aerobic exercise program, ensures adherence to same, and modifies procedures as necessary to improve services.

- Performs duties of instructor in response to work load and staffing demands. In doing so, prepares aerobic exercise classes, selects music, leads classes, provides instruction in proper form and technique, and so forth. Instructs at least 3 hours of aerobic and conditioning classes weekly.

- Performs related duties such as conducting periodic staff meetings, presenting in-service sessions, maintaining logs and reports of incidents and activities, and so on.

Knowledge, Skills, and Abilities Required

- Requires the knowledge normally gained in 2 to 3 years of education or training after high school and 3 to 5 years of previous experience plus approximately 3 to 6 months of on-the-job experience.

- CPR certification required within the first 6 weeks of employment.

- A moderate level of analytical ability is required. Work is performed in accordance with standard procedures and requires basic technical knowledge or in-depth, experience-based knowledge in order to analyze and interpret information.

- A significant level of communication skills is required in order to explain policies or otherwise communicate in situations requiring sensitivity and tact.

- Work is not completely standardized. Assignments are often received in the form of results expected, due dates, and general procedures to follow.

- Work requires the ability to lead and instruct various levels of aerobics classes, walk or stand for an hour or more at a time, lift or carry objects weighing 5 to 20 pounds (2-9 kilograms), and use a keyboard to enter, retrieve, or transform words or data.

- Work conditions include working with equipment or performing activities where carelessness would probably result in minor cuts, bruises, or muscle strains.

Reporting Relationships

- Reports to the program manager.
- Responsible for supervising the work of approximately 10 to 20 employees.

Fitness Instructor

The **fitness instructor** is responsible for assisting members and nonmembers who have health and special needs. The fitness instructor performs individualized fitness consultations, equipment orientation, and continued follow-up, and also assists and develops, coordinates, and implements fitness-related programs and education presentations and special events as directed by the supervisor.

Corporate Philosophy

It is the obligation of each employee to abide by and promote the mission and values of the corporation to ensure that excellent services are delivered with compassion.

Principal Duties and Responsibilities

The following duties and responsibilities are all essential job functions.

- Provides individualized fitness consultation to members and nonmembers with health and special needs in order to assess their overall fitness level. Prescribes exercise programs in accordance with established fitness consultation protocol. Provides continual follow-up services.

- Proactively assists members with exercise programs, instructing orientation to equipment, group exercise, and wellness classes.

- Instructs group exercise classes for healthy and special needs members and nonmembers.

- Develops, coordinates, and implements clinical, fitness, and member motivational programming and special events as directed by supervisor.

- Contributes in the development and administration of the budget and program plans of fitness programs as directed by supervisor.

- Monitors quality, progress, and success of members and nonmembers engaged in fitness programs and assists with medical members.

- Develops wellness educational lectures and presents to members at hospital locations and to the community.

- Contributes to the member service of the center by completing face-to-face interactions with members on a daily basis.

Knowledge, Skills, and Abilities Required

- Requires a bachelor's degree in exercise science or a closely related field or any bachelor's degree plus a nationally accredited certification. (Degree may be in process with completion within 2 years of employment.) A minimum of 1 year of previous fitness specialist experience is preferred. Excellent customer service skills are required.

- CPR certification required within the first 90 days of employment.

- A moderate level of analytical ability is required. Work is performed in accordance with standard procedures and requires basic technical knowledge or in-depth, experience-based knowledge in order to analyze and interpret information.

- Relatively high levels of communication and customer service skills are required in order to lead, teach, and persuade others and interact effectively with others in difficult situations.

- Work is not completely standardized. Assignments are often received in the form of results expected, due dates, and general procedures to follow.

- Work requires the ability to walk or stand for an hour or more at a time, lift or carry objects weighing more than 45 pounds (20 kilograms), and assist members with exercise workouts.

- Work conditions include working in an area that is somewhat unpleasant due to drafts, noise, temperature variation or the like, and working with equipment or performing activities where carelessness would probably result in minor cuts, bruises, or muscle strains.

Reporting Relationships

- Reports to the fitness supervisor at the center where majority of hours are spent working.

- Has no responsibility for leading or supervising the work of others.

Corporate-Based Fitness Organizations

Corporate-based fitness organizations provide convenient, cost-effective, customized, and flexible plans to meet the demands of a company. As health care costs continue to rise, companies are investing in their employees' health and well-being, which is increasing work productivity and decreasing physician visits. By offering health promotion and screening programs, employees can benefit from more balanced living, including exercise and improved self-monitoring of adverse health symptoms such as stress and mild depression. Through well-organized programs and ongoing promotion of the facilities' activities, increased participation is realized. Not only does heightened awareness result in increased membership enrollment, but the facility helps foster a positive workplace mind-set. The facility becomes a healthy environment through which employees' health and well-being are nurtured and improved.

Corporate facilities take into account all pertinent influences on the employees' health, from tangibles such as family medical history, eating habits, and cholesterol levels to intangibles such as life satisfaction, stress, and work–life balance. The employee on the verge of a breakdown appears no more at risk on the outside than any other employee does. While companies are containing health care costs and reducing medical claims, their employees are addressing pertinent work and life issues and participating in a healthier way of life. Together, they make the every-day work experience more productive and positive, establishing the company as a progressive leader in healthy, effective change.

A sample wellness model

- targets healthy populations;
- improves exercise participation to relieve stress and increase self-esteem;
- provides social structure outside the work-place, lowering incidence of mild depression from job or life burnout;
- reports progress with systematic and accurate diagnostic measurement, resulting in greater motivation and sustained participation; and
- alerts chronically at-risk populations (for example, those who smoke or are obese, depressed, or hypertensive) to seek medical care in conjunction with lifestyle programs.

Figure 2.5 is an organizational chart for a corporate-based facility. Two of the key positions are described in the material that follows.

THE BOTTOM LINE

A successful corporate-based facility needs a comprehensive wellness tracking system to report the overall health of its employees. Improving health conditions will increase productivity in the workplace, and this information can increase the likelihood of corporate memberships at the facility.

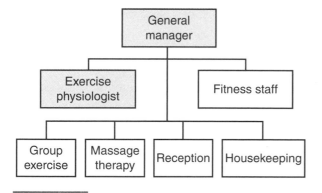

Figure 2.5 Organizational chart for a corporate-based facility. Shaded areas indicate positions that are described in the text.

Reprinted by permission.

General Manager

The general manager reports directly to the corporate management team.

Minimum Requirements

- Master's degree required.
- Minimum of 3 years management experience and experience in teaching customer service techniques with a sensitivity to maintaining staff relations and cohesiveness required.
- Must have an outgoing personality with the ability to effectively communicate, teach, and motivate a variety of people.
- Must have personal commitment to a fit and healthy lifestyle.
- Must be professionally dressed at all times, maintaining a well-groomed appearance.
- Proficient computer skills required.

Job Description

- Responsible for managing all aspects of operations, marketing, and financial reporting of the center.
- Ensures the highest level of customer service and fiscal success.
- Provides an organized leadership role, including ongoing staff training, club programming, and new business development.
- Reviews all financial reporting for accuracy, monitors all purchasing practices to ensure expense controls are sufficient to meet budget, and prepares staffing plans and pricing policies to achieve club operating budgets.

Job Responsibilities

- Know and understand all company and club policies and procedures and direct the operating affairs of the club within these parameters.
- Establish a staffing plan that efficiently achieves the operating standards of a first-class club operation, including appointing department heads, creating job descriptions for all positions, and developing work schedules to optimize successful club programs. Positions could include assistant manager, fitness staff, or housekeeping.

- Establish a personal schedule that provides high visibility at peak operating times, such as managing the club and walking the exercise areas at busy times to meet and greet members.

- Manage daily operations to achieve the financial and operational objectives as described in the annual operating budget.

- Create a cohesive and seamless delivery of services and operational standards to maintain a high level of member satisfaction.

- Establish and implement monthly marketing strategies, membership policies and procedures, and club programs to maximize club revenue.

- Become familiar with and direct personal efforts to monitor and participate in business, athletic, and cultural events that will result in new opportunities for business development.

- Learn and present the wellness programs and services offered by the company.

- Advise, guide, direct, and authorize staff to complete club events, housekeeping standards, and member service standards that are consistent with established policies, ownership's expectation, and annual budget of the club.

- Become familiar with and use the club operating system, billing system, collections process, membership utilization, and other management systems necessary to achieve the operating standards and annual budget for the center.

- Establish and maintain an effective system of communication throughout the organization, including staff, members, and management.

- Conduct interviews and assist department managers with budgeting, interviewing, supervising, and staff training. The general manager is responsible for maintaining all employee policies and procedures as defined in the employee handbook.

- Report any actions, rumors, allegations, or negative insinuations made by any employee, member, or person that may detrimentally affect the operations of the club.

- Support and protect the interests and views of all employees as they pertain to enhancing the best interest of the company and their personal development.

- Monitor proper maintenance of all club equipment, furnishings, and fixtures, and make sure that written diaries of all preventive maintenance and repairs are maintained.

- Continually review the operating results of the club, compare these with established budgets, and prepare and compile the month-end financial report and executive summary, including an explanation of any variance in operations exceeding 10%. Recommend steps to ensure appropriate measures are taken to correct any unsatisfactory results.

- Assist the marketing and sales staff with the implementation of corporate and individual membership campaigns and provide creative suggestions to continually improve these programs and membership enrollment.

- Monitor department managers and their staff for customer service and satisfaction levels.

- Conduct employee performance reviews on an annual basis and maintain current employee files.

- Ensure the completion of and contribute to the membership newsletter.

- Coordinate and conduct biweekly staff meetings.

- Approve and track club expenses and work cooperatively with the accounting department to facilitate purchase order processing.

- Process semimonthly staff payroll.

- Perform other duties as assigned.

Supervisory Responsibilities

- Implement marketing strategies in keeping with overall company philosophy.

- Monitor tracking of sales related to club operations.

- Respond to the needs, questions, suggestions, or complaints of members and staff.

- Maintain a facility standard of excellence and cleanliness.

- Ensure implementation and professionalism of all programs and promotions.

- Maintain a positive environment for all employees.

- Share values according to ownership's desires.

- Continually improve, reorganize, and redefine systems.

Exercise Physiologist

The **exercise physiologist** reports directly to the general manager and occasionally to the corporate management team as requested. During MOD hours, the exercise physiologist is an extension of the authority of the general manager.

Minimum Requirements

- Bachelor's degree in exercise physiology (or related field) required.
- Clinical exercise testing experience required.
- Current CPR certification and national training certification required.

Job Description

- Responsible for the supervision, safety, and cleanliness of the fitness floor.
- Assists members with exercise programs and provides clinical testing.
- Monitors workouts and exercise routines, provides guidance on proper form and technique, and answers questions as necessary.

Job Responsibilities

- Health Profile and Heart Risk Assessment
  - Have a working knowledge of all aspects of the testing system and evaluation standards.
  - Have knowledge and competency in exercise testing, including screening for potential contraindications.
  - Interpret results and design safe, appropriate, and enjoyable individualized exercise prescriptions.
  - Complete and maintain all member files in accordance with the fitness manual.
  - Contact every member for 6-month reevaluations.
  - Compile and analyze data from the testing system for group reports and specific groups with identified risk factors.
  - Correspond with members after evaluations for the purpose of continued education, awareness, and answering questions.
- Orientation
  - Review the exercise prescription and data provided by the health profile and heart risk assessment and detail a personalized exercise prescription for every member.
  - Implement a personalized cardiorespiratory and strength program.
  - Give a detailed orientation on how to properly use each piece of equipment.
  - Encourage interaction between members and fitness staff, as well as the responsibility of members to contact fitness staff for questions and concerns.
- Floor Supervision
  - Monitor equipment maintenance needs and advise the general manager immediately of any developing problems.
  - Clean each piece of equipment daily per manufacturer specifications.
  - Assist, motivate, and educate all members on the use of machines and personal fitness goals.
  - Be proactive and approach every member to ensure proper training techniques are followed.
  - Provide routine blood pressure and heart rate checks.
  - Maintain a safe, productive, and inviting exercise environment for members and guests.
- Health Promotions
  - Assist in the implementation of all health promotion, medical screening, and educational programs.
  - Contact special populations from previous member files and the testing system for upcoming events.
  - Develop creative strategies for encouraging participation.
  - Assist in the development of specific interventions that serve the needs of members and subsidiaries.
  - Work with the member services staff in implementing health fairs.
- Personal Training
  - Motivate and educate participants.
  - Follow specified guidelines and personal training services as stated in the fitness manual.
  - Conduct complimentary training sessions for new members.
  - Assist in the development and implementation of marketing initiatives designed to

generate awareness of personal training programs.

- Other
  - Ensure that aerobics staff members are present and on time for all scheduled classes. Report any tardiness or missed classes to the general manager.
  - Prepare all assignments and correspondence in a neat, timely, and professional manner.
  - Keep all business-related interests, resources, and correspondence well-organized and neat at all times.
  - Maintain a high level of professionalism at all times.
  - Remain active in industry associations and education.

- Work well with others and maintain professional working relationships with all employees.

THE BOTTOM LINE

For a fitness professional who loves interacting with members, creating or revising job descriptions is not a top priority. Who wants to sit behind a desk when you can be touching people's lives with education? However, if you want to start your own health club or become a manager for a health club, the probability of employee, facility, and overall success will be improved by creating clear, concise, and comprehensive job descriptions.

KEY TERMS

corporate-based fitness organizations

customer service

exercise physiologist

finance development executive

fitness director

fitness instructor

for-profit commercial facilities

general manager

health and wellness director

hospital-based fitness centers

I-fees

membership consultant

membership director

nondues revenue

not-for-profit community facilities

organizational design

personal trainer

referral program

subtenant

third-party nationally accredited certifications

REFERENCES AND RECOMMENDED READING

American College of Sports Medicine (ACSM). 2007. *ACSM's health/fitness facility standards and guidelines*. 3rd ed. Champaign, IL: Human Kinetics.

Centers for Disease Control and Prevention (CDC). 1999. *Promoting physical activity: A guide for community action*. Champaign, IL: Human Kinetics.

Gerson, R.F. 1999. *Members for life*. Champaign, IL: Human Kinetics.

Grantham, W.C., R.W. Patton, T.D. York, and M.L. Winick. 1998. *Health fitness management*. Champaign, IL: Human Kinetics.

International Health, Racquet, and Sportsclub Association (IHRSA). 1998. *Why people quit*. Boston: IHRSA.

———. 2000. *Why people stay*. Boston: IHRSA.

———. 2004. *Guide to membership retention*. Boston: IHRSA.

———. 2006. *Profiles of success*. Boston: IHRSA.

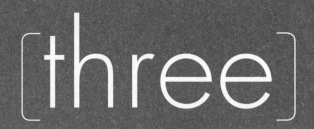

Recruiting the Best Staff for Your Facility

Kevin Hood

LEARNING OBJECTIVES

After studying this chapter, the reader will be able to

- identify and use critical industry and marketplace employment benchmarks to positively influence strategic planning for recruiting and hiring;

- identify essential internal review processes so that appropriate personnel adjustments can be made by reorganizing, creating, or replacing positions;

- define the criteria for creating purpose-driven job descriptions to form the framework for successful personnel management;

- understand and implement efficient recruiting processes that identify qualified candidates and ensure the greatest possible buy-in from current employees;

- create organization-specific standards for screening and reviewing applications and résumés to ensure the best candidates move on to the interview stage;

- learn to apply a wide range of interviewing techniques to best bring out the talents, skills, experience, and work style of candidates for long-term retention and productivity; and

- ensure that the hiring process provides a solid foundation for both the business and the new employee with regard to legal, operational, and cultural orientation.

Bob, the front-desk manager at XYZ Club, was desperate to get someone to cover the front desk in the middle of the busy season. Two of his best people were on vacation and he was covering too many shifts himself. He had placed an advertisement in the newspaper and received a large number of messages about the job, but he was so busy covering the desk and performing his usual management tasks that he was becoming frustrated at not being able to get back to the candidates. After several days of phone tag with a few candidates and extensive phone conversations with people who turned out to want more money than the club was able to offer, he had a good conversation with a young nursing student and made a hurried appointment with her for the next day. Bob's schedule was so tight that he decided to interview the candidate during a slow time while he was covering the front desk.

The candidate showed up a little late but was well dressed and seemed articulate and energetic. After a short conversation, during which he was distracted several times by member questions at the desk, Bob decided the candidate was worth a try, thinking to himself, "If I could just get a warm body in here, I might be able to get caught up." Two weeks later, after spending considerable time training the new employee, she turned in her resignation because she had been accepted to a nursing school in another state. Bob thought she had said she was already in nursing school, but she had just been applying. He hadn't thoroughly looked at her application or followed up on the references because he was so busy. Bob called the newspaper and restarted the ad, thinking to himself, "When am I going to get off this merry-go-round?"

Those who are responsible for recruiting and hiring staff have one of the most important roles in any organization. Think about it—in almost all circumstances, businesses are successful or fall short based on the performance of their employees. The recruiting and hiring process serves as the foundation for ensuring that organizations have the greatest chance of success. This chapter covers a range of techniques and tactics designed for those who are charged with recruitment and hiring.

The first section of this chapter deals with analyzing staffing needs so that the recruiting efforts match the needs of the organization. The next sections explain how to formalize and refine job descriptions in a practical way so that they can be used in developing quality interview techniques. The latter sections provide information on positive profiling and the important interview questions that can come from the profiling exercise. Finally, strategies for selecting the best candidate for the job will be discussed.

Analyzing Staffing Needs

One of the most important jobs for any manager is to understand the personnel requirements necessary to get the job done. The goal of managing is to ensure that the right number of people are assigned to any given task and that those people produce the best work possible in the most efficient and effective way. Understanding the mission and vision of the organization, the appropriate salary ranges based on selected **benchmarks** for the fitness industry, and the overall marketplace is necessary to achieve this goal. Wage and salary benchmark categories include comparing similar and different types of clubs (e.g., fitness, multipurpose, women's only, personal training) based on jobs with similar responsibilities, hours, and comparative benefits. Understanding the wages, benefits, and other forms of compensation that competitive clubs offer helps to shape an offer that motivates quality candidates. This information also helps to evaluate past, current, and predicted future trends so they can be put into perspective and necessary actions planned and undertaken. Some of the important questions to answer before beginning the recruiting process include the following:

- How many people need to be hired to accomplish the job? Staff–member or supervisor–frontline employee ratios may need to be evaluated from a productivity, customer service, or legal standpoint (e.g., state and federal laws that prescribe ratios regarding the maximum number of infants per day care provider).

- What are the appropriate marketplace comparatives in terms of hourly wages for the position?

- What is the availability of trained and untrained labor in a given market?

- How do the answers to the previous questions affect the chosen market **wage position** (setting salaries toward the high, average, or low end of the market) for a specific job type so that qualified candidates are attracted to the position?

There are several sources of answers to these questions, including trade associations such as IHRSA, which provides detailed information on salary ranges for a variety of positions along the full spectrum of club types from large multipurpose clubs to small studios. Professional associations such as the National Strength and Conditioning Association (NSCA), the American College of Sports Medicine (ACSM), and the American Council on Exercise (ACE) also can provide salary data for different types of positions in the fitness field.

The staffing needs of every organization invariably evolve over time. Employees may accept a position in a different organization or an advancement opportunity within the organization, or the employer may choose to terminate them because of poor performance or personnel reorganization. The exact amount of turnover in specific positions throughout each organization that is ideal versus acceptable versus damaging is somewhat hard to define; however, it is clear that the general trend of employee attrition is proportionately related to member attrition (IHRSA 2006). Simply speaking, the more employees leave the organization, the more members will be departing. Therefore, the ability to hire and retain high-performing people is critical to the success of any health or athletic club.

However, some employee turnover is inevitable. New employees who are selected through an appropriate recruiting and hiring process can bring a number of positive benefits, including the following:

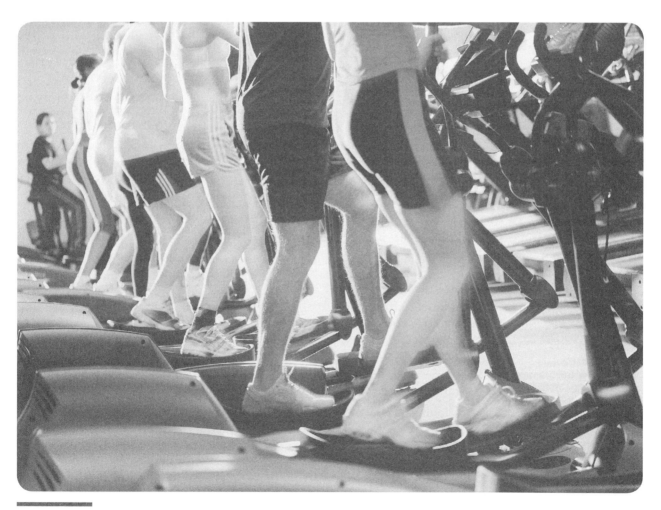

An exercise floor filled to capacity is only one factor of a club's success; of equal importance is the staff–member ratio. If a club is understaffed, customer service will suffer.
© BananaStock

- New employees frequently approach business challenges in a refreshing way, bringing new perspectives to solving old problems and new ideas to keep the business energized.

- The natural evolution of employees seeking more challenging opportunities in other organizations can be a healthy indication of a stable company where upward movement may be limited because of long-tenured and productive employees.

- Turnover in organizations can simply mean the evolution of high-performing employees moving out of one position into another of more responsibility, creating the need for additional personnel.

- Seasonal requirements can also contribute to the need for hiring new employees on a regular basis.

Because of these and many other positive benefits that new employees bring to a club, the investment in time and energy to ensure quality hiring practices is well spent.

Regardless of the circumstances surrounding the need to replace a position, it is almost always essential to ask the question, "Is it possible to redesign the personnel organization chart to better handle the responsibilities associated with the position?" There are several methods for covering the responsibilities associated with the vacated position and changing the way the position is oriented in the organization, including the following:

- Change the supervisory **reporting structure** or move the position to a different department.

- Combine the responsibilities into one or more positions that are already filled (this may or may not mean the opportunity to advance or promote someone from within the organization or change compensation structures).

- Hire contract or temporary employees to fill the position for the short, medium, or long term.

- Reorganize the position by changing it to full or part-time, adding or deleting job responsibilities, changing the pay rate, adding or removing benefit opportunities, and so on.

Formalizing Job Descriptions

In the recruiting and hiring process, the **job description** is the starting point for defining the skills and attributes that are outlined in an advertisement or job availability notice. In addition, the general and specific tasks covered in a detailed job description should form the basis for the creation of specific questions designed to determine the candidate's ability to deliver the necessary performance. For example, one section of the **performance expectations** portion of a job description for a front-desk job might look something like the following:

Constant attention to creating the highest level of proactive customer service, including all aspects of service delivery such as appropriate phone etiquette (greetings, transferring calls, voice tone, and grammar), is essential to creating the consummate member-focused environment. A warm and friendly communication style that facilitates a personalized relationship with each member and yet is respectful of the member's sense of formality (e.g., the desire on the member's part to be addressed by the first or last name) and familiarity is a necessity.

Questions designed to reveal a candidate's ability to deliver the kind of personalized service listed in this description might include the following:

- Describe situations in your professional or personal life where you've experienced excellent customer service. What specific staff behaviors did you notice that created the customer service excellence?

- What businesses or organizations do you feel have a reputation for providing great customer service? Explain why you think they either deserve or don't deserve this reputation.

- What books or articles have you read that deal with delivering great customer service?

- If you were going to coach a new group of receptionists for the club, what would you describe to them as the critical elements of answering the phone? Include how you would instruct them to handle a situation in which a member is signing up for a program at the desk when the phone rings and no one else is available to answer it.

- What are some examples of **defined behaviors** that front-desk personnel could display that would be consistent with the highest levels of customer service?

Later in this chapter we will cover a broader range of questions for interviews.

Formalizing a job description for every position is one of the most important personnel tasks any manager can undertake. Job descriptions form the framework for training, resource planning, wage and benefit decisions, and establishment of job performance criteria. See Key Elements of Job Descriptions below for some of the factors to consider.

Key Elements of Job Descriptions

A good job description contains key elements that are important to both the organization and the employee. In clarifying its needs for recruiting and hiring, the organization should address a number of issues that pertain to each key element.

Qualifications

- *Importance to organization*—The organization needs to define the criteria by which it will choose the candidate who has the greatest chance of being successful.

- *Importance to employee*—Workers can determine if a job is appropriate for them and what training, experience, or education might be necessary to become eligible for the position.

Issues to Address

- Education
- Experience (overall and specific to the industry)
- Special skills
- Commuting distance
- References

Wages and Salary

- *Importance to organization*—Salaries and wages often represent the company's highest operating cost. Any opportunity to ensure that the highest wage value is being received for the money spent is essential to the long-term financial success of the company. Positioning wages appropriately within the marketplace is also critical in determining the quality of employee candidates the company attracts. Organizations can decide to pay more than average in the marketplace for some specialty positions and may choose to pay less than average for others that it deems less critical to its success. This process of comparing pay rates to the marketplace is designed to position the company to compete for employee talent and is called **external equity**. Another important process is to ensure that employees' salaries are positioned proportionately within the club based on levels of responsibility and accountability.

- *Importance to employee*—Defining pay guidelines creates logic in employees' minds about the structure of the company and their current place within the hierarchy. Additionally, guidelines for pay advancement give workers clear pathways to increase their compensation.

Issues to Address

- Compensation methods and wage classification (hourly versus salary; full versus part-time; performance-based compensation with opportunities for commission and bonus versus base wage; opportunities for overtime; 90-day, semiannual, or annual reviews)
- Internal versus external equity
- Benefits status (vacation eligibility, accrual schedule, personal time off versus vacation and sick days)
- Starting wages as low as possible without demotivating employees in order to provide room for adjustments and setting expectations for range and timing of increases

(continued)

(continued)

Performance Expectations

- *Importance to organization*—Allows organizations to review how all jobs fit together to ensure the most efficient and effective personnel structure for creating the product. Establishes framework for supervisors to structure performance coaching and goal setting for those they supervise.

- *Importance to employee*—Provides tangible direction for priorities and removes uncertainty at performance review sessions.

Issues to Address

- Performance review structure, including objective, subjective, results-based and process-based types of performance criteria
- Time frames for achieving goals and objectives
- Appropriateness of tying performance goals to potential salary adjustments and bonus rewards in cash or other perks (e.g., vacation)

Management Support Structure and Number of People to Supervise

- *Importance to organization*—Puts managers and supervisors on notice as being responsible for the development of workers and for being accessible to those they are supervising. Helps confirm that the number one job for those in management is to support those being supervised by providing personal accessibility and material and information resources.

- Importance to employee—Provides a framework for knowing who and where to go for answers regarding critical aspects of the operation. Defining the chain of command allows all employees to understand the resources they have access to and how their job fits into the organization as a whole.

Issues to Address

- Training provided by the organization in the form of internal or external opportunities
- Appropriate chain of command to facilitate effective and efficient communication
- Making sure people don't have too many subordinates reporting to them (typically, 5 to 10 is a good number of direct reports)
- New-employee orientation or mentoring program to help new workers acclimate to systems, people, and procedures

Career Advancement Within the Organization

- *Importance to organization*—Allows supervisors to tailor training needs for workers who are able to communicate their desire for advancement. Also contributes significantly to the attractiveness of a given position by adding future value to a job that may not initially meet the ideal requirements of candidates who are slightly overqualified.

- *Importance to employee*—Gives employees a picture of how they might advance through the organization.

Issues to Address

- Potential timing of opportunities for career advancement
- Qualifications for next-step jobs

Personal Appearance Standards

- *Importance to organization*—Provides clear standards that enable managers and supervisors to train and enforce a high standard maintained by all employees. These standards can be challenging to define and contribute to the culture of the organization and the type of person attracted to the position.

- *Importance to employee*—Clear communication of company standards reduces unnecessary conflict and helps employees maintain an appropriate standard by providing clear and concise guidelines regarding what kind of attire is acceptable and what is not.

Issues to Address

- Jewelry, body piercings, and tattoos
- Clothes
- Posture and body language
- Makeup and hair styles

Physical Requirements

- *Importance to the organization*—Thoughtful consideration of the physical demands of the job helps companies recruit workers who are suited to the job and can increase employees' longevity and productivity.
- *Importance to the employee*—Candidates and employees must understand the physical nature of the job. Physical limitations that are unexpressed could lead to underperformance or even injury, so it's best to be up front if there are limitations and see if there are ways to mitigate some of the physical requirements of a job.

Issues to Address

- Analyzing a job and being direct about physical expectations (for example, "Front-desk work requires extended periods of up to 2 hours of uninterrupted standing")
- Putting away leftover weights (heavy loads) in the weight room (fitness personnel)
- Bending, twisting, kneeling, and lifting throughout the course of the day (housekeepers)
- Working outside in the heat or cold or exposure to chemicals by working in the maintenance department or around a pool

Refining Job Descriptions

Is there a certain type of candidate that has proven to be good for certain kinds of positions? Managers can grow comfortable with a particular mixture of personal and professional assets for a given position, but it is important that other qualified applicants are not automatically overlooked in preference for the type that has become the most familiar. Defining important qualifications in the job description can help managers determine which candidates are personable and have familiar behavior patterns but may not meet the experience, skill, or education criteria.

Some forms of profiling are illegal as well as immoral and unfair. In the United States, the Civil Rights Act of 1964 and the Equal Employment Opportunity Act of 1972 cover the types of profiling that are illegal. These two pieces of legislation form the foundation of employment protection provided to Americans, and the information and laws associated with them should be part of the knowledge base for managers and owners of clubs.

The U.S. Equal Employment Opportunity Commission (EEOC) is charged with enforcing federal law against discrimination based on race, color, national origin, sex, age (between the ages of 40 and 70), disability, veteran status, handicap, and religion. Another law to be aware of is the Equal Pay Act of 1963, which requires that men and women receive equal pay for equal work.

However, some kinds of **positive profiling** can be helpful. For example, certain skill sets (e.g., people who have spent time in other countries for clubs that entertain an international clientele), educational backgrounds (e.g., preference for a degree program focusing on a specific need of the organization), or career stages (e.g., adults in school preparing for a second career) are categories that may be helpful when defining characteristics of successful candidates for certain positions. For example, receptionists frequently need to relate to the members and therefore life experience that mirrors the maturity level of the customer can be helpful. Candidates in formal career transitions who have commitments that are relatively predictable (e.g., part-time graduate school for the next 3 years) can be great assets in positions where long-term employment is challenging to maintain anyway, such as positions at the front desk, in housekeeping, or in food service.

Including preferences for these kinds of helpful characteristics in the job description can help managers ensure they are identifying appropriate, fair, and legal types of characteristics that contribute to further refinement of the job description.

Selecting the Appropriate Recruiting Vehicle

It's important to make conscious recruiting choices that lead to appropriate responses along the continuum of two possible extreme recruiting outcomes. At one end of the continuum, you have a large and relatively less qualified pool of applicants, and at the other end you have a small number of respondents whose qualifications are specifically matched to the predefined needs of the job. Five variables to consider in choosing the appropriate recruiting vehicle are as follows:

1. Technical nature of the skill set required—How likely is it that the target audience of the recruiting vehicle will have the technical skills and other requirements of the position being advertised? Are the skills relatively common or hard to find?

2. Available recruitment budget—Is there a large or small budget?

3. Urgency of hiring need—Does the position need to be filled in 60 days or 60 minutes?

4. Geographic reach—Is it important for people to live close to work? Might the candidate relocate as a result of taking the job?

5. Compensation range—Do the pay parameters of the job vary depending on the qualifications of the applicant?

Table 3.1 lists a number of recruiting vehicles, their advantages and disadvantages, and their costs.

The most effective advertisement maximizes the number of highly qualified respondents and minimizes the responses of those who are less qualified, perfectly matching the candidate with the job. Information that should be included in an advertisement to ensure a high percentage of qualified respondents includes the following:

• *Managing response*—In general, an advertisement should be designed to either limit the number of respondents by tightly defining the parameters of the opportunity or to encourage the largest possible response in the hopes of engaging candidates who might typically be screened out. Sometimes through conversation or review of résumés unlikely initial candidates become worthy of consideration.

• *Number of words*—The number of words is directly related to the cost of all print ads; therefore, brevity means money saved. However, being penny-wise and pound-foolish by not adequately describing the job circumstances can lead to an inadequate response. Newspaper ads typically range from 50 to 200 or more words. Use active words to describe work responsibilities in order to inspire greater response to the ad and to clarify key responsibilities.

• *Headline*—Headlines differentiate ads and help attract appropriate candidates, so keep them interesting.

• *Section*—Choose the section of the want ads (e.g., service, housekeeping, reception) that is most appropriate to the position.

• *Contact method (phone, fax, e-mail, or regular mail)*—Giving candidates several ways to respond to ads can increase response. However, be careful when using a phone number as a response option. Being swamped by phone messages from unqualified candidates can mean wasted time in sifting through a large haystack of applicants to find the needle. For jobs requiring phone skills, it may be appropriate to get a first impression of candidates by having them respond to the ad by phone; just make sure to include enough information to limit the calls.

• *Necessary skills*—It is essential to describe in adequate detail the skills that are required. If computer and typing skills are important, mention that. If the job requires a degree in exercise science or professional certifications, be sure to include the requirement in the ad.

• *Required experience*—Response to ads can be increased or decreased simply by using the word *preferred* or *required*. If there are no modifying factors that would trump a requirement of a certain amount of experience, listing that requirement will decrease the number of responses to the ad.

• *Wage (salary or hourly) and benefits*—Depending on the type of position, providing specific wage information for the ad can be important. Phrases such as "compensation commensurate with experience and education" can broaden the spectrum of response and allow for negotiation toward an appropriate compensation package. Providing a

Table 3.1 **Sources for Recruiting Candidates**

Type of recruiting vehicle	Pros	Cons	Cost
Regional newspaper (want ads)	Provides exposure to large population.	Hard to target a specific audience. Can be cost prohibitive.	$200-$600
Local newspaper (want ads)	Low cost. Targets specific geographical audience.	Quality of the publications sometimes doesn't adequately represent the standard of club.	$100-$300
Trade journals and associations	For technical jobs this vehicle can be very effective. Examples include IHRSA, Club Success, *Club Business*, and *ACSM Journal*. Many trade or professional associations provide Web-based job postings as part of or as an alternative to their journal print ads.	Cost can be prohibitive. Unless the journal is local in its distribution, may attract applicants who have to relocate.	$400 and up
Temporary labor companies	Can provide an effective bridge when unable to fill a certain position.	The significant efforts required to train temporary workers for short-term needs may outweigh advantages. Basic manual labor tasks may be best choice for this kind of help.	20%-30% more per hour than regular employees
Job fairs	Can be great for seasonal hiring when a relatively large number of employees need to be hired at the same time (lifeguards, camp counselors).	Timing of available fairs may not match the need of the organization.	Variable
Recruiters	Can be a good investment for essential positions or for positions that require statewide or nationwide searches.	Can be very costly.	10%-50% of annual salary for the position
Staff referrals	Can be a low-cost and reliable method of getting people. Requires positive employee culture.	Can create friction if referrals aren't hired.	Monetary incentive (e.g., $50)
Current employees	Elevating or moving a current employee from a different position can keep existing employees excited about their jobs and learning new skills.	May eliminate opportunity to get new ideas and perspective. Can produce the need to hire someone else to fill a different spot.	Small thank-you gift or no cost
Member or customer referrals	Customers can be great sources of referrals. They understand the frontline needs of the business and generally are invested in the success of the business.	A mishandled referral can leave a bad taste in the customer's mouth. Make doubly sure hiring processes are top-notch to leave good impressions.	Referral gift to member (e.g., product or service)
Vendor referrals	This is an underused segment of the referral world. Venders may be hiring and have too many qualified applicants for a position or may be downsizing.	Any potential poaching of employees from a company with which the club does business could jeopardize the relationship with the company.	Complimentary service or product (can help build relationships)

(continued)

Table 3.1 *(continued)*

Type of recruiting vehicle	Pros	Cons	Cost
University newspapers and Web sites	Almost all universities have a career services center where jobs are posted on a Web site or bulletin board, which can be a great location for finding moderately priced, flexible labor.	Depending on the type of position, college students may only provide medium-term solutions because as they graduate, they may move on to jobs that better match the focus of their degrees.	Often free
State employment office or community job boards	County, city, or state employment offices provide no-cost brokerage of applicants who have been screened on the basis of work experience, education, and some psychological testing.	Doesn't always produce the most qualified pool of candidates.	Free
Web-based search engines	Web-based advertising can include links to employment section of the club's Web site and electronic methods of completing applications or testing devices related to employment (aptitude, IQ, personality style, technical knowledge and skills).	May produce more response than is necessary (overkill). Can overrun a manager's e-mail account.	$100-$6,000

range of wage or salary options is also appropriate, as is using the phrase "to start" to indicate room to increase the wage as the employee increases tenure or value with the organization. If there is an absolute wage that the job pays (e.g., $8.50 an hour), be specific about that wage.

- *Work schedule*—Being specific about the days of the week and the hours available is essential to getting a qualified response to the ad.

- *Number of days to run ad*—Pricing is usually based on the number of days the ad runs. The best value in terms of cost per day is typically an ad that runs approximately 7 to 10 days. It is usually possible to stop the ad and recoup some of the cost if at some point enough résumés, calls, or applications are received.

- *Which days of the week*—Saturdays and Sundays are the days when people who are employed typically look for new jobs. However, Saturdays and Sundays are also the most expensive days to run ads. Starting with a Saturday and running the ad for a week can provide exposure to the most readers early in the run of the advertisement, giving you an opportunity to evaluate the response and make decisions about continuing the ad during the weekdays.

- *Special touches*—A number of techniques can make an ad more noticeable, including bold lettering, underlined portions of copy, an outline or frame around the ad, and increased font size. Each of these requires additional cost. Choosing the most compel-

ling aspect of the ad to highlight can be effective in increasing qualified response. Table 3.2 offers two examples of print advertisements that are more and less effective.

Another important part of the recruiting phase is to clearly set expectations for the way applications and résumés will be processed and what kind of response will be made to candidates. For example, if candidates are calling in response to an ad, you might want to leave a voice mail recording like the following:

Thank you for calling XYZ Company and expressing an interest in employment. Applications and résumés are being accepted by fax at 303-772-1235 and in person at 1234 Bellevue Drive. The deadline for receipt of applications is August 25. We are in the process of reviewing applications and will be responding to applicants by September 1. If you do not hear from a company representative by that date, you can assume that you were not selected for further evaluation in the process of hiring for this position. Thank you for calling XYZ Company.

If candidates are responding in person, a written note similar to this message could be provided.

Developing Interview Questions

In preparation for the interview phase of the hiring process, it is essential to develop thoughtful ques-

Table 3.2 **Sample Print Ads**

Less effective	More effective
General help wanted: Club seeks night custodian. Experience preferred. Applicants should call Jan @ 918-555-8926.	Janitorial: Prestigious ACME Health and Fitness Club hiring hardworking, self-motivated night housekeeper. Full-time, Sun-Thurs 9 p.m.-5 a.m. shift. Min 2 yrs professional cleaning experience pref. $10/hr to start; paid vacation & additional benefits provided. Qualified applicants apply in person at 1234 Broadway Ave., Cleveland, OH 97241, or mail résumé to Jan.
General help wanted: Front-desk help needed—greeting customers & opening club, wage negotiable, several shifts available, fax résumé to 818-555-9858.	Customer service: XYZ Athletic Club is hiring friendly, fitness-focused, outgoing, people-oriented, energetic reception desk service specialists for Sat & Sun 6 a.m.-2 p.m. Benefits include use of club facilities, uniform, free parking, & shift meals. $8.50/hr with opportunities for advancement and wage increase with outstanding performance. Respond by faxing résumé to 720-555-1666 or mailing or applying in person @ 3465 Cherry Lane, Denver, CO 80224.

tions that bring out the characteristics, skills, and experience that have been identified in the job description.

The process of developing interview questions can be a way of team building with existing coworkers and creating buy-in with regard to the hiring process. As a general rule, current employees who have been involved in the hiring process are more committed to ensuring the greatest chance of success for a new employee who needs to fit in with the team. In some situations, such as where a group of coworkers is relatively dysfunctional or where the current culture of the organization is not representative of the ultimate direction of the company, it may not be appropriate to involve existing employees in the development of interview questions. Existing employees who are at odds with the organization may seek to disrupt the hiring process or take the well-intentioned efforts of other, more positive employees off track.

In most cases, however, conducting a brainstorming session among current employees to develop quality hiring questions can be a positive process. Start by choosing the group of employees to be involved in the project either by asking for volunteers (if there is no concern over who might volunteer) or by using criteria that allow the manager the necessary control to choose employees best suited for the task. For example, the manager can choose a few employees to help develop a draft of questions, thus controlling the efficiency of the process. The manager can then create effective buy-in from the rest of the staff by reviewing the questions with them to refine the questions and address input or concerns.

Involving the existing employees in the review of job descriptions that are related to their position or are the actual description of a job they are already doing can help remind existing coworkers of expectations for job performance. It can also give you feedback from frontline staff on updates that might be necessary to keep job descriptions cutting edge.

Job Preview

A crucial task in developing a recruiting strategy is to identify the skills, attributes, and personal characteristics that provide the candidate with the greatest chance of being successful in the job. This helps to ensure a good fit between the organization and the candidate. A **job preview** gives the candidate a snapshot of what it might be like to work at the company and allows the company to observe the response of the candidate to these preexisting conditions that could be **deal breakers.**

It's much better to communicate these deal breakers up front, such as personal appearance. For many companies, for example, nose rings are unacceptable. If candidates are significantly attached to their nose ring, that standard is going to be a deal breaker. If shifts are only available in the early morning and there is little likelihood of that changing, it is better to communicate that information up front so everyone understands the boundaries going in. When jobs are fairly intense and have little opportunity for downtime, such as working the front desk, you should clearly communicate those circumstances before initiating the more comprehensive parts of the interview. Identifying deal breakers through the job preview can streamline conversations in person or via the phone and reduce the amount of wasted time for the candidate and the employer.

Types of Questions

Whether developing interview questions with a group or individually, questions should solicit information that can be compared with the criteria listed in the job description. There are several types of questions that should be included in an interview.

Open Ended Versus Closed Ended

Open-ended questions require candidates to frame their answer in more than a single-word response. Open-ended questions invite people to expand their answer and cover a range of potential issues related to the question. There are, however, situations where **closed-ended questions** are appropriate. For example, if you're asking someone about the ratio of compressions to breaths involved in performing CPR for an adult, the answer is straightforward and does not require explanation. The following are examples of open- and closed-ended questions:

• *Open ended:* Tell me about the systems you used to track member utilization in your last job as front-desk supervisor. What level of input did you have in the design of the system? What did you think were particularly effective components of the system and what do you think could have been improved?

• *Close ended:* How many coworkers did you have working for you? Is your CPR certification current? What, in millimeters of mercury, is the definition of borderline high blood pressure?

Discussion Versus Question and Answer

Discussion-style interviewing provides an environment that feels like a conversation. This style can help the candidate feel more relaxed and provides a more natural flow to the interview. A question-and-answer style, on the other hand, tends to be more structured and formal.

Experiential Versus Situational

Experiential questions draw on people's experience and ask them to relate how they handled some problem in the past. **Situational questions** create circumstances that candidates must react to and can give clues to the problem-solving abilities of candidates.

For examples of questions to ask applicants for specific positions, see Interview Questions Relevant to Specific Positions on page 53.

Suggestions for General Interview Questions

The following questions are grouped by general category and could be applied to a range of positions. Remember, questions can be situational or experiential. Generally, using a balance of both types of questions is most effective.

Past Experience

- Describe your professional experience and how it might apply to this position.
- Give some examples of jobs or experiences you've had that require you to successfully (insert task).

Motivation

- What is it about this position that makes you interested in the job?
- How do you see this position contributing to your career aspirations?

Work Ethic

- What was the hardest (physically, emotionally, or mentally) job you ever had and why?
- Are you interested in overtime hours if they are available?
- What's the best job you've ever had? Why?

Customer Service

- Give an example of a situation where you provided service that was significantly more than was expected by the customer.
- A member has approached the front desk and is upset because the whirlpool has been out of order for 5 days. She is aggressive and threatens to quit her membership. How do you handle this situation?
- What have been some of the biggest customer service mistakes you've made, and what did you learn from them?

Personality Type

- Would you say that your personality tends to be more outgoing or more reserved? Give an example of when this has been an asset and when it has been a liability.
- Give an example of a personal characteristic that you would like to be different about

Interview Questions Relevant to Specific Positions

The questions asked during a job interview are directly related to the performance criteria and skills needed to perform the job.

Front-Desk Personnel

- *Job performance criteria*—The ability to multitask is essential to this position. Candidates who are able to maintain a positive and upbeat customer-centered approach in an environment that requires a constant shifting of attention will be the most successful.
- *Skills and characteristics associated with this task*—Making an appropriate amount of eye contact, being unflappable, being patient but energetic, and having a quick mind are all important in this task.
- *Sample question*—Give me examples of situations where you've successfully dealt with multiple tasks in a time-intensive manner and maintained a high level of customer service.

Fitness Specialist

- *Job performance criteria*—The ability to administer a variety of health screens and use the resulting information to determine participant goals and establish an appropriate exercise prescription is crucial.
- *Skills and characteristics associated with this task*—Knowledge of anatomy, kinesiology, physiology, and special health conditions and the ability to develop rapport are essential.
- *Sample question*—A new member is a 40-year-old man with diabetes and arthritic knees. He is 30 pounds (13.5 kilograms) overweight and wants to lose 20 pounds (9 kilograms) in the next two months in preparation for his high school reunion. Explain how you would approach this situation and develop appropriate exercise recommendations.

Membership Salesperson

- *Job performance criteria*—Must be able to perform a needs analysis as part of the sales process to determine the prospect's motivation for considering membership at the club.
- *Skills and characteristics associated with this task*—This job requires an engaging personality, the ability to mirror a client's energy and personality style, and familiarity with specific techniques associated with needs analysis.
- *Sample question*—Explain the concept of needs analysis and its importance in selling club memberships.

Housekeeper

- *Job performance criteria*—Candidates must be able to be on their feet for extended periods of time, lift up to 40 pounds (18 kilograms), travel up and down stairs, and bend, twist, and reach in association with the tasks of vacuuming, dusting, trash collection, and window cleaning.
- *Skills and characteristics associated with this task*—Good physical condition, including strength and flexibility, is required.
- *Sample question*—Provide examples of physically demanding jobs you've had in the past, including the specific tasks associated with the job.

yourself and how you're working toward changing it or have become comfortable with not changing it. In what types of situations do you notice this characteristic, and how do you handle yourself?

- In a year from now, if we're sitting around having a cup of coffee, what will I say surprised me most about you that I would have never guessed from meeting you during this interview?

Teamwork

- Give an example of a conflict you had with a coworker and how you contributed to resolving it. If it wasn't resolved, explain why.

- Give an example of a poor boss that you've had. Explain why the person was not a good manager and what strategies you used to manage your relationship.

- Give some examples that demonstrate your ability to successfully contribute to a team project or effort.

Problem Solving

- The air conditioning is not working, it is 7 p.m. on a Sunday, and you're the shift manager. It's getting very hot in the cardio room and members are complaining. What do you do?

- A member complains after coming out of the whirlpool that he feels light-headed and nauseous. While talking to you, he collapses, unconscious. What do you do?

Timeliness and Ability to Work Early, Late, or Weekend Shifts

- Give examples of jobs, activities, or hobbies that indicate you're someone who can consistently be on time for early-morning shifts.

- Why is the late-night (early-morning, weekend) shift attractive to you?

Passion

- Give examples of things in your life that you're passionate about. If I were to watch you engaging in these things, what sort of behaviors would I see that would convince me of your passion?

- Is there someone in history, sport, politics, or your personal life that you admire because of that person's passion for something? Explain why you admire this person.

Commitment to Personal Growth

- What kinds of reading or other forms of professional education have you recently completed or are currently involved in?

- What accomplishment in your life are you most proud of? Include at least one professional example and include personal examples if you desire.

One of the most important questions to ask is if the candidate has any questions. The type and depth of questions offered by the candidate can provide information on the preparation the candidate has done for the interview. Another good wrap-up question is, "Is there anything that I haven't asked or that you'd like us to know before we conclude the interview today?"

Quality of Answers

Managers should spend as much or more time thinking about the right answers to questions as they do the questions themselves. Some general basics about evaluating the quality of answers to interview questions include categories such as

- answered succinctly,
- stayed on track,
- probed for more information to improve the quality of the answer, and
- weren't afraid to say when they didn't know.

Interviewers should take the time to answer the questions they plan to ask the candidate. This exercise can help you consider follow-up questions that better illustrate the kinds of qualities or expertise the ideal candidate should possess. For example, let's say the interviewer is planning to ask the applicant the following question:

Please tell me about situations where you've had to deal with a disgruntled customer.

As part of the interview preparation process, the interviewer has identified the ideal components associated with the answer, which include the following:

- Apologize for how the customer feels.
- Acknowledge the customer's perception of the problem.
- If the answer to the problem has several options or is uncertain, ask for the customer's preferred method to solve the problem.

- Proactively offer a reasonable range of solutions to the problem.
- If uncertain about how to fix the problem,
  - brainstorm with the customer, or
  - seek out another employee who might be able to help.
- If the problem is a condition of the business (e.g., club doesn't open until 5:30 a.m. or no shaving allowed in the steam room), state the reason for the policy as a commitment the company has made to the membership and community at large and that making occasional exceptions reduces the credibility and consistency of the company's overall image and product.
- Confirm by reflecting back the customer's feelings and specific concerns. Go on to confirm how you will fix the problem if possible and how you will follow up with the customer.

Identifying these components ahead of time clarifies the ideal answer for the interviewer.

Selecting the Best Candidate for the Position

The procedure for assessing the applicants generally follows these steps:

1. Initial review and sorting of applications into priorities for phone contact
2. Phone screening
3. In-person interviews
4. Background checks
5. Comparison of candidates
6. Job offer

Review of Applications and Résumés

It is advisable to ensure that all candidates fill out a **job application** regardless of whether they provide a formal résumé. The job application provides a standardized list of requested information and compels the person who's filling it out to tell the truth. Many applications explicitly state that fabricated information on the application is a specific reason to not be hired and after hire could be cause for immediate termination of employment. It is important that clubs consult with a reputable labor attorney to ensure that all federal and state regulations are complied with in developing an appropriate form. Many consulting firms work with small businesses to provide wide-ranging advice on applications such as where to get them, what information should be included, why candidates have to fill them out, and legal protection for the company. Other important reasons for using an application is that it allows the personnel manager or hiring supervisor to compare the content of the application with the résumé to ensure that the information is accurate and consistent.

It can be helpful to have a checklist of qualifications to review with each application. You can also use this checklist for comments or questions with regard to some aspect of the application since notes should never be taken on the application (if the candidate is hired, it needs to become part of the employee file). The notes can also be helpful in managing a stack of résumés to ensure the pertinent information from each résumé is summarized for review later. The checklist is a great place to note where one candidate's experience may be more applicable to the position or where a graduate degree is more compelling than an undergraduate degree. This initial **paper screening** should sort applications into two or three categories such as excellent, possible, and disqualified.

Phone Screening

Once the initial paper screening has been completed, the next phase is typically **phone screening** for the priority candidates. Getting the chance to evaluate a candidate's phone etiquette and phone presence is valuable by itself, and the time saved compared with meeting all applicants face to face is helpful. The purposes of the telephone interview include the following:

- Confirm candidates' interest in the job and the information listed on their application. Reconfirm potential deal breakers that could sabotage the second interview, such as basic pay range, work hours, work environment, availability of the candidate (sometimes candidates may not be available by the time you need them), professional certifications or education, and ability to perform critical job tasks. By expanding on the information provided in the job advertisement, managers can screen out a few candidates that look good on paper but would be a waste of time to see in person.

- Ask the applicants a couple of questions from the list that has been developed from the job description. It's important to ask all the applicants essentially the same questions so all have a similar chance of demonstrating their competence. If inspired by the answers to questions, managers should feel comfortable asking follow-up or clarifying questions.

- If it becomes apparent early in the conversation that the candidate is not right for the position, don't feel the need to drag the conversation out by going through the motions of a more thorough phone interview. Thank such applicants for their time and let them know that this a preliminary phone screening of potential job candidates and that if there is interest the applicant will hear back by phone within a certain time period, such as 1 to 2 weeks.

If you've identified good candidates, find out if they're involved in employment conversations with any other companies. If they anticipate having to make a decision regarding another opportunity before the time you're prepared to make an offer, try saying something like, "I understand that you may be entertaining an attractive job offer sometime soon. At this point, given our relatively brief conversation and the early stages of our company's interviewing process, I would classify you as a very good candidate for the position we have available. Before making a final commitment to another company, would you consider giving me a call so that I could try to speed up our process to take advantage of your availability? That way, if we determine we'd like to make you an offer, you'd potentially have a choice of employers."

In-Person Interviews

Remember the circumstances presented in Tales From the Trenches at the beginning of this chapter? The interview environment the manager created was poor and he therefore risked making a bad impression with the candidate by being distracted. He also missed essential information, which led to an ineffective hiring decision. The first interview is not only a chance for the applicant to make a first impression, it is also a chance for the company to define itself as a serious, business-oriented organization that takes the hiring process seriously by establishing a professional environment in which to conduct thorough interviews. The ideal environment and circumstances for an interview include the following:

- Private, quiet room that is neat and tidy (well organized)
- Comfortable furnishings, including a table and at least two chairs

- Beverages to offer the candidate (some will be nervous, which can lead to a dry mouth)
- Adequate time (a typical first interview could range from 5-30 minutes)
- No interruptions from phones or other personnel if at all possible

With regard to the ideal number of interviews, as a general rule, the more opportunities to interview a candidate, the better. The frequency with which a candidate demonstrates timeliness, appropriate appearance and body language, and consistent, targeted, and accurate responses to interview questions is confirmation of a quality potential hire.

Using a variety of interviews can also be an effective strategy. Table 3.3 describes different interview types and their purposes.

Concluding the interview by offering thanks for the applicant's time and providing an outline of the process for the future are important. Let the candidate know how long it will be before the company makes a decision and the necessary steps and approximate time frame for completing the process if a job offer is made.

Background Checks and Reference Reviews

Before making a final hiring decision and a job offer, many companies require **background checks** for employees. Background checks range from criminal conduct reviews to financial credit checks to drug and alcohol screens. Candidates must provide their consent to have their background checked. There are a number of companies that provide background checks as part of their service as payroll management companies (e.g., Automatic Data Processing, Inc.; Paychex Payroll Services; and Kelly Management Services). Other forms of checking candidates' information include requiring university transcripts and documentation of professional certification and following up with references. Some companies require three professional references, and others require contact with one or more former employers to confirm employment history.

Defining the value of and seeking out meaningful **references** can be a challenging task. The average candidate is not going to supply references that don't have a high likelihood of being positive, so one might wonder if references are truly important. One of the reasons references are important is that they provide confirmation of the impressions and beliefs you have developed during the interview process. They also confirm that the information listed on the résumé is accurate. Candidates who play loose with the facts in listing their length of employment, job title, responsibilities, or pay rate may not be fully trustworthy as an employee.

One of the most important aspects of references is those that are not listed. Frequently candidates may choose to not list their most immediate past employer

Table 3.3 Types of Interviews

Type	Description	Purpose
One on one (supervisor directed)	This is a typical interview scenario with the supervisor meeting personally with the candidate.	Allows the manager to control all aspects of the interview process.
One on one (support personnel directed)	This type of interview is conducted by a member of the team with whom the applicant will be working or the manager of a department that works closely with the department where the job is located.	Allows the manager to see the degree to which the applicant fits in with other personalities. This style can also create buy-in and provide the manager with additional perspectives of the applicant.
Group or committee	This type of interview may involve a group of the applicant's potential peers or a committee composed of a cross section of current employees charged with vetting candidates.	Demonstrates a candidate's ability to be consistent and perform in a group environment.
Trial	This type of interview involves having the candidate perform some of the functions associated with the job. The trial could take the form of role-play with a supervisor or could involve part of an actual shift working directly with customers or existing employees. Paying applicants as contract labor may be necessary for interviews that use a several-hour trial in an actual working environment.	This interview provides a realistic picture of how a candidate will respond. Because of the time involvement, this sort of technique is typically limited to the best candidates.

because their job search is confidential. They may not want to alarm their current employer or place their current job in jeopardy. References should, however, be available for at least one or two of the candidates' last few employers. If those references are not made available, it could be a red flag that there are problems the candidate would rather not have exposed. As part of the interview process, don't be afraid to ask for references that have not been readily made available on résumés or applications. Even though the people who were directly involved in supervising or working with the applicant may no longer be employed, dates of employment and other information can be confirmed, lending credibility to the applicant's résumé and experience.

In these times of increased litigation, companies are sometimes reluctant to give out detailed information about anything other than if the candidate was employed and the specific dates of hire and termination. However, it is important to ask for detailed information if someone is open to providing it. Questions for references can be general (e.g., about work ethic, timeliness, punctuality) but should also be related to the job for which the candidate is applying. For example, if a candidate is applying for a position performing preexercise health screenings and exercise prescriptions, confirmations of the candidate's technical skills may be appropriate. Asking the supervisor's opinion about the candidate's ability to perform accurate blood pressure readings may be a good question. Remember, though, that you may be better able to test a candidate's aptitudes on technical issues during the interview process and not have to rely on someone else's judgment. Therefore, sticking with questions that confirm characteristics that are not as concrete, such as ability to work with others and work ethic, may be more appropriate for references.

Comparison of Candidates

One dimension of comparing candidates may include **scoring** their responses to questions or standards related to the hiring process. Scoring the candidate can be very helpful when companies use several interviewers or have a committee-based process for candidate selection. Agreeing on most criteria for job selection in advance (e.g., undergraduate degree preferred) is necessary if this method is to be employed. Additionally, creating a point or ratings system associated with preferred characteristics and skills can be time consuming but can also be valuable by refining the areas that are critical to making the best hire. An example of a rating system for applicants would ask

interviewers to rate the candidate using a scale of 1 to 5, with 1 representing *poor* and 5 representing *excellent*, on the following areas:

- Appearance
- Relevant past experience
- Likelihood of the candidate being long tenured
- Relevant education
- Technical skills
- Personality characteristics
- References

Total the scores received (or average them) so that each candidate has a rating.

Rating systems add a degree of objectiveness to a process that many times can feel fairly subjective. These types of systems can be particularly useful when several candidates are very close in terms of their perceived potential as employees. The scores can serve to highlight the differences, create helpful conversation about important differences between similar candidates, and eventually can contribute to a better final decision. A small twist to the system is to rank the criteria listed so that all those involved in the interviewing process understand that one attribute is more important than another. For candidates who are close in total score or average, reevaluating the scores with a focus on the most important criteria may provide a tiebreaker.

Job Offer

Some companies choose to make a job offer in writing. This form of job offer usually stipulates certain conditions such as the candidate's ability to successfully pass background or drug and alcohol tests.

Most companies have a **new-hire packet** that supervisors and managers use to streamline the process of hiring and to ensure the necessary paperwork is completed. In the United States, the standard new-hire forms include W4 (tax-related information), I-9 (confirmation of citizenship), payroll information and information for direct deposits to personal bank accounts, some form of welcome letter, and a booklet containing the general policies of the organization (e.g., sexual harassment, drugs and alcohol, safety, payroll, benefits, vacation, sick days, paid holidays, dependent care savings). Other processes that need to be dealt with at point of hire are the assignment of a time card for hourly paid positions, distribution of a uniform and name badge as necessary, and formalization and agreement of a work schedule.

KEY TERMS

background checks

benchmarks

close-ended questions

deal breakers

defined behaviors

experiential questions

external equity

job application

job description

job preview

new-hire packet

open-ended questions

paper screening

performance expectations

phone screening

positive profiling

references

reporting structure

scoring

situational questions

wage position

REFERENCES AND RECOMMENDED READING

American College of Sports Medicine (ACSM). 2007. *Health/fitness facility standards and guidelines*. 2nd ed. Champaign, IL: Human Kinetics.

Arthur, D. 2006. *Recruiting, interviewing, selecting, and orienting new employees*. 4th ed. AMACOM Books, Div. of Am. Management Association.

Chambers, H.E. 2001. *Finding, recruiting and hiring peak performers: Every manager's guide*. Cambridge, MA: Perseus Books Group.

Harvard Business School. 2002. *Hiring and keeping the best people*. Cambridge, MA: Harvard Business School Press.

International Health, Racquet, and Sportsclub Association (IHRSA). 2006. *Profiles of success*. Boston: IHRSA

McTague, T.S. *Hiring in good times and in bad: A guide to entry level staffing*. Boston: IHRSA.

U.S. Small Business Administration. 2004. *Human resource management*. Washington, DC: Small Business Administration.

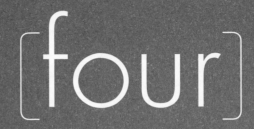

Training and Developing Staff

Brenda Abdilla

After studying this chapter, the reader will be able to

- use training as a powerful management tool,
- perform a training needs assessment,
- choose training topics,
- develop a training strategy,
- deliver training material effectively, and
- justify training investment.

Excellent club managers learn quickly that the only way for clubs to succeed in this intensively customer-focused business is through the employees who interact with the members. People in management usually have reached that level by providing excellent customer service, using effective communication, and mastering the skills of their job, but it does little good if the manager is the only person to possess these qualities. The desire to have others behave in a certain way drives most managers to invest time and resources in staff training and development. The ability to influence the behavior of others becomes a critical element of effective club management. Even the most skilled manager has a limited number of ways to influence the behavior of others.

Developing the skills and changing the behaviors of the team can be one of the most interesting and rewarding duties of club managers. Training requires a tremendous amount of planning and work, but the outcome can be remarkable. There are few actions a manager can take that will be more effective than delivering training with the intent of changing someone's approach to a skill. If handled properly, the manager will see increased confidence in the staff as well as a better appreciation for the aspect of their job that the training covered. Quality training can help attract and recruit excellent staff as well as help the club retain current staff. Although a warm personality and bright smile can only be hired, nearly any other skill can be trained with the right effort.

Training and development can get results and deliver consistent behaviors among staff in any department, including sales, hospitality, group exercise, housekeeping, and more. Used properly and over the long term, training and development can help staff develop a **career path,** which promotes employee retention and professional growth. Furthermore, training can benefit employees by providing additional job skills and intellectual stimulation. Finally, regular training provides a forum for communication of important information on an ongoing basis.

THE BOTTOM LINE

The world's best managers maximize the impact of training by developing employees' strengths rather than trying to improve upon their weaknesses (Buckingham and Coffman 1999).

Five Steps to Creating Internal Training Programs

Successful internal training programs are created through a five-step process. The steps include committing to a **needs analysis,** choosing the topics to be included in the training, choosing a strategy, delivering the material, and creating accountability.

Committing to a Needs Analysis

Starting a training program in the club setting is easier than most managers think. The best way to start the process is to commit to an observation period, such as 2 weeks. Managers can easily continue to perform their regular duties during this observation period by labeling file folders with every department name and topic in the club that needs enhancement. They should keep the files in a nearby drawer and get into the habit of filing anything that comes into view that applies to the analysis process. Items to consider could be a memo, an article, a sticky note with a thought that comes to mind, notes from a speaker or program, advertisements from local seminars on a particular topic—anything. Later, when it is time to put together a training program or delegate training to someone else, a collection of discussion items will be at hand.

Begin by making files for departments. Examples of departments include the following:

- Fitness
- Group exercise
- Hospitality desk
- Sales
- Housekeeping (cleaning)
- Maintenance (fixing and upkeep)
- Aquatics
- Child care
- Café or restaurant

Next, move to general topics that may affect multiple departments. Examples of general topics include the following:

- Customer service
- Dealing with difficult situations
- Cross-training
- Member retention
- Leadership
- Selling
- Special populations (seniors, members in postrehabilitation)
- Grassroots marketing
- Technical skills (electronic cash register, computers, pool maintenance)

During the 2-week observation period, it will be important to assess current needs within each department. This process takes about an hour for each department. It is easiest to start with the four departments that have the greatest impact on customer satisfaction and the bottom line—sales, hospitality,

housekeeping, and fitness. This assessment is best done after the manager has worked in the department or spent some time observing the department in action while answering the questions in the Departmental Training Needs Assessment on page 64.

Choosing Topics

Once the needs analysis is complete, the manager should take some time to read the notes made during the process and sort training needs into three categories:

- Urgent need
- Short-term need
- Long-term need

Urgent training needs should be met within 30 days of the needs analysis, short-term needs within 90 days, and long-term needs within 6 months to 1 year, if possible. See table 4.1 for a sample list of training topics and level of need. At the same time, the manager should determine if there are basic elements where training would be beneficial to the entire staff or if the basic elements are all in place and the more urgent needs are department specific. For example, if poor communication or marginal customer service was present in most of the departments analyzed, then perhaps the general topic of customer service excellence is an urgent need that must be addressed before specific training occurs within departments. On the other hand, if the observations revealed impressive levels of staff communication and customer service, then more specific training might come first (e.g., point-of-sale training for the front desk or training in how to perform fitness evaluations for the fitness team). For a more complete list of topics, see the Club Training and Development Planner on page 65.

Choosing a Strategy

After coming up with a clear idea of training needs, managers can go to work finding resources to help with the training process and decide on a training strategy for each need. First, however, it should be noted that completion of the needs analysis and topics list is more than just a management process. Having a clear idea of training needs (even if the list is long) can provide tremendous stress relief for a manager who has been observing bothersome behaviors on the part of the club team. Also, awareness of specific needs often stimulates thoughts, ideas, and connections in the manager's mind that can lead to resources and strategies to get the training done.

Departmental Training Needs Assessment

Date _____

Evaluator name _____

Department name _____

1. List the top 3 to 5 critical tasks of this department.

   _____

2. List the names of the people who perform these critical tasks with expertise, consistency, and professionalism (if any).

   _____

3. If you were working the department yourself, what would you do differently?

   _____

4. What efficiencies are present in this department?

   _____

5. What inefficiencies are present in this department?

   _____

6. On a scale of 1 to 10, how would you rate the overall success of this department, with 1 being poor and 10 being excellent?

   _____

7. If applicable, from a financial perspective, how does this department rate (over budget, under budget, understaffed, profitable)?

   _____

8. What elements could be added to this department to make it more financially viable or to save costs?

   _____

9. General observations about the department's current condition:

   _____

From M. Bates, 2008, *Health Fitness Management*, 2nd ed. (Champaign, IL: Human Kinetics).

Choosing a strategy requires answering the questions *who* and *where*. (The *what* and the *when* have already been determined in the needs assessment, and the *how* will be covered in Delivering the Material on page 68.)

Who Will Provide the Training?

For each of the training topics, managers must determine if they are planning to deliver the training themselves, if there is someone on staff who can deliver the training (both of these are considered internal), or if an outside resource is necessary (external). With some topics, such as CPR, pool care, or even sales training, an outside resource may be a necessity unless the manager also holds teacher certifications or special expertise in these areas. However, with many of the topics there are training options. Sometimes the budget is so limited that it is necessary to keep all training internal for

Table 4.1   Sample Topics and Level of Need

Training topic	Level of need	Departments to receive this training
Customer service	Urgent	All staff
Point-of-sale system	Urgent	Hospitality desk, personal trainers
Team building	Short term	All staff
Sales training	Urgent	Sales team, personal trainers
Cross-selling skills	Long term	All staff
Telephone skills	Short term	Desk staff, sales staff, personal trainers
Personal training for special populations	Short term	Personal trainers
Pool supplies and chemical safety	Urgent	Housekeeping, maintenance staff

Club Training and Development Planner

Your training programs will likely focus on specific areas of need. Here are some suggestions for topics to cover in each area, along with ideas for delivering the training.

Safety and Compliance

• *Topics to cover:* Occupational Safety and Health Administration (OSHA) regulations, sexual harassment, CPR and AED, bloodborne pathogens, facility safety, first aid, water safety, personal training certifications, and lifeguard certifications (check state laws for positions that require drug testing or background checks as part of the hiring process)

• *Ideas for training:* Consider outsourcing this training or purchasing an e-learning program; make certain classes mandatory for all employees and schedule them quarterly or more often; call the local fire or police department and schedule drills for fires, bomb threats, first aid, and safety.

New-Associate Orientation

• *Topics to cover:* Company standards, cross-training for all departments, benefits, service strategies and policies for uniforms, grooming, benefits, and so on

• *Ideas for training:* If the club's orientation is outdated, schedule a half-day brainstorming session with all department heads to commit to a new agenda and method of delivery. The ideal orientation is concise, upbeat, and has a test for maximum effectiveness.

Basic Management Skills

• *Topics to cover:* Recruiting, interviewing, budget process, goal setting, organization, schedules, uniforms, basic coaching skills for managers as well as discipline approach and policy

• *Ideas for training:* Ideally this course is given for any associate who manages one or more persons. These skills are critical for new managers to be successful. The general manager can perform training with the human resources and finance departments or bring in a trainer.

Leadership Skills for Experienced Managers

• *Topics to cover:* Building a team, time management, leadership versus management, crisis prevention, advanced coaching, forecasting and accountability systems, inspiring others to serve, influencing others, and how leaders think.

(continued)

(continued)

- *Ideas for training:* Consider bringing in a professional speaker for this program once managers have mastered the basic skills. Also, consider enrolling everyone in a public seminar and making a day of it. Have all participants present what they learned. Also, see Taking Training to New Heights on page 75.

Team Building

- *Topics to cover:* Structured or skill-focused topics such as goal setting, mind mapping, wealth building, personal health and nutrition, and life balance; unstructured or fun-focused activities such as bowling, outdoor activities, weekend getaways, theme parks, ropes courses, awards dinners, movies, theaters, or trips
- *Ideas for training:* Unless the club has an expert on the team, it will likely have to pay someone to provide this training. Try to do some things that are completely unexpected by the team. Have some fun and be sure to block out the time without any interruptions. (Also be sure to avoid anything that is physically dangerous or that may be religious or personally offensive to team members.)

Sales Training for New Reps

- *Topics to cover:* Industry-specific topics such as competition, selling intangibles versus tangibles, product knowledge, needs versus interests selling, informational calls, following up, lead tracking, tours, and referrals
- *Ideas for training:* Start a training file today and fill it with articles, memos, and any relevant information a new rep will need. Next, see what books, tapes, and materials industry experts have published and start a library. Schedule new reps for 30 minutes of training with each department.

Sales Training for Experienced Reps

- *Topics to cover:* Personal development subjects such as dressing for success, time management, organization, wealth building, nutrition, and life balance; advanced sales skills such as prospecting strategies, grassroots marketing, business-to-business selling, and networking
- *Ideas for training:* Keep an eye open for relevant books to read as a team. Register everyone for the next full-day business rally that comes to town or invest in a speaker or trainer. Ask the group what they are interested in learning and provide it for them.

Personal Trainers

- *Topics to cover:* Safety training, updated information on exercise science, selling skills that focus on the needs assessment of the member plus closing the sale, time management, communication skills, and referral generation
- *Ideas for training:* Try to hire trainers who can sell; trying to teach this skill can be an exercise in futility. That being said, credibility is critical here. This group needs someone they can believe in to teach them new skills. A person with a background in exercise plus proven business skills is ideal.

Customer Service

- *Topics to cover:* The greeting, telephone etiquette, handling difficult clients, behavior toward coworkers, service expectations, technical training, and cross-selling
- *Ideas for training:* If the club doesn't currently have a solid program, put the department heads to the task and supplement the program with tapes and videos that reflect club expectations. Periodically take groups on field trips to see local businesses that offer top-notch service and then discuss the trip. If the club wants to go big, consider Disney University, a program that is available in several cities and has more than 500,000 graduates.

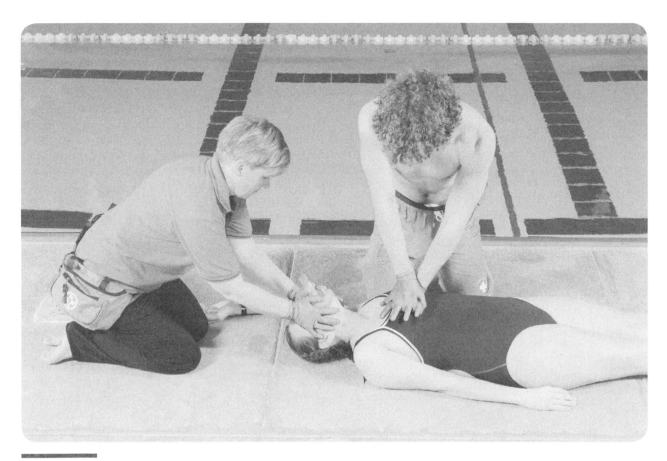

Determining who will present the training and where the training will be delivered are important considerations. Is there someone on staff who is qualified to present the training or should an outside resource be used? Is there enough space to present the training inside the facility or will an off-site location be necessary?

the time being. If budget permits, the best strategy is a combination of internal and external training resources since no one resource or person usually has all of the answers. (A list of outside resources to consider is presented later in this chapter.)

Where Will the Training Take Place?

Choosing a training venue is important in creating a productive learning environment. Seemingly nonessential factors like room temperature or outside noise can have a negative impact on how the training is received. If the venue of choice is inside the club, the manager should be sure to have comfortable seating, tables, materials, and lighting suitable for learning. The in-club training venue should be free of member traffic and should not be conducted within earshot of members—often a tall order for busy clubs with limited space.

Budget constraints need not limit venue options for staff training if **trade-outs** (i.e., countertrades or contras) are an option. Many local hotels would gladly take free guest passes in exchange for a conference room, audiovisual materials, and even meal service. Taking the **off-site training** one step further would be staff retreats.

Staff retreats, where the club takes part or all of the team off site for a training experience, are increasing in popularity in the business world. Typing the words *corporate retreats* in a popular Internet search engine returned over a million results. Staff retreats can range from something as simple as taking the staff bowling to hiring a company to take the team on a ropes course or rafting. Hosting and planning an outing that is outside the norm for staff can be useful in the following situations:

- If the staff (or department) is very advanced and has seen it all
- As a reward for excellent performance
- If the goal is for staff to think differently and change their problem-solving approach to solve a dilemma

- To establish a team spirit with a team that needs to be more supportive of each other in order to succeed
- To facilitate transitions such as new ownership, staff changes, and so on
- To simply try something new
- If the budget allows it or a trade-out exists with a facility or organization

For some employees, the concept of a staff retreat or team-building event is exciting and a welcome departure from the ordinary. For others, it can be perceived as highly uncomfortable and a waste of time. Keep this in mind during the planning and decide in advance how much to tell the team about the upcoming event. It might help to involve several members of the team in the planning process. As with all training, begin with the end in mind. Ask what outcome is wanted and then go about planning the special event. Consider the following key elements:

- How much social interaction is wanted?
- Is there a theme?
- Will internal or external facilitators be used?
- Does anyone in the group have any physical limitations?
- Are there safety considerations?
- Are there any liability concerns?
- What is the duration of the retreat? Will there be an overnight stay?
- How will success be determined?
- What is the total budget for the event?

THE BOTTOM LINE

When a management team, staff team, or executive team holds a corporate retreat or off-site business meeting, the investment of time is significant. The question is how to make the most of this limited and extremely valuable time (Withrow 2007).

Delivering the Material

Possibly the most critical element of effective training is the method of delivering the information. Many different generations of employees work in clubs, and they all receive and process information in different manners and have different comfort levels with technology. Also keep in mind differences in learning styles when considering areas of the current training program that could use some serious updating.

Anyone who has attended a professionally prepared seminar or training class likely experienced an organized, well-thought-out program with a variety of learning modalities and a clear beginning, middle, and end. The standard for in-house training is much the same as professional training and many of the same qualities can be present with time and preparation.

Keys to Developing Effective Training Programs

Developing effective training programs is a matter of using the following keys:

- *Keep the focus narrow.* If the people selected to conduct the training have not had a lot of experience putting together training material, they will want to allot a large period of time in a quiet environment for this task. Now is the time to peruse the notes and items filed in folders to help determine specific topics to cover in the upcoming training. When putting together a training program on any topic, it is important to keep the topic narrow and to focus on a skill rather than a concept. If time is limited, it is better to focus on a few aspects of a larger topic than to try to lump all of one topic into one training session. For example, when preparing training sessions on delivering customer service, it is better to focus on a few related topics like handling member complaints and dealing with difficult situations in one session than to also try to include telephone skills, scheduling, and snack bar sales in the same session. It is better to cover narrow topics deeply than to cover wide topics broadly.

- *Begin with the end in mind.* The next step in preparing the training program is to think about the desired outcome. The following three questions should be asked:

  1. What specific skills should the group come away with?
  2. How will their knowledge be apparent?
  3. What words, body language, or results will be present after the training that are not consistently present now?

- *Break it down.* Virtually any skill can be broken down into steps or important concepts. The trainer should come up with at least five steps or concepts that will help the audience absorb the material. For example, if the topic is dealing with difficult member situations, come up with the steps necessary to handle the situation.

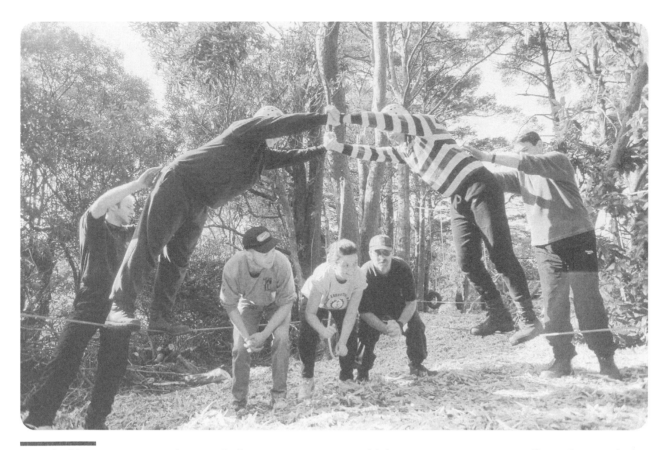

Team-building activities, such as a challenge course, can establish a team spirit among staff members and also prompt a change in the staff's usual approach to solving problems.
© Modron/Laif/Aurora Photos

1. Listen carefully to the member (using both eyes and ears).
2. Remove distractions and pause before reacting to the member's words.
3. Calmly repeat the member's words back to the member for clarification.
4. Decide how to respond—call reinforcements if needed, but keep the member informed of pending actions.
5. Take responsibility to resolve the situation.

This process can be applied to any skill that the trainer is attempting to impart to the group. Once the steps are in place, the next process is breaking down each step and deciding what the best approach is to teaching each step.

• *Bring training material to life.* Many people think that the most difficult part of training is the public speaking (see Tips for Delivering Training Material on page 70). However, anyone who has ever developed a training program knows it is the preparatory work of making ideas and training goals come to life that is the most difficult. If getting people to change their behavior were easy, then simply circulating a memo containing the training information would change the way staff deal with difficult members. It is difficult to change human behavior and habits, and that is the crux of training and development—getting people to change. The only measure of effective training is whether it is changing the way people act and think. The goal of change requires a combination of good material and an effective teaching method.

THE BOTTOM LINE

We learn by example and by direct experience because there are limits to the adequacy of verbal instruction (Gladwell 2005).

Selecting Interactive Exercises

Now that the training steps have been outlined, it is time to come up with a teaching method for each step.

Tips for Delivering Training Material

It is perfectly normal for people delivering training material to feel nervous or self-conscious even though they may know the audience well. The key is to focus on the material and the desired result instead of personal appearance or nervousness. Presenters should immerse themselves in the material they want to impart and the rest will fall into place. Keep these seven tips in mind.

1. Never start with a joke unless you are a professional comedian. In the old days the advice for nervous speakers was to always start with a joke. This can be a mistake on a number of levels, including difficulty pulling it off if the trainer is a bit nervous, political incorrectness, and repeating a joke that the audience has already heard.

2. Practice makes perfect. Rehearse until the message is committed to memory—that way, the material won't be lost to nerves. Practice, practice, practice!

3. Use the word *excited* instead of *nervous*. How the presenter internalizes thoughts about the upcoming training program affects performance. Make actions and thoughts positive. Also, do something positive before speaking (work out or meditate) and avoid anything that might be upsetting (watching the news, checking voice mail).

4. Focus on the material. Trainers should focus on the material instead of on how they will be perceived by others. If the material is good and the delivery is decent, the speaker will be well perceived.

5. Ignore insignificant distractions. People sneeze, cough, move around, talk, and even fall asleep in training sessions. If someone requires disciplinary action, take care of it later. While presenting, focus on the material and ignore distractions.

6. Plan each moment. Trainers should take time to write down everything they will say and proceed in a step-by-step fashion. Not only will this help with delivery, it can help if they get sidetracked. Also, it will help with timing the length of the program.

7. Start on time, end on time—every time! Begin as close to the starting time as possible (this often requires reminding staff of the starting time in advance). If given the choice, go short rather than long and leave the audience wanting more. Never exceed the time allotted. There is nothing worse than having the audience looking at their watches and wondering, "When is this going to end?"

Interactive exercises keep the group interested in the material and can have a dramatic impact on the retention of information. Myriad interactive exercises and training games are available; the important thing is that the exercise is related to the topic (icebreakers are the only exception). The most effective training programs include a combination of modalities.

Icebreakers   Icebreakers are the only activities that do not need to be directly related to the subject being trained. The purpose of icebreakers is to set the mood for the training and help the attendees get to know each other. The most common icebreaker is having everyone go around the room and introduce themselves. However, the possibilities for breaking the ice are endless.

A fun twist on the typical icebreaker is to have everyone fill out a name tag when they come in that includes their first name and their favorite color, food, or hobby. Another idea is to have everyone stand up and tell the person next to them something nobody would ever guess about them. Be sure to keep the icebreaker brief and make sure everyone feels included.

Fill-in-the-Blank Handout   This modality is perfect when the training topic is something that the audience does not know or understand. The fill-in-the-blank element keeps the group guessing until the trainer covers the answers to the blanks. For example, if covering CPR in a training setting, the handout might read:

The number of compressions for an adult victim is _____ to every _____ breaths.

Reading Aloud   If the trainer wants to emphasize a certain part of the training such as the company mission statement or a case study, having group members read aloud can be helpful. In spite of harkening back to school days, reading aloud can keep the group on their best behavior as they feel empathy for the person reading in addition to some natural trepidation that they might be selected next.

Case Studies   **Case studies** can be a powerful tool, especially when the step or process is complicated and there is more than one right answer to the problem. A case study should be designed to get the participants to think through a problem and to have a lasting impact on those involved. Sample Interactive Exercise Using a Case Study below is designed to help the group develop empathy for difficult members. However, this goal should not be immediately apparent to the participants.

Team Brainstorming   Similar to the case study, the team brainstorming session involves the entire room and has no guaranteed outcome. Many topics can be presented as brainstorming in a training environment. However, it is important that only a portion of the session be devoted to brainstorming since it can wear on the group after a while.

Brainstorming is usually done with the trainer standing next to a flip chart, dry-erase board, or laptop computer. The basic rule with brainstorming is that all ideas are good ideas; therefore, a topic that is open for discussion should be selected. Ideally, the ideas from the group would be saved or typed up and distributed later.

Live Demonstrations or Skits   This can be a fun, serious, or poignant part of a training session and can be achieved in many ways. One idea is to choose some people in the group who have already mastered the particular step that is being taught (such as overcoming an objection in sales) and ask them to playact for the group.

Another strategy is for the trainer to demonstrate without rehearsal (improvise) the skill to the group. For example, the trainer could ask the group to give their worst member complaint.

An additional element that can be entertaining is to preplan and rehearse an actual skit with some key staff members ahead of time. With some exaggerated behaviors and a bit of humor, a whole host of awkward and frustrating subjects can be handled (e.g., associates on the Internet during

Sample Interactive Exercise Using a Case Study

Lucy Blankenship has been a club member for about 15 years. Her husband died suddenly last year in a car accident. When Mrs. Blankenship tried to remove her husband's name from the membership statement, the accounting department had an internal miscommunication and for a variety of reasons 3 months passed before we were able to correct our error.

Last fall Mrs. Blankenship's personal trainer of 6 years left the club to move to another state to care for her ailing mother and we have had trouble meeting Mrs. Blankenship's special needs with any of the trainers on our staff.

Mrs. Blankenship has lost her temper with our desk staff several times in the past few months. Seemingly small mistakes, like not having change for a dollar or the club opening a few minutes late, are causing her to complain loudly about the club, the service, and the staff.

Discussion Points

- What, if anything, should be done about Mrs. Blankenship?
- How long is a club expected to pay for its mistakes?
- Is Mrs. Blankenship's anger justified in any way?
- Is there ever a time when a club should ask a person to quit the club? When?

Debriefing the Case Study

The trainer should divide everyone into small groups and then allow time for them to read the case study and discuss the points listed. It is best if a group leader is assigned the task of making sure that all group members get a chance to express their thoughts and opinions. Once everyone has had a chance to speak, the trainer should ask for feedback from each group leader. When one of the group leaders or participants has a response that shows empathy or has an empathic idea or strategy, the trainer should expand on that thought and involve the entire group in that line of discussion. This exercise also allows the trainer to make mental note of those with an open mind for solutions and, conversely, those who have a deeply entrenched negative view of members.

work, cell phone usage, lax attitude, lack of attention to detail).

Sources for Other Interactive Exercise Ideas for other types of interactive exercises can be found in the following recommended books (see References and Recommended Readings at the end of the chapter for more information):

- *Games Trainers Play* by Edward E. Scannel and John W. Newstrom
- *The Complete Games Trainers Play* by Edward E. Scannel and John W. Newstrom
- *The Big Book of Team Building Games: Trust-Building Activities, Team Spirit Exercises, and Other Fun Things to Do* by John W. Newstrom and Edward E. Scannel
- *The Big Book of Humorous Training Games* by Doni Tamblyn and Sharyn Weiss
- *The Big Book of Customer Service Training Games* by Peggy Carlaw and Vasudha K. Deming
- *The Big Book of Motivation Games* by Robert Epstein and Jessica Rodgers
- *Team-Building Activities for Every Group* by Alanna Jones

Be aware of copyright laws when using the published material of others. Most copyright laws apply internationally. The U.S. copyright is a form of protection provided by the laws of the United States to the authors of original works, including literary, dramatic, musical, artistic, and certain other intellectual works. This protection is available to both published and unpublished works. Using copyrighted material without permission is plagiarism, and you can be sued by the copyright owner for damages. More information is available at www.copyright.gov.

Creating Accountability

The final step in this process is to create elements that test the effectiveness of the training and provide information or data to help justify training expenditures in the future. Although there are several ways to test effectiveness, sometimes the mere knowledge of accountability makes the training more effective. In other words, the fact that the group knows they will be tested at the end of a course (or asked to role-play) makes them pay more attention and therefore makes the training more effective. Training effectiveness can be measured in a variety of ways:

- Testing—The most common strategy for measuring the effectiveness of a training program is to test participants after each section of material is presented. The test can be written or verbal, formal or informal.
- Role-playing—A more intensive form of testing is to ask several or all of the participants to explain what they have learned and use it in a simulated situation. This **role-playing** can be done privately after the training is complete or in the group setting.
- Written follow-up—After the session is complete, trainees are asked to summarize what they learned and how they plan to apply it. This assignment should have a due date and associates should receive some feedback based on what they wrote.
- Impromptu testing—These tests are conducted after the session and require the manager to approach staff members in an impromptu fashion and ask them to explain or demonstrate the new skill learned in the training.
- Financial tracking—If the training was designed to increase profits or save on expenses, the manager can do a simple analysis by measuring the same line item before and after training.

Also be sure to include some type of feedback mechanism after presenting or hosting a training program. Feedback can be as simple as a short form (see the Training Feedback Form on page 73) that asks participants what they learned and what they would change about the program. You could also ask each participant to write a synopsis of the program and hand it in or e-mail it.

THE BOTTOM LINE

The half-life of newly learned material is 3 days. If learners don't use it immediately, they lose it (Cross and O'Driscoll 2005).

Outside Resources for Training and Development

Combining do-it-yourself programs with proven, professional programs is an ideal combination for any business. The resources to select from are endless. Here is a partial list:

- *Industry-specific expert.* This person has a specific area of expertise that can be of great benefit to

Training Feedback Form

1. Which program did you attend?

   _____

2. What was your favorite part of the program?

   _____

3. What was your least favorite part of the program?

   _____

4. What was the best thing you learned today?

   _____

5. Is there anything you would change about the program?

   _____

6. Do you have any comments about the speaker?

   _____

Thank you for your time!

From M. Bates, 2008, *Health Fitness Management*, 2nd ed. (Champaign, IL: Human Kinetics).

the team. Some of the topics include sales, service, and personal training. If you have not heard of the expert, be sure to check references from past clients and take the time to work out the details of the program far in advance of the training date. Check industry resource manuals and associations for recommended speakers. An ideal place to preview industry experts is at conferences and trade shows held worldwide. Also, many industry experts have tapes and books available for purchase to add to the club library.

• *Professional speaker.* This person either has a general area of expertise (e.g., life balance, motivation) or a specific one, though not specific to a particular industry (e.g., sales, service, finance). A professional speaker should be polished and prepared and can be a wonderful adjunct to the annual staff get-together or special event. Be sure to clarify all fees, including travel, with a speaking professional. One great international resource is the National Speakers Association (NSA) (www.nsaspeaker.org).

• *Professional training company.* Several training organizations are available that will handle club training on a large scale. Ideally, the company would be local to save on travel costs. This is generally a

big investment, so be thorough in researching and in outlining your expectations. Usually professional training companies sign on for at least 1 year.

• *Public seminars.* A public seminar is any training program or speech that is made available to the general public for a per-person fee. The quality can range from poor to awe inspiring, so be sure to check them out in advance. Sometimes the speaker is well known, but often you will register based on the topic or title (e.g., coaching tips for new managers) and will not know the quality of the material or the speaker until attending. Public seminars can be a wonderful, low-cost way to add training to the club; however, one downside is the (sometimes) shameless focus on selling of additional training materials from the speaking platform. Most professionals subtly mention their materials during their presentation, but hawking materials throughout the program is considered in bad taste and is a waste of audience time.

• *Local networking events featuring speakers.* Many local networking groups invite local businesspeople to present a topic at their regular events. These can be excellent sources of information and can serve as networking events for the club as well. Call the local chamber of commerce and inquire about networking events and local speakers.

• *Compliance programs and special certifications.* Laws on CPR and AED requirements vary by state and country, so check to see if the club is in compliance. Check with the local chapter of the Red Cross to see what programs they offer. Additionally, check with industry associations for a list of specific certification providers, such as certification in personal training, lifeguarding, whirlpool maintenance, water safety, Pilates, and so on.

• *Online learning.* Online learning is commonly known as **e-learning.** It encompasses any type of training or information exchanged via the computer. *InformationWeek* magazine estimates that the number of providers of e-learning systems has grown from 67 to 113 in the past 2 years. Although many companies think that online learning saves on training costs, some experts say that this is often not the case and caution companies against using this training medium to save money. However, it does appear to be worth the money invested: According to an *InformationWeek* survey, 46% of respondents already see a return on investment, but 21% say it will take a year or more to see a return on their programs (Swanson 2001).

It seems the primary reason for adding e-learning to training programs is increased penetra-tion of the information. Simply put, more people will have access to the information because it does not require an instructor to teach it and associates can view it on their own schedules. However, experts encourage e-learning as one part of a program instead of the only vehicle because only so much can be communicated via computer screens and talking heads. Mark LeBlanc, vice president of the NSA and president of Small Business Success, supports e-learning: "Do not underestimate the value of e-learning. Successful organizations are already taking advantage of this important medium. It is the ideal complement to regular training vehicles, supports the learning process, and helps put ideas into action" (M. LeBlanc, personal communication).

Assessment of Training Costs

Many managers are reluctant to invest in training because it can be costly and there is always the risk that the club will invest in training and then the employee will take this newfound knowledge and find better work. However, this belief is contrary to the position of many experts who agree that training and development help retain employees. Also, as mentioned, employee retention has been tied to

Instant Staff Training Idea

Training does not always have to happen in a class setting. An excellent way to get started with team training and development when time is short is to read the same book as a group. Reading a book together opens the lines of communication, creates a forum for discussion, and gives everyone common knowledge on a subject. Another benefit of reading a book together is that it takes pressure off managers who have not led training sessions before. The book can be read with a specific department or with the entire team at once. Choose a book that has universal appeal and a clear message. Self-help books are a great place to start; team members are more likely to read them since it may help with their personal lives as well. Be sure to read the book before buying it for the group in order to make sure it is appropriate. These timeless self-help books are recommended for staff reading (see References and Recommended Readings at the end of the chapter for more information):

• *Think and Grow Rich* by Napoleon Hill (wealth, positive thinking)
• *How to Win Friends and Influence People* by Dale Carnegie (kindness and good deeds)
• *The Seven Habits of Highly Effective People* by Steven Covey (life balance, life mission, time management, relationships with others)
• *The Power of Your Subconscious Mind* by Joseph Murphy (positive thinking, affirmations applied to work and everyday life)
• *The Alchemist* by Paulo Coelho (inspiring parable of a boy in ancient time who goes on an adventure and finds his true value)
• *The Monk Who Sold His Ferrari* by Robin Sharma (fable about fulfilling your dreams and reaching your destiny)

customer retention. When people grow personally and professionally through training and development programs, they often become more loyal to their employer and feel more competent in their work. They are more able to plot their own advancement within the larger framework of the company's growth. All of these factors help justify the costs involved in staff training and development.

When budgeting for training and development costs, be sure to consider the following:

- Learner's time away from the job
- Cost of job coverage during training
- Training materials (e.g., books, handouts)
- Electronic equipment (e.g., computers)
- Audiovisual aids (e.g., flip chart, overhead projector)
- Licensing fees, where applicable
- Training venue or facility costs
- Fees and expenses of instructor, including travel expenses
- Support materials for follow-up
- Meals and refreshments

Untrained staff can have many negative effects on a club. One of the most significant is the impression that untrained staff can make on club members. Other costs of not training staff include the following:

- Potential liability from mistakes can be costly.
- Untrained employees can take up to six times longer to perform their tasks.
- Coworkers may spend extra time helping with routine tasks that could have been trained.
- Employee retention is not as high as it could be.
- A 4-year study by the American Society of Training and Development (ASTD) shows that firms that spend $1,500 per employee in training compared with those that spend $125 per employee experience on average 24% higher gross profit margins and 218% higher income per employee (Avatech Solutions 2007).
- Just a 2% increase in productivity has been shown to net a 100% return on investment in outsourced, instructor-led training (Avatech Solutions 2007).
- A person being paid $50,000 per year who is wasting just 1 hour per day costs the organization $6,250 per year (Wetmore 1999).

Taking Training to New Heights

Anne Nolen, training manager for the Houstonian Hotel, Club, and Spa, believes staff training is the answer to every problem and the key to achieving nearly any goal. Many top-rated employees join the enormously successful Houstonian Club based on its commitment to training and development. Training and education are used not only for improving critical skills toward profitability, like sales and customer service, but also for recruiting and for saving money through safety compliance (litigation avoidance) and reduced turnover.

The Numbers Speak for Themselves

The club portion of the Houstonian Hotel, Club, and Spa will achieve $26 million in gross revenue on its own for 2005 with approximately 5,700 memberships. The spa (Trellis) will achieve $5 million in total revenue by itself with 17,000 square feet (1,579 square meters) and 19 treatment rooms. Houstonian Lite, a small subchain started by the Houstonian, has grown to two clubs with a third on the way, each 15,000 to 18,000 square feet (1,394-1,672 square meters). The two clubs combined have a total of 1,400 members.

The first step in training at the Houstonian is to make sure new associates understand and absorb the club values, or what they refer to as their *compass*. Even though the values may seem simple, the Houstonian takes them seriously and incorporates them into every training session, staff interaction, decision-making process, and disciplinary action. There are six Houstonian compass values:

- Dignity
- Trustworthiness

(continued)

(continued)

- Accountability
- Continual improvement
- Personal and professional balance
- Friendliness

The Ultimate Commitment

In 1996, the Houstonian sent three of its managers to be certified by FranklinCovey in the famous program titled *The Seven Habits of Highly Effective People.* "This process requires that the Covey people approve your organization for licensing and comes with a high-priced ticket and a commitment to the people you send since they cannot, by law, teach the training at any company other than yours," explains Nolen. The managers spent about a week in Salt Lake City, Utah, learning the program and learning to deliver the material. After the managers attended the program, they were required to teach segments to the group. "At first you wonder if you are going to be worthy of the material and then you realize that the material speaks for itself," says Nolen.

"The reason we are committed to this body of work is that it outlines a remarkable way of managing relationships. It is a common human condition to not be able to handle everything in your world and to need to make good choices. You must take care of your relationships. If you are trustworthy, then you have people's trust. To share that information and have that common language and connection with our entire staff is priceless. It infiltrates everything we do here," says Nolen. The Houstonian runs the FranklinCovey program approximately five times per year and encourages all staff to attend. They offer the program in English and Spanish and encourage all employees of the company, including part-time and even substitute employees, to attend as many times as they like.

Training Programs Offered at the Houstonian

- *Customer service training*—All associates attend this required course once per year. "It is critical that you get together and talk about service and about relationships—why we are really here," explains Nolen.

- *Management development*—The Houstonian uses a Dallas-based training group to teach cutting-edge management strategies to their busy management team. Topics focus on the latest research in learning styles and effectiveness.

- *New-manager training*—Also for newly promoted managers, this is an orientation-style training facilitated internally by each senior manager in that discipline. Hiring, corrective action, financials, and so on are covered. This is a coordinated effort through the training department and happens a few times per year.

- *New-hire orientation*—This program covers the compass values (see page 75 and above) in detail. After orientation, each new hire is assigned to a peer partner, a coworker who is not in a position of authority but can help the new associate. "It's like the buddy system," says Nolen. "They help them get oriented and have a friend and the peer partners take pride in having been selected. Peer partners get some special attention, too, and it helps develop their career. They do it voluntarily." A peer partner is often rewarded with additional training and development.

- *Specialized department training*—This is often taught by an outside expert and covers the needed legal compliance for that department (e.g., CPR and AED certification, bartender certification, sexual harassment training) or continuing education needs (e.g., bringing in a special yoga instructor to teach a master class).

- *Speaker track*—Outside experts are brought in to inspire and teach management-level employees.

- *Tuition reimbursement*—The Houstonian also reimburses outside education for its employees.

KEY TERMS

career path

case study

e-learning

interactive exercises

needs analysis

off-site training

role-playing

staff retreats

trade-outs

REFERENCES AND RECOMMENDED READING

Avatech Solutions. 2007. Training return on investment: The real cost of not training. Retrieved April 19, 2007, from www.avat.com/training/trainingroi.asp.

Buckingham, M., and Coffman, C. 1999. *First break all the rules.* New York: Simon & Schuster.

Carlaw, P., and Deming, V.K. 1998. *The big book of customer service training games.* New York: McGraw-Hill.

Carnegie, D. 1990. *How to win friends and influence people.* New York: Pocket.

Coelho, P. 1993. *The alchemist.* San Francisco: Harper.

Covey, S. 2004. *The seven habits of highly effective people.* New York: Simon and Schuster.

Cross, J., and T. O'Driscoll. 2005. New American workplace. *Training Magazine,* March 2005.

Epstein, R., and Rogers, J. 2001. *The big book of motivation games.* New York: McGraw-Hill.

Gladwell, M. 2005. *Blink: The power of thinking without thinking.* New York: Little Brown.

Hill, N. 1987. *Think and grow rich.* New York: Random House.

Jones, A. 2000. *Team-building activities for every group.* Richland, WA: Rec Room.

Murphy, J. 2001. *The power of your subconscious mind.* New York: Bantam.

Newstrom, J.W., and Scannell, E.E. 1997. *The big book of team building games: Trust-building activities, team spirit exercises and other fun things to do.* New York: McGraw-Hill.

Scannell, E.E., and Newstrom, J.W. 1980. *Games trainers play.* New York: McGraw-Hill.

———. 1994. *The complete games trainers play.* New York: McGraw-Hill.

Sharma, R. 2004. *The monk who sold his Ferrari.* New York: Element.

Swanson, S. 2001. E-Learning branches out. *InformationWeek,* 26 February 2001.

Tamblyn, D., and Weiss, S. 2000. *The big book of humorous training games.* New York: McGraw-Hill.

Wetmore, D.E. 1999. Price of not training. Retrieved April 19, 2007, from www.balancetime.com.

Withrow, B. 2007. Corporate retreats: How to get the most out of them. Retrieved April 19, 2007, from www.facilitators.com/corporate_retreats.htm.

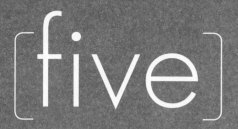

Managing Staff Performance

Bud Rockhill

After studying this chapter, the reader will be able to

- identify the role of the manager in influencing staff performance;
- clarify job expectations;
- recognize the importance of the job description;
- provide performance feedback;
- address performance problems; and
- understand the importance of recognition, rewards, and incentives in influencing job performance.

The manager of a luxury hotel once encountered an employee who took little pride in his job as a dishwasher. This employee thought that he was making no contribution to the overall purpose of the hotel, which was known around the world for its exceptional service, luxury accommodations, and elegant spa.

"I don't think you understand," the hotel's general manager told him, "how important your job really is. If the dishes are not cleaned properly, then either a guest will become ill or the health department will issue a violation. We could be shut down, or business could decrease due to word of mouth. So even though it seems to you that your job is only about washing dishes, you're really a critical link in the chain to make sure that we uphold the highest standards of cleanliness and safety and continue to enjoy our well-established reputation."

Perhaps the dishwasher did not enjoy the tasks required by his job any more than he did before the conversation, but he went about them with a new sense of purpose and pride, knowing that he was truly making a contribution to the larger organization.

Managing performance is the ultimate test of a manager's skill and the reason that the manager's job exists in the first place. **Performance management** is the process of achieving the business goals by building and working with your staff. It is not simply a matter of conducting performance appraisals annually—it encompasses virtually everything in this textbook, from hiring to business strategy development to financial management, and requires the manager to integrate staff, strategy, and business objectives.

Performance management is not separate from the other managerial areas; it is the outcome of being effective in these different areas and integrating them smoothly. The ultimate measure of a manager's skill at performance management is the final score—the financial results—as well as the more qualitative and subjective staff satisfaction.

Just as a successful new product or service generates buzz—that sense of excitement that attracts customers—the successful organization will have an intangible feeling of excitement and energy, the kind of environment that makes people want to go to work every day, where new ideas are valued and where people take responsibility for their own job performance. This isn't a theoretical utopia or limited to textbook narrative—it's possible to achieve in virtually any organization. But it takes a willingness to embrace the building blocks of performance management and use them consistently. As with most aspects of business, it requires a willingness to do the small things well and consistently, and it requires the manager to focus on the achievement of the organizational goals rather than personal glory. When the team is winning, the spirit is contagious—success breeds success.

Role of the Manager in Staff Performance

In traditional management classes, the role of the manager has often been defined as planning, organizing, directing, and controlling. Although these areas of responsibility usually are part of what a manager does, they don't provide a particularly instructive or insightful understanding of the job.

The management role could also be defined as organizing and directing resources to achieve the goals of the organization. This definition is more focused on results than the specific tasks and addresses the need to manage resources, including people, money, and time, but it isn't specific to performance management. To help make the topic as understandable and usable as possible, it may be more instructional to use sport analogies and terminology, given that most people involved in fitness management have some degree of experience in organized sport.

Therefore, the reference point for the effective performance manager is that the manager is the coach. A performance-oriented manager needs to address the same things a coach would:

- What's the game plan and does everyone understand it?
- Are the right players on the team and in the right position?
- Do the players know what is expected of them and how their performance will be measured?
- Are players given feedback during the game so they know how they're doing and what they could do better?

- If they're doing something well, let them know.
- If they need to make a change, let them know.

Developing a Management Style

New managers or managers trying to improve their effectiveness often look for the magic pill to management, or the best way to manage. In truth, there is no one best way, though there are fundamental principles and concepts that can and should be applied in most management situations.

The most common mistake made by inexperienced managers is to become overassertive and try to dominate. In many situations, less is more, and this is no exception. Everyone in the organization already knows who the manager is, whether it's the position of general manager, department manager, or frontline supervisor, so there is no need to constantly remind people who the boss is. In addition, managers who try to assert their authority by bullying, yelling, or telling people what to do are rarely respected, often resented, and usually do not achieve their goals.

That said, there are some basic approaches to management style:

- Managers should play to their strengths. There is no one best style, and it is not possible to become a different person through some magical management transformation. Some people are naturally more outgoing and enthusiastic than others, some are more analytical.
- Keep the focus on the goals, and try to link all performance—individual, departmental, and club—back to the goals, both financial and strategic.
- Limit the number of tasks, projects, or outcomes to a manageable number. It's far better to pick 3 items and do them well than to develop a 40-item list that is perceived as overwhelming and doesn't allow staff to understand the priorities. The other 37 items can be maintained separately on a list of things to be done while you continue to focus on the top 3 items.
- Effective managers can tailor their approach to the individual staff member. Some people thrive with a detailed review of what's expected whereas others only want to know the expected final result and prefer to determine their own route to success. Some people want and need daily contact, whereas others prefer more autonomy and a weekly review.

Managing With an Open-Book Philosophy

As stated earlier, most people are sincerely interested in making a contribution and doing a good job, and the more they understand how their position contributes to the goals of the organization, the more effort they're willing to make. One way to ensure that this type of work environment is created is to share information. In addition to providing specific feedback on the job performance of individual staff members, it is helpful and motivating to share information about business performance.

An article about last night's soccer game in today's newspaper most likely would not read, "It was a beautiful, warm night, and the grass was green, and the players looked crisp in their uniforms . . ." Instead, the article would first talk about the final score and then describe the key activities in the game that affected the outcome, along with highlights of the scoring or particularly brilliant defensive plays. After reading the article, everyone would know what happened.

In some businesses, including clubs, there is a tendency at times for managers to not want to share the results. As a result, the players don't even know if they won the game or not. Confidentiality is certainly understandable, but several key numbers that affect the result could be shared with virtually everyone. Sales, termination rate, and performance results of profit centers could be shared in a simple scorecard format (see figure 5.1) with virtually all staff, and then that information could be reinforced with explanations about how each position in the club can affect the key numbers.

At the level of department manager, there should be comfort in sharing more in-depth information. This may be referred to as **open-book management,** but it may also just be considered common sense.

Succeeding Through the Success of Others

A helpful way to visualize the role of performance management might be to remove barriers that prevent others from doing their job. The job of the manager is to ensure the achievement of club goals through the most effective and efficient use of resources, including people, money, and time. It's not about the manager, it's about the organization.

If there are obstacles preventing people from doing their job well, one aspect of the manager's job is to remove those barriers to allow the staff to be successful. This perspective, focus, and willingness

Club Scorecard

	Month actual	Month budget	Variance	YTD actual	YTD budget	Variance
Sales	125	115	10	560	540	20
Termination rate	3.2%	3.0%	–.2%	3.5%	3.0%	–.5%
Average dues	$83	$85	$2	$82	$85	$3
Personal training	$4,356	$4,000	$356	$34,578	$35,000	$422

Figure 5.1 Key performance numbers that can be shared with staff.

to derive satisfaction based on the success of others and to share the credit are the most critical factors for a manager to be successful.

Some people want to be the star, but the most successful organizations are built more on the **servant leadership model.** The most successful managers are those who are willing to base their success on the success of others and share the credit. A book that elaborates on this perspective and supports the theory with quantitative research is *Built to Last* (Collins and Porras 1994).

Determining the Identity of the Facility

In sport, everyone on the team knows the objective—to put the puck in the net, to score runs, to get the ball across the goal line. And most of the players on the team understand the purpose of their position and how it relates to the objective, whether they are a defensive lineman, goalie, or power forward. Each team will have a specific style of play based on its strengths, such as a running team, a passing team, a defensive team, and so on. Thus, everyone knows the objective and knows the type of play that's expected.

The first task for the performance-oriented manager is to establish the club's competitive strategy and business goals so everyone knows what the purpose is and what the club is trying to accomplish. Every club has several things that it does (or should do) better than the competition. These things may relate to programming, such as tennis, kids' fitness, or group fitness, or they may relate to the target market, such as families, seniors, or singles. In business school, this might be defined as the *unique selling proposition*. For the performance-oriented manager

who is focused on simplicity and results, it might better be described as, "What are we famous for?"

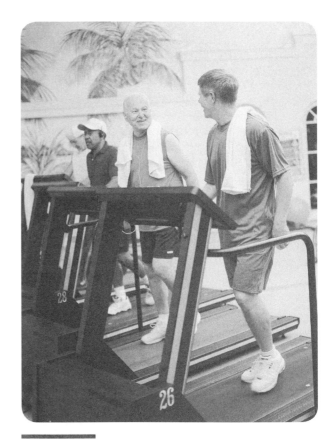

If a club's target market is seniors, the performance-oriented manager will make sure that all employees are aware of that objective so that they can work toward building a unique identity for the club.

© Getty Images/Bruce Laurance

Once it is determined what the club should be famous for, it needs to be constantly communicated to staff so that everyone is clear about the club's identity. Unfortunately, in many businesses people often come to work with an understanding of the specific tasks they must do, but they don't understand the club identity or its competition and how their job supports the club identity and positioning.

Front-desk associates working in an upscale club with an affluent membership base, for example, may think of their job as checking membership cards, answering the phone, and making sure guests fill out a guest register. They don't realize that they are the club's first impression on potential members, guests, and members, and that their enthusiasm and energy help make the club a club instead of just a building with facilities and equipment.

Again, most people want to do a good job and make a contribution, but they need to know what the rules of the game are and what their position is expected to contribute.

Steps in Managing Performance

Performance management can be the most challenging yet often the most rewarding of all the responsibilities undertaken by a manager, and it is one of the most critical in ensuring the continued financial and strategic success of the organization. Performance management integrates all the different facets of supervising people, including defining the job, interviewing to find the best candidate, orienting the new hire, setting goals, providing performance feedback, offering recognition and incentive compensation, and building a team committed to achieving the goals of the club.

Clarifying Job Expectations

The first step for a manager to help an employee become successful is to clarify the expectations for the specific job, both in terms of expected results and the ongoing responsibilities and tasks.

Depending on the size of the club and whether it's part of a larger organization, many job descriptions are written in somewhat formal language or so-called corporate speak that makes it difficult to understand how the job fits into the business and what its overall purpose is. Alternatively, other job descriptions are overly task oriented and present a laundry list of daily responsibilities, which provides a checklist approach to the job but again neglects to demonstrate how the job fits into the overall organization and what results are desired.

As discussed in chapter 2, the job description is the perfect opportunity to define why the job exists, how it fits into the rest of the organization, and its primary objectives. Ideally, it is the foundation on which the organization is built, and each individual job description must fit together to provide a solid base on which the club can stand.

A well-written job description, in addition to defining why the job exists and what the expected results are, will identify the experience and skills needed for someone to fulfill the job. Thus, it provides the basis for any job postings or advertisements and the types of questions that should be asked during the interview process, as described in chapter 3. It also is the foundation for training new hires, establishing performance goals, and providing performance feedback.

For all of these reasons, it is essential for the performance-oriented manager to look at the job description as the first step in building an organization that's focused on results rather than the administrative tasks of the job. If the job is not properly defined, it will never be possible for employees to see beyond the tasks and understand how their job contributes to the purpose of the company.

Controller Job Description A below is for the controller position in a club that is 60,000 square feet (5,574 square meters) and has 3,000 memberships. It is a fairly standard approach to a job description. Controller Job Description B is for the same position, but it places greater emphasis on how the position fits within the company and the expected results. The tasks, while important, will be covered during the training process.

For specific information on hiring, please refer to chapter 2.

Controller Job Description A

Primary Focus

- Ensure the development of annual budgets and periodic forecasts that support the achievement of company growth objectives.
  - Supervise the preparation of annual budgets, using the company budget development procedures and providing support to club managers as needed.
  - Supervise the preparation of periodic forecasts, providing support to club managers as needed.
- Ensure that financial and management data are provided to club managers on a timely and accurate basis.
  - Consolidate and prepare monthly financial statements for all operations.
  - Create monthly financial package consisting of profits and losses, balance sheet, cash flow statement, financial analysis of operational results, variance reporting, and key business indicators.
  - Provide owner, bank, and investors with required financial information.
  - Manage credit and collections to ensure the timely receipt of cash and minimization of bad debt loss.
- Ensure the development and maintenance of company financial policies and procedures to ensure integrity and accuracy of data.

Detailed Listing of Controller Duties

- Prepare annual budgets.
- Aid in periodic forecasting process.
- Manage, train, and develop accounting and office management staff.
- Assist club personnel with accounting.
- Consolidate and prepare monthly financial statements for all operations.
- Create monthly financial package consisting of profits and losses, balance sheet, cash flow statement, financial analysis of operational results, variance reporting, and key business indicators.
- Provide owner, bank, and investors with required financial information.
- Perform internal audits for fitness clubs.
- Handle all preparation for and daily interaction with corporate auditors.
- Prepare reports required by regulatory agencies, including tax compliance and estimates.
- Maintain compliance list to ensure filing of all tax returns, corporate reports, and so on.

(continued)

(continued)

- Oversee human resource and insurance (employee and commercial) concerns.
- Process payroll.
- Manage cash on weekly basis and sweep excess into investment accounts as needed.
- Manage account reconciliations.
- Manage records retention.
- Manage all bank accounts and signature cards, including reconciliations.
- Sign checks as necessary.
- Manage accounting system.
- Manage credit and collections.
- Manage accounts payable.
- Manage fixed assets.
- Continually evaluate practices for improvement opportunities.
- Execute, review, and revise accounting policies and procedures as necessary.
- Assist club managers with return on investments and benefit–risk analysis.

Controller Job Description B

Great Lakes Fitness, Inc., based in Centerville, is looking for an experienced controller whose experience includes work with multisite operations and who enjoys the environment in a small company.

Great Lakes operates six commercial fitness clubs in suburban locations of Centerville. The company is focused on a well-rounded approach to fitness, sport, and wellness and targets the family market.

The controller position is an integral part of the senior management team and will participate in all major planning and reporting activities, including financial reporting, forecasting, budgeting, and business performance analysis. The controller will lead a small accounting staff that is responsible for generating the financial statements for each club, consolidating the reporting, and working with club managers on an ongoing basis to review financial performance and identify opportunities for improvement. The position reports to the CFO of the ownership group and has frequent contact with the owner.

In addition to accounting and financial expertise, the person in this position must have a management mind-set and enjoy working with the club managers in a support role to ensure that they continually receive the reports, data, and analysis that enable them to improve business performance. The position requires excellent communication skills, the ability to work effectively with club managers not located in the same building, and a hands-on approach.

Key responsibilities include the following:

- Oversight of and responsibility for preparation of monthly financial statements, including income statements and balance sheets, preparation of variance analysis, completion of account reconciliations for balance sheets, and participation in management review of performance
- Leadership responsibility for preparation of the annual budget for each club and consolidated clubs, which involves a hands-on role and frequent discussions with club managers to develop the detailed operating assumptions needed to support the line-item budget
- Responsibility for preparation of a detailed business forecast on a quarterly basis
- Management of credit, collections, cash, and payroll
- Preparation of tax returns and oversight of auditors

(continued)

(continued)

Position Requirements

The person filling this position should meet the following qualifications:

- 10 to 15 years experience in accounting supervisory and management positions, including as a controller
- Certified public accountant (CPA)
- Preferably experience in working with businesses that have multisite operations such as hotels, restaurants, fitness clubs, or retail; service business or nonmanufacturing experience desirable
- Good analytical skills and a demonstrated ability to proactively identify problems and opportunities for improvement, supported by clear analysis and recommendations
- Temperament to enjoy and succeed in small-company work environment with only five people in the office
- Excellent communications skills and the ability to establish productive rapport with managers in different locations

Hiring

Hiring the right person for the right job is the second step in managing performance. As discussed in chapter 3, this process begins with the job description and determining the skills, experience, and personality characteristics that are necessary to ensure the greatest likelihood of success in the position. Once these have been defined, specific questions should be developed that will enable the manager to determine if the candidate meets the job requirements. For some positions, such as accountant, maintenance director, or personal trainer, there are specific technical skills or educational requirements that are mandatory. But for other positions, attitude and enthusiasm may be equally or more important than any specific experience.

In the National Football League (NFL) in the United States, one of the most important activities each year is the draft, the day on which each team selects graduating college football players to join the team. There are two different approaches to this—draft to fill a specific position or draft the best athlete and then find a place. In larger clubs or multiclub organizations, it is possible to draft the best athlete, so to speak, and find a place for that person. In a smaller organization, such as a single club, the payroll is limited and it's important to hire the person with the skills, experience, and attitude to do the job.

Regardless, clubs are a hospitality and service business as much as a fitness and health business, so hiring people with the right attitude and enthusiasm will make it much more possible to achieve the desired results.

For specific information on hiring, please refer to chapter 3.

Training

Even if the right person is hired for the right job, it is the responsibility of the manager to create the

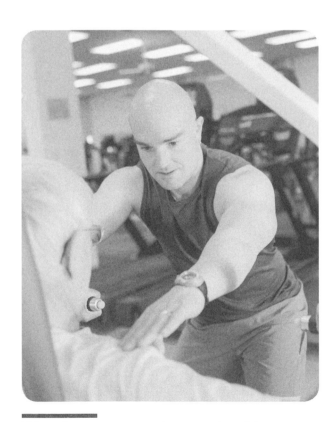

When hiring a personal trainer, the club manager should consider not only the candidate's technical skills but also his or her attitude, enthusiasm, and ability to get along with clients.

© Getty Images/Marc Romanelli

opportunity for the person to be successful. This goes back to the core definition of the manager as a person who is willing to succeed through others. Some managers, often because they are so focused on the day-to-day operations or responding to the crisis of the moment, adopt a sink-or-swim attitude toward new staff. However, this approach will only result in the manager having to spend more time in the reactive mode later, either having to hire a replacement when the new hire gets frustrated and leaves or having to correct performance problems that result from a lack of clear direction.

The new employee provides the manager with a fresh opportunity to instill the values of the club, share its strategy and vision, and ensure that staff understand the basic purpose of the club, its target market, its competition, what it does well, and how this job fits into the whole. If employees understand the purpose of the organization, its values, and its market position, along with how their job fits in, they are much more likely to do a better job. It can't be said enough—people want to feel like they're making a contribution and using their skills while still fitting into the whole, but they cannot do so if their job is positioned as part of an assembly line by strictly emphasizing tasks, or they have no sense of how they contribute to the end result.

The most effective time to make this impression on a staff member is during the training period after hire. For more information on new-associate training, please refer to chapter 3.

Measuring Job Performance

For each position, the expectations for the job should be reflected in some type of measurement standards. The intent is not to micromanage or patronize the staff; it is to help everyone understand what is expected and how performance will be measured.

The worst outcome for a manager would be to evaluate an employee and find out that the employee had no idea that the results expected by the manager were entirely different than what the employee thought was important. Front-desk associates, for example, might think the most important part of their job is checking membership cards, handing out towels, and collecting guest fees, and thus might adapt a policing demeanor in an attempt to make sure that members do not think they could sneak in with a guest or forget their card. The manager, however, might think the job is the crucial point of creating a first impression with members, guests, and potential members and expect the associate to convey an entirely different demeanor.

This situation could be avoided with a clear job description that explicitly states the importance of the position in creating a sense of hospitality and welcome, as well as some simple goals that explain how job performance will be measured.

Set Goals With Employees

As a coach, the manager is trying to make sure that the employees are going to be successful and that ultimately the club will win—achieving its financial, strategic, and service goals. To keep people focused on the priorities that support the overall goals of the club and move it forward rather than maintain the status quo, the effective performance manager will work with employees to establish individual goals. **Goal setting** is generally most effective when the manager uses the goals of the club as the starting point to provide an organizational framework and then discusses how the employee's position can contribute to the organizational goals. Most people find it motivating to understand how their performance can affect the direction and results of the organization, and this understanding also helps create more teamwork and integration across departments.

There is a difference between the ongoing tasks that people must perform on a daily or weekly basis as part of their job and the goals that help improve overall business performance. For example, daily cleanliness inspections of the club are important, but they are part of someone's ongoing responsibilities. A goal for a supervisor responsible for club housekeeping might be to improve member satisfaction as measured in the annual member survey from a score of 8.3 to over 9.0.

Goals, as opposed to ongoing job responsibilities, should be

- specific,
- measurable,
- achievable,
- relevant, and
- time based.

This can be remembered by the acronym *SMART*.

To develop goals that are effective for the employee and the organization, follow these steps:

1. Start with the job description, focusing on the 3 to 5 main responsibilities for the position.
2. For each area of responsibility, list the ongoing accountabilities and tasks. This same list can

be used when training new employees. The purpose of this step is to identify what the employee must do on an ongoing basis and to clearly segregate these tasks from any performance goals on which incentive compensation or recognition will be based.

3. Develop performance goals that are not part of the ongoing responsibilities or tasks. These are results that move the business forward and are not part of day-to-day responsibilities. They are most commonly used as the basis for salary increases, promotion, or incentive compensation.

Provide Performance Feedback

Once the right person has been hired and provided with orientation and training, the role of the manager is to monitor performance and provide ongoing feedback to ensure that the person is successful. Again, the emphasis is on helping staff members succeed, not on catching them doing something wrong. Positive feedback is just as important as corrective feedback.

Many organizations and managers believe that **performance feedback** is an annual event, conducted in a formal setting as a performance appraisal or performance evaluation. Although it is necessary to have a formal evaluation once or twice each year, it is usually much more effective to also provide staff with ongoing, frequent feedback.

If a manager were coaching a sport team instead of a club and one player in the middle of the game seemed to be out of position, making errors, and not executing the appropriate tasks, the manager would provide corrective feedback on the fly, or no later than immediately after the game. Coaches certainly don't wait until the end of the season to give feedback!

Many managers, fearing a confrontation or negative experience, quietly accumulate ammunition for the performance appraisal and unload on the employee during the evaluation meeting. This then becomes a negative experience rather than a learning opportunity, if for no other reason than the employee is usually caught off guard because the manager has not provided any previous feedback about performance behaviors that needed to be addressed. It is an indicator of bad management if the feedback provided in a formal review comes as a surprise. Remember, this is a review, which means anything discussed in the formal evaluation should have already been talked about.

Providing staff with feedback is an important and challenging responsibility of a manager. It can be difficult for any manager, from the new supervisor to the experienced senior executive, to provide feedback that is likely to be interpreted as criticism. But by not doing so, the manager is not fulfilling a basic job responsibility to the company or to the employee, who may not be aware of certain needs to improve performance.

Most organizations have a formal process for performance evaluation. This is always a good management system to have in place, if for no other reason than it imposes some discipline on the organization and forces managers who might otherwise be reluctant to provide in-depth feedback to do so. In most cases, an organization will use a specific form and may use one form for part-time staff and a different form for full-time staff. The form should be viewed as a guideline to drive the process, not the endpoint. The most important aspect of the process is the discussion between the manager and the employee.

A sample form, Nonexempt Performance Review, is provided on pages 89–91.

Components of a typical **performance evaluation form** include the following:

1. The first section often consists of discussion items or questions intended to help the manager and employee talk about different qualitative aspects of job performance, the company, and the work environment. Typical items included in this section are as follows:

- Overview of employee strengths
- Areas in which the employee needs to improve or needs training
- Ability to work as an effective member of the team
- Problem-solving ability
- Willingness to take initiative

2. Next come overall skills and attributes that relate directly to the job description and may vary by position.

- Technical knowledge for the job
- Customer service
- Meeting deadlines

3. The third section usually focuses on performance results for specific goals that were assigned for the measurement period, also related as specifically to the job and the job description as possible. These goals should form the basis for decisions regarding salary increases or promotion and should link to the overall strategic and financial goals of the club. Goals should, wherever possible, include measurement standards and target completion dates, as in the following examples:

Nonexempt Performance Review

Name: _____ Today's date: _____
Club: _____ Date of hire: _____
Reviewing manager: _____ Date of last review: _____
Job title 1: _____ Job title 2: _____

Definition of Ratings

D = Distinguished (4 points): Consistently exceeds standard expectations.
E = Exceeds expectations (3 points): Frequently exceeds standard expectations.
M = Meets expectations (2 points): Regularly meets or occasionally exceeds accepted standards.
R = Requires improvement (1 point): Occasionally meets expectations, but frequently performs below standard.
U = Unacceptable (0 points): Rarely performs at accepted standard; improvement essential.
N/A = Not applicable

Job Performance

		Comments
Displays thorough knowledge of job.	4 3 2 1 0	_____
Completes expected quantity of work.	4 3 2 1 0	_____
Completes expected quality of work.	4 3 2 1 0	_____
Performs work efficiently.	4 3 2 1 0	_____
Works well without close supervision.	4 3 2 1 0	_____
Works well under pressure.	4 3 2 1 0	_____
Offers practical suggestions to management.	4 3 2 1 0	_____
Shows initiative; solves problems that arise.	4 3 2 1 0	_____
Team player.	4 3 2 1 0	_____

Job Performance Points _____

Job Skills

		Comments
Administrative	4 3 2 1 0	_____
Communicative	4 3 2 1 0	_____
Organizational	4 3 2 1 0	_____
Technical	4 3 2 1 0	_____

Job Skills Points _____

Service and Attitude

		Comments
Complies with customer service standards.	4 3 2 1 0	_____
Always pleasant to members.	4 3 2 1 0	_____
Works well with other associates.	4 3 2 1 0	_____
Shows interest and enthusiasm for job.	4 3 2 1 0	_____
Shows respect for supervisor.	4 3 2 1 0	_____
Reacts well to feedback.	4 3 2 1 0	_____
Demonstrates pride in company.	4 3 2 1 0	_____

Service and Attitude Points _____

From M. Bates, 2008, *Health Fitness Management,* 2nd ed. (Champaign, IL: Human Kinetics). Reprinted by permission of Wellbridge Fitness-Wellness-Sports-Fun. Wellbridge is one of the leading health club chains in the USA today.

(continued)

(continued)

Work Habits

			Comments
Maintains a clean and organized work area.	4 3 2 1 0		_____
Respects company property.	4 3 2 1 0		_____
Adheres to company dress code for position.	4 3 2 1 0		_____
Complies with company policies.	4 3 2 1 0		_____
Accurately logs work hours.	4 3 2 1 0		_____

Work Habits Points _____

Job Development

Place a checkmark next to each training class required and completed (based on position). Rating based on the following:

Distinguished (4)—All four of the required training sessions must be complete and additional outside and WU training or certifications.

Exceeds (3)—All four of the required training sessions must be complete and additional WU training or outside certifications.

Meets (2)—All four of the required training sessions must be complete and certifications current.

Requires improvement (1)—Fewer than four of the required trainings completed or certifications expired.

Unsatisfactory (0)—Fewer than three of the required trainings completed and certifications expired.

Required training
* All 4 classes are required for a rating of 2.

_____ Team

_____ Bloodborne pathogens (exp. date   )

_____ CPR/AED (exp. date   )

_____ Sexual harassment (exp. date   )

Additional training

_____ _____

_____ _____

_____ _____

_____ _____

PT/group exercise required training and certifications
* Current certification is required for a rating of 2 (in addition to required training sessions).

_____ Personal training certification 1 _____   Exp. date _____

_____ Personal training certification 2 _____   Exp. date _____

_____ Group exercise certification 1 _____   Exp. date _____

_____ Group exercise certification 2 _____   Exp. date _____

Job Development Score _____

	Total points		# of indicators		Individual section score		Weight		Points
Job performance		/	9	=		×	.30 (30%)	=	
Job skills		/	4	=		×	.15 (15%)	=	
Service and attitude		/	7	=		×	.30 (30%)	=	
Work habits		/	5	=		×	.15 (15%)	=	
Job development	N/A	/	Varies	=		×	.10 (10%)	=	
							Total points		

From M. Bates, 2008, *Health Fitness Management*, 2nd ed. (Champaign, IL: Human Kinetics). Reprinted by permission of Wellbridge Fitness-Wellness-Sports-Fun. Wellbridge is one of the leading health club chains in the USA today.

Overall Performance

Score: _____

Letter rating: _____

Areas for Improvement

Strengths

Overall Performance Summary

Signatures

Reviewing manager: _____ Date: _____

Next level supervisor: _____ Date: _____

Human resources: _____ Date: _____

Associate: _____ Date: _____

From M. Bates, 2008, *Health Fitness Management*, 2nd ed. (Champaign, IL: Human Kinetics). Reprinted by permission of Wellbridge Fitness-Wellness-Sports-Fun. Wellbridge is one of the leading health club chains in the USA today.

- Ensure achievement of annual sales budget of 980 memberships for the year.
- Ensure front-desk staff are trained on hospitality, emergency procedures, and problem resolution.
- Ensure that 80% of new members receive a fitness orientation and personally meet with at least one member of the fitness staff within 2 weeks of joining the club.

There is no doubt that this form is important—it is highly valued by many employees as a tangible indication of their value to the club and to the manager—but the discussion process and how it is handled are equally or more important.

The most effective way to start the process is for the manager to meet briefly with the employee and let the employee know that the manager would like to meet to discuss performance, to get some feedback in a more formal way on how the employee is liking the job, and to look ahead to the next year for the club and what the employee would like to accomplish. The manager should then provide the employee with the form in advance and ask the employee to fill it out and bring it to the meeting for discussion. Both the manager and employee should come to the meeting with the form filled out and use it as the basis of discussion; this gives the manager the opportunity to make modifications based on the discussion.

After the meeting, the manager should finalize the form, which is a formal document that becomes part of the employee's employment record, and have a final brief review with the employee. This is another opportunity to reinforce the employee's strengths and value to the club, to discuss areas needing improvement and what both the manager and employee can do to help address them, and to outline the employee's specific role in contributing to the goals of the organization. Both the manager and employee should sign the performance evaluation. Each should keep a copy, and another copy should be placed in the employee records.

Addressing Performance Problems

Despite the best intentions and following the appropriate steps for defining the job, hiring a person, and providing feedback, there will inevitably be situations in which an employee continues to have performance problems and is not achieving the

Guidelines for Providing Effective Feedback

- *Focus on success.* The goal is to help employees succeed in their job and achieve their specific performance goals. The job of the manager is not to look for problems or find fault, it's to help employees be successful. If workers are not fulfilling the requirements of the job description or not meeting their goals, they are not succeeding, and it's the manager's job to figure out how to help them win. Few people do not want to do their job well.

- *Request employee input and involvement.* This is a two-way conversation. Before a formal performance review, the manager should ask the employee to come prepared to discuss major accomplishments, strengths, areas needing improvement, goals for the next year, and assistance requested from the manager, including specific training.

- *Find the appropriate setting.* Select a setting in which you can have an uninterrupted conversation. There should be no phone calls and no walk-ins, the door should be closed, and so on.

- *Start with positive feedback.* Effective managers look for opportunities to compliment their staff and make this part of their ongoing management style. If positive comments are not provided on an ongoing basis, suddenly doing so in a performance discussion will seem insincere or forced.

- *Provide frequent, informal feedback.* This is not a shooting gallery. Don't store up ammunition and then unload. More frequent, informal feedback is far more helpful and much less threatening.

- *Less is more.* For corrective feedback or behaviors requiring performance improvements, limit the criticism to one or two items. Don't attack—the other person will not be able to process the criticism, and it will feel personal. The goal is not to have the person feel beat up; the goal is to correct the problem and improve performance.

- *Be specific.* Generalities are not helpful (e.g., "You really annoy the other people in the office").

- *Recent history is more helpful.* Use recent examples, not situations that are months old. Memory fades, and the situation being used as an example may no longer be relevant.

- *Have an open dialogue.* Ask if the person agrees that the specific result or behavior is a problem. If the person doesn't agree, bring the discussion back to the result or behavior, try to link it to the job description, and continue until there is agreement or perhaps the manager finds out some underlying explanation. Open dialogue is helpful for everyone, including the manager.

- *Define specific corrective actions.* Define the actions to be taken to improve performance, how the results will be measured, and when there will be another conversation. Don't leave these actions vague or up in the air.

- *Offer to help.* You're in this together. Offer to provide assistance and support as needed (and as appropriate).

- *End on a positive note.* Provide encouragement and reinforce that you want the person to be successful.

---

expectations for the position. The first reaction in this situation should not be to assign blame to the employee; instead, effective managers will try to take an objective view of the situation and include themselves as a potential source of the problem.

Questions to ask include the following:

- Have the expectations for the position been made clear?
- Can the performance problems be solved by training or coaching?
- Could this person be more successful in another position?
- If not, is it necessary to make a change?

Offering Recognition

Some managers, especially people new to supervisory positions, may think that the job of the manager is to correct performance problems or identify things that an associate is doing incorrectly. However, many effective managers operate under the opposite philosophy, looking for an associate's strengths and examples of positive performance and recognizing these to provide positive reinforcement.

When training a puppy, the most important thing to remember is to use positive reinforcement. Dogs want to do the right thing; they just need to know what that is. The use of positive reinforcement is conveyed through simple gestures and words, such as "Good boy," an enthusiastic tone, a treat, or a hug. Believe it or not, managing effectively includes many of the same elements—a little bit of recognition and praise pays off in better performance and a more civilized and fun workplace.

Many managers think it's unprofessional, inappropriate, or a poor use of time to go out of their way to thank people for their work. But if people don't receive some type of recognition or acknowledgement for a job well done, why should they bother? Some managers think that's what the employees are getting paid to do. But in a free country, people can vote with their feet. Thus, effective managers use recognition (and bonuses, as discussed next) as part of their ongoing management. Make it fun, recognize performance, and add a little competition to the workplace.

There are many ways to let staff know how much they're appreciated and to recognize good performance. Guidelines for effective recognition programs are similar to some of the guidelines for performance feedback:

- Make it specific to an individual achievement or action.
- Make it timely.
- Personalize it.
- Make it meaningful.

There are endless ways to let staff know how much they're appreciated. Examples include the following:

- Say "Thank you."
- Send a card or note.
- Remember birthdays or work anniversaries.
- Provide tickets to a ball game or movie.
- Buy lunch for the person and a few coworkers.
- Give a book that relates to work.
- Offer longevity awards (for 1 year, 3 years, 5 years, 10 years, and so on).
- Give a gift certificate for a local restaurant or a favorite store.

- Provide a staff lunch—let a different person pick each month.

Nearly all of these cost less than $50, but they can have an amazing payoff, and they demonstrate that employees' work is appreciated and that the manager cares. A club with 1,000 members and $40 average dues could allocate $250 per month for little thank-yous—less than half of 1% of revenues.

The delivery is as important as the item. Don't just hand someone tickets and say something like, "I have these tickets left over and thought you might be able to use them." Instead, use the opportunity to reinforce your appreciation for the specific work results and to mention how valuable the person is to the team and to the club. Depending on the achievement or circumstance, this can be done on a one-on-one basis, in front of the person's department, or in front of the whole club. Recognition can also be used for an entire team or department and can be an effective team builder. An excellent book on this topic is *Managing With Carrots* by Adrian Gostick and Chester Elton (2001).

Providing Incentives and Compensation

Like it or not, money is a powerful motivator, and it has been used for years as the most successful motivator of sales staff. It doesn't always have to be a lot, but it makes the game more fun, more competitive, and more rewarding.

Incentive compensation plans tied directly to the club's financial performance can be a powerful motivator and engage people in the results, treating them more like an owner. People want to make a difference, they want to do a good job, and they like to be rewarded. Ideally, an incentive plan is in sync with employees' individual goals, and it supports the company or business unit goals. The targets should be structured so that if all team members do their job and the company or club does well, the people who contributed to success get rewarded.

At the level of department manager, some type of annual bonus plan is often created that pays a percentage of salary if the club achieves a certain level of profitability. General manager bonuses tied to annual profitability may range from 10% to 25% of base salary, and department manager bonuses may range from 5% to 20%. Although these are appropriate and can be effective, it can be difficult for such compensation plans to be motivating on an ongoing basis because the payout is so far in the future.

In structuring an incentive plan, there are several steps:

1. *Determine the approximate amount to be paid.* This includes both the amount in dollars and as a percentage of salary or total compensation. For example, a club may have an annual budget of $1 million in revenues and $150,000 in operating profit. In setting the budget, the club may determine that an operations manager earning a salary of $30,000 is eligible for a $3,000 bonus (10% of base salary) if the club achieves its operating profit. This $3,000 expense would be included as an expense in the budget and must be covered for the club to achieve its operating profit goal.

With additional analysis and calculations, the general manager or club owner may determine that if membership sales at the beginning of the year exceed the plan, the termination rate can be improved by 0.5%, and the personal training business can be improved, it may be possible to earn $180,000 in operating profit. This would be a $30,000 improvement, 20% more than the budget. The question, then, is how much of that $30,000 the owner is willing to share with the key staff members who made it happen. There is no defined formula, although in many businesses the owner would be willing to share between 10% and 30% of the upside. If so, that would create an extra $3,000 to $9,000 that could be allocated to key staff. In the case of the operations manager, who will earn a $3,000 bonus if the club achieves its budget, perhaps an additional $1,000 to $2,000 might be available if the club exceeds its goals by 20%. In this way, managers are motivated and compensated to think like an owner and push beyond the budget target.

2. *Determine the timing of the payment.* The shorter the time frame for the target, the more focused the staff remain. This is a fundamental principle of sales compensation, and it is why many sales staff members are compensated on monthly or weekly targets in addition to being paid on each sale. There is a sense of immediate gratification. The risk of shorter time frames is that a bonus or incentive payment could be made for a shorter amount of time, yet the club might not hit its annual target.

3. *Make it simple.* The bonus calculation should not rely on a complicated formula or calculation; otherwise people will not be able to keep score and realize whether or not they've won.

4. *Make it within the participant's control.* An incentive plan is motivating only if participants feel that they have the ability to influence the results.

For example, a bonus based only on total club financial performance may not be especially motivating to a front-desk supervisor. Even though such workers may be appreciative if a bonus is awarded, they will most likely be unable to determine which job performance behaviors or outcomes should be changed to influence the bonus. It would be more effective to have specific compensation criteria that link directly to the job, even if part of the bonus depends on total club financial performance or the club must hit its goal for everyone to be eligible for a bonus.

5. *Make it self-funding.* Incentives should be self-funding, especially if they're based on profitability. This means that a dollar amount for incentives should be included in the budget so that achievement of the profit goal has covered the cost of the incentive. For example, if a club had $100,000 in revenues and $80,000 in expenses for a certain period, the operating profit goal for that period would be $20,000. If club ownership decided that they were willing to pay total incentive compensation of $2,000 for achieving that original $20,000 target, then that $2,000 expense should be added to the original expenses. Now expenses are $82,000, and management is willing to pay $2,000 for achieving $20,000 in operating profit. This means that revenues must be $102,000 to achieve the $20,000 profit.

In setting the budget, the expected expenses for the incentive compensation are included as an operating expense under payroll, which means additional revenues must be generated to cover the expense and still hit the operating income goal. Instead of a budget with $100,000 in revenues and $80,000 in expenses, the budget will now state $102,000 in revenues and $82,000 in expenses. The result is a **self-funding incentive program,** and everyone wins.

Incentives for Nonmanagement Staff

Many companies provide annual or quarterly bonus plans to management staff, but the rest of the staff is sometimes overlooked, even though the power of the incentives may be even greater for part-time or lesser-paid employees. The impact of daily, weekly, or monthly incentives with sales staff is well documented and used in many clubs. In most cases, sales staff are paid a relatively low base salary and relatively high commissions or bonuses.

Successful managers offset the challenges in being a salesperson—making 20 to 30 calls per day, lots of rejection, uncertainty while potential members make up their mind—by using daily, weekly, or monthly incentives to make it more of a game. Examples might include $50 for anyone who makes five sales in a week or $20 for the first sale of the day. From the outside, it looks like it's just about the money, and although there's no denying the power and value of hard dollars, it also brings an element of fun and competition.

However, many managers and nonsales staff end up resenting sales staff and their compensation.

Instead of creating resentment, perhaps it would be more effective and useful to learn from what works and apply it elsewhere. There are a variety of ways to apply incentive compensation, rewards, or contests to other positions in the club.

- Make it a game—people like contests and competition.
- Determine whether the incentive is based on individual results or team results (such as an entire department).
- Include the compensations in the budget to make them self-funding and avoid the "it's not in the budget" argument. And even if they aren't in the budget, there is usually a way to find at least a couple hundred dollars to motivate and reward staff.

Examples of Incentive Compensation

Following are some examples of incentive plans and contests for staff. Regardless of the department or the specific criteria, the act of setting aside additional money for incentive compensation and taking the time to recognize the efforts of staff members can be a powerful management tool that has long-lasting results.

Retention-Based Incentives for Fitness Staff   The purpose of this type of incentive plan or contest is to focus fitness staff on the ultimate measure of success for their job: the ability to help members integrate exercise into their lifestyle and to achieve results. This will result in member retention, which is the most profitable business outcome for a club—keeping an existing member is much less expensive and more profitable than getting a new member.

One way to create a self-funding incentive program is to develop an annual budget based on the expected member termination rate (the percentage of members who terminate their membership). After calculating operating profit for the expected budget, try some different assumptions for termination rate and note the improvement in operating profit. For example, in a club with 2,400 memberships, $75 average dues, and a 3.2% monthly termination rate, a reduction of the termination rate to 2.7% per month yields an improvement in operating profit of approximately $50,000.

Knowing this, a club might be willing to allocate some of this potential increased profit to the fitness staff (and any other staff who should focus on member retention) for incentive compensation. If the club were willing to share at least 15% of the incremental profits—which will only be paid if the member termination rate decreases and the club generates the additional $50,000 in operating profit before payment of any bonuses—then $7,500 would be available. In a club with a fitness director and several full-time fitness staff members, $3,000 of that $7,500 might be allocated as a bonus for the fitness director and the remainder divided among full-time and part-time staff in a fair manner.

Contest for Staff Who Answer the Phone   The purpose of this contest, Friendliest Voice in the City, is to focus front-desk staff on answering the phone in a friendly, welcoming manner. Sometimes the staff members responsible for answering the phone consider it to be an interruption. However, potential members usually call before they come in, and the front desk is responsible for the all-important first impression. In addition, members want to feel that they belong to a club, not just a building with facilities and equipment, and a friendly, welcoming voice on the other end of the telephone can help reinforce this club atmosphere.

This contest can work with a multiclub operation or a single club as long as there is a minimum number of different employees who answer the phone. Criteria should be established in advance, such as phone answered in three rings or less, friendly tone, answering the phone according to club standard, and knowledge about questions. Judges can be management staff, family members of management staff, or members.

A contest with a prize—or better, several prizes—of $500 or $300 is usually enough to get the staff focused on telephone etiquette and provides a terrific reward.

Contest for Housekeeping Staff   Most industry surveys rank cleanliness as the most important club attribute to both current and potential members, although the housekeeping staff usually does not receive as much management attention and positive reinforcement as other departments in the club. One way to include them in the incentive compensation plan or recognition program is to create a contest such as Cleanest Club in the City.

It is important to establish evaluation criteria. Most clubs already have a detailed inspection list for the manager when walking through the club. The club could either be evaluated by doing a walk-through and comparing it to other clubs in the market, or a baseline ranking could be established by the general manager from doing a walk-through on a specific day, possibly before announcing the contest. Then, either by conducting evaluations of other clubs in the market (by the general manager, hopefully accompanied by the housekeeping supervisor) or an evaluation of the club on a date designated in advance to give everyone time to focus, the rating is completed. An improvement by a designated amount could win the contest, or having a higher score than the other clubs in the market could win the contest.

For this type of contest, it might be more effective to directly ask the supervisor responsible for housekeeping or some of the staff members themselves what would be most motivating, such as a bonus, gift certificate, party, or dinner. Money is always welcome, but another activity that makes a lasting impression can also be effective and creates the chance for staff to remember the great time they had and that they were appreciated and recognized by the club management.

Employee Termination

Regardless of how well a manager performs from the hiring process to providing ongoing performance feedback to recognition, there will undoubtedly be times when it is necessary to terminate an employee. Reasons for termination may include a business downturn that requires staff reductions, the employee's failure to meet performance expectations, or some type of behavior problems on the job.

The manner in which the process is handled depends on the circumstances that have resulted in the decision to terminate the employee. In any case, the conversation with an employee about termination is something that should be planned in advance so that the discussion goes as smoothly as possible and minimizes the possibility of legal action or any type of physical altercation. It can be an emotional event for both participants, so it is critical that the conversation be scripted in advance and possible reactions anticipated.

The purpose of this section is to provide a general overview for handling the termination process and is not intended to be specific to any particular situation. Each situation will have its own circumstances and requires consideration of the factors outlined here. Employment laws vary by country and state, and it is important to check with a human resources expert or legal representation before terminating an employee so that you ensure compliance with legal requirements. (Note: The material on procedures for employee termination is based on a publication written by Mountain States Employers Council, Denver, Colorado.)

Recognizing the Importance of Ongoing Feedback

The performance-oriented manager will provide ongoing feedback to each associate, both formally and informally. This is particularly important when there are performance concerns and an employee is not meeting the expectations for the job. As a result, the employee should not be surprised when the discussion about termination takes place; if the employee is surprised, it usually means that the manager's job has not been carried out appropriately.

That is why, in the course of providing performance feedback and documenting the discussions, it is necessary for the manager to make it clear to the employee that termination is a likely or possible outcome if there are not specific changes in performance outcomes or behaviors. It would be unfortunate for employees, upon hearing of their termination, to justifiably respond, "I had no idea I could be fired for this." In addition to being a sign of ineffective management, it could be a cause for legal action, which is nearly always expensive, time consuming, and demoralizing.

Preparing for Termination

Terminating an employee should be a last resort, not a knee-jerk reaction to a performance problem. When a performance problem with an employee is first identified, questions the performance manager should ask include the following:

- Have I made the expectations for this position clear?
- Have I provided the training necessary for the person to do the job?
- Is this person in the right position? Might the person be more successful in a different job?

If these questions have been addressed, then the communication process between the manager and the employee needs to be reviewed. There are two reasons for this. First, most managers want to do the right thing with staff and make sure every effort has been made to let the employee succeed. Second, by doing the right thing, the chances of legal action will be minimized. Thus, whenever a performance or behavior problem with an employee is encountered, written summaries of all conversations, preferably signed or initialed by the employee, should be maintained to verify that the termination was not the first notice an employee received.

Before proceeding with the final decision to terminate, questions managers should ask of themselves include the following:

- Has the expectation been made clear to the employee regarding the performance, standard, or policy?

- Is the expectation, standard, or policy reasonably related to the employee's job?

- Have there been previous discussions with the employee about the problem, and has any warning or notice been provided?

- Was it made clear that the consequences of a failure to meet the performance or behavior expectation could result in termination?

- Did the employee have a chance to explain?

- Are the same expectations in place for other employees in the same position, and are similar performance problems handled the same way?

- Is there anything in the employee handbook that contradicts the performance or behavior standard or that could be used by the employee to argue against the decision to terminate?

Meeting With the Employee

Before the meeting, the person who will have the discussion with the employee should prepare a script of what to say. Now is not the appropriate time for a casual or ad-lib meeting. At the same time, the manager should try to anticipate how the employee will react. Possible reactions could include the following:

- The employee may expect to be terminated and will be relieved.

- The employee may get emotional and either cry or refuse to talk.

- The employee may get upset and leave the room.

- The employee may get angry, make threats, or even become violent.

Do not begin the meeting with small talk or do anything that avoids the main purpose of the meeting. Begin by stating that the employee is being terminated, and explain the reasons as clearly and briefly as possible. Even if the employee does not agree with the decision, it is important for ethical and legal reasons that the person understands the reasons for termination and that it is for business reasons, not personal reasons.

Depending on the experience and level of the person being terminated, it may be prudent to have one other person present, although doing so may indicate the purpose of the meeting. The space in which the meeting is held should be as private as possible so that nothing can be overheard and the employee is treated respectfully. The meeting should be held at a time when it is possible for the employee to leave quietly and without upsetting other employees; late afternoon is often an effective time. If possible, it may be thoughtful to avoid terminating an employee late on Friday, which then gives the employee the weekend to rehash everything; instead, early in the week provides the opportunity to begin a job search and do something proactive.

In the meeting itself, follow these eight guidelines:

1. Keep it brief (less than 10 minutes). This is not a discussion.

2. Get to the point. Avoid preambles and the temptation to recount history and previous discussions.

3. Speak decisively but calmly, without anger or frustration.

4. Accept personal responsibility for the decision; don't blame it on a higher level manager or the club owner. That will simply worsen the situation.

5. Be respectful and empathetic, but without signaling that there is any chance that the decision could be reversed.

6. Be willing to listen, but do not get into a discussion or debate.

7. Provide any final paperwork, depending on company, state, or country legal requirements, as well as any compensation due.

8. After the meeting, document what was said and add it to the file.

Termination should never be the desirable outcome, but sometimes it is inevitable, and it is important to handle the situation appropriately. The manner in which it is conducted will reflect on the manager and the organization and may have legal and economic implications as well.

KEY TERMS

goal setting

incentive compensation plan

open-book management

performance evaluation form

performance feedback

performance management

self-funding incentive program

servant leadership model

REFERENCES AND RECOMMENDED READING

Collins, J.C., and J.I. Porras. 1994. *Built to last*. New York: HarperCollins.

Gostick, A., and C. Elton. 2001. *Managing with carrots.* Salt Lake City: O.C. Tanner.

Stack, J. 1992. *The great game of business*. New York: Bantam Doubleday Dell.

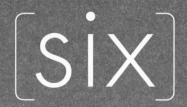

Developing a Compensation Program

Mike Bates

After studying this chapter, the reader will be able to

- understand the importance of compensation policies and staff accountability,

- identify compensation needs,

- construct and implement a compensation plan, and

- be aware of the different forms of compensation and when each one is most appropriate.

Tales From the Trenches

Jamieson was a new manager who was taking over a club that had been in operation for 15 years. The previous manager, Debbie, had been in place for the last 10 years. During Debbie's tenure the club had performed well, but not to its full potential. One of the other major challenges at the club was employee turnover. One of Jamieson's biggest tasks would be reducing employee turnover and standardizing compensation practices.

During Jamieson's first few weeks on the job, he spent a lot of time meeting with staff and reviewing key financial statements and employee files. He found the following situation:

- The majority of employees were paid based on the length of time they had spent with the company.
- Many staff felt they were underpaid based on what their friends made at other clubs.
- There was resentment among many employees who felt they were contributing more to the club but were being paid the same or less than others in similar positions.
- The sales staff in particular were unproductive and rarely hit their monthly sales quotas.
- Staff members were not aware of what they could do to increase their compensation and did not know when this increase would happen.

Jamieson understood the importance of performance-based pay, standardized practices, and knowing what his competitors were paying. Based on this information, he met with the owners and made the following suggestions:

- Immediately implement a performance-based pay system that would reward staff based on the goals they achieved. He also outlined specific educational opportunities staff could take advantage of that would allow them to increase their rate of pay. All staff members would have the opportunity to increase their pay rate based on the goals that were set for them.
- All competitors were analyzed and information was collected on their pay rates. Based on this information, some employees were immediately given raises while others were told what they would need to do in order to make a higher wage. In some situations, competitors were simply paying more than what Jamieson's club could afford. He told the staff why this occurred and highlighted some nonfinancial benefits of working at his club. These were things that other clubs did not do, like pay for educational courses, cover the costs of staff uniforms, and give extra vacation time.
- Jamieson spent a significant amount of time educating his staff on the benefits of a performance-based pay system. A handful of staff members did not like this new system and decided to leave.
- Jamieson met with all of the sales staff and told them how important they were to the bottom line. During this discussion he stressed the importance of hitting their monthly sales quotas. New pay systems were put in place that rewarded staff for hitting their quotas. In addition to the new pay systems, sales staff had the opportunity to win prizes, like free personal training systems, extra vacation days, and gift certificates to their favorite establishments. Jamieson was careful not to give the sales staff an unfair advantage over other staff, but he was also aware of their unique importance.
- Yearly evaluations were implemented. All staff members knew exactly what they needed to do in order to increase their pay.

After only 4 months there was a marked improvement in staff morale and the overall performance of the club. There were some increases in compensation, but the overall increases in revenue more than made up for it. The owners attributed a large part of this to Jamieson's standardized approach to compensation.

Even though the health and fitness industry has undergone major changes over the last decade, most organizations are still compensating employees the same way they did 25 years ago. Standard merit pay raises, length of service, and organizational rank are still the norm. However, creative managers are attempting to modify existing pay systems to fit their changing environments. For some organizations this could include such things as performance-based pay, retirement benefits, or bonus plans. Whatever the situation, the challenge with pay systems is to keep them flexible and focused on meeting the needs of the employees and the business.

In this chapter, we explore the basics of compensation programs and how to develop one to fit your program. Further discussion centers on the various elements of compensation, surveys and job pricing, job evaluation, and pay-for-performance issues. Finally, we discuss the most common pay practices in the industry today.

The health and fitness business is a customer service–driven industry. Adhering to the needs and expectations of members and guests requires a skilled and knowledgeable staff. Human talent is the most important resource a club has in today's competitive market, and managers should consider it an asset. Successful managers realize that no matter how state of the art the facility, sophisticated the equipment, or extensive the services, businesses cannot survive without highly motivated employees.

To attract and retain the caliber of people needed in the health and fitness field, you need a well-designed and properly implemented compensation plan. Organize the plan to show the value of all employees and reward their contributions to the organization. All too often employees feel a lack of recognition for the work they perform. For this reason, it is the responsibility of every owner or manager to ensure that the compensation package is fair for both the employee and the employer.

THE BOTTOM LINE

Whether or not managers can substantiate employees' feelings of underappreciation, these feelings can have a negative impact on employee morale if left unattended.

Compensation and Management

Compensation is a vital component of management. It contributes to the success of any health and fitness operation and provides the mechanism to compensate employees for their productivity. Because compensation is a part of management, the management style must be reflected in the method of compensation. Does the compensation plan consist of salaries and hourly wages only, or are performance-based incentives, benefits, or bonus plans included? Addressing these issues reflects management's commitment to employees.

Five Compensation Suggestions

A well-developed compensation program can have an impact on the success of a health and fitness organization in a number of ways: It can set you apart from the competition, assist in recruiting candidates for employment, help retain existing personnel, and contribute significantly to employee morale. To create a compensation plan that contributes to the success of the operation and is supported by employees, consider these five suggestions:

1. *Make certain that pay is competitive with similar positions in the field.* With the increasing number of health and fitness facilities and the decreasing number of hourly wage employees, more attention has been directed to the competitiveness of pay. Industry surveys are now available listing national salaries and wage scales, so you can compare similar positions in the field. Managers should monitor comparable facilities within their community to maintain a competitive pay scale. As the industry has matured, the price paid for labor has increased along with the demand for additional services and facilities.

2. *Recognize that employees are income-producing assets.* View each employee as a major contributor to the overall success of the organization. Because health and fitness are not considered tangible products, it is the responsibility of every employee to assist in creating the overall value or image associated with belonging to the facility. For this reason, managers in all settings must recognize that compensation has to do with acquiring and using a club's most important asset—human talent.

3. *Balance payroll costs with employee productivity.* Unfortunately, traditional accounting practices have impeded the way most managers view personnel. On a balance statement employees are considered liabilities, and on an income statement they are treated as an expense. Rarely do you hear managers talk about the income-producing potential of employees; instead, emphasis focuses on wage cost containment. With this view, there is inevitably an overemphasis on cutting payroll and little emphasis on increasing the output per payroll dollar.

4. *Manage payroll costs, not just pay rates.* The single largest expense in the health and fitness industry is payroll. Currently, salaries and wages, benefits, and payroll taxes represent 35% of the total expenses of a commercial fitness center. For this reason, you should manage payroll costs like any other expense, even though payroll costs are not like other expenses. For example, if a successful member-retention program is the result of trained and enthusiastic employees, management should seriously consider the negative impact of reducing payroll or eliminating training and development programs. In this scenario, if management reduces payroll costs, then the overall business will suffer. Payroll management involves weighing the impact of payroll cost against the financial results of the business.

5. *Consider payroll costs as an investment in the future.* An accountant views every dollar of payroll as an expense. Although this is seen as sound accounting, a good manager considers other factors when determining appropriate compensation. If, for example, a club compensates employees by paying a straight wage, this is considered a direct expense: pay for time worked, regardless of the output of the work. However, if the club decides to incorporate profit sharing as an incentive for employees to receive higher pay while contributing to the increased profits of the business, this is considered an investment opportunity for the business as well as the employee. Although both options are recognized compensation plans, one is considered an expense and the other is an investment.

THE BOTTOM LINE

Controlling compensation means optimizing the margin between output and payroll costs.

Compensation Policies

Once management has developed its views and strategies on compensation, establish policies that reflect the values of the organization. Identify and address compensation concerns to ensure all personnel are treated fairly and consistently during their employment. Basic policy issues that you should address include the following:

- What should be the pay for jobs compared with similar positions in the field?
- What is the policy with respect to pay for performance?

- Is there a standard policy for performance-review pay adjustments?
- Will the organization provide health and retirement plans? If so, what will the employee contribute?
- What will be the compensation policy differences for full-time employees, part-time employees, and independent contractors?
- As a form of compensation, are employees able to use the facilities without charge? If so, when are acceptable times of usage?
- Which positions will be designated salaried, hourly wage, commissioned, or payment per class?

Although in every setting there are additional compensation issues that you must address, these seven items represent the major policy concerns for most health and fitness organizations. The compensation policies that evolve from answering these questions should meet certain requirements. First, they should be specific enough to act as a screen. When an employee makes a proposal regarding a certain action, you can screen it against the policy statements. Policies must be the basis by which supervisors or department heads make decisions about compensation matters. Finally, policies must be both specific and comprehensive enough that they become an important communication tool.

Accountability to Employees

Part of being a health and fitness manager is providing accountability when necessary, including accountability to employees. Answering compensation-related questions by saying, "I'm sorry, but that's our policy," might have worked 50 years ago, but not as we enter the 21st century.

Because pay is such a personal matter, managers have the obligation to justify, report, or explain any issue relating to compensation. Being accountable means having the authority to act if needed. If, for example, an employee brings up a policy that is deemed unfair among other personnel, management has the responsibility to investigate and act on the concern in a timely manner.

Being accountable to employees is not meant to restrict or dilute the manager's position. The final decision maker in any compensation issue is always the manager. However, being accountable enforces that the organization wants to show fairness and a commitment to its employees.

Compensation Program Basics

Every health and fitness setting is unique not only in terms of the type, size, location, and services offered but also in more subtle ways. For example, some settings have different management styles: Tasks are performed differently and decisions made in various ways. As a result, managers of each setting should tailor its compensation programs and practices to fit the specific situation.

Successful compensation plans are simple in design, yet adaptive to the management philosophy. The procedures for providing employee pay should be easily understood and implemented by the payroll administrator and be flexible enough to facilitate the employees' needs. New employees should be able to register easily into the plan, and existing employees receive appropriate remuneration. For example, managers will often cross-train employees to work in two or more divisions of an organization. The pay associated with working in separate divisions may differ; consequently, the compensation program must be flexible enough to identify the areas worked and provide the appropriate pay. This is just one example of the importance of a payroll system that is adaptive to the needs of the organization.

Grouping Employees

Before establishing a compensation plan, make a list of every employee position. This list assists in determining how to group employees in various divisions. A sample employee position list for a commercial health and fitness setting is provided in figure 6.1.

Employee Positions

1. Ownership group
2. General manager
3. Administrative assistant
4. Accounting or business office manager
5. Accounts payable services
6. Member accounts services
7. Accounts receivable coordinator
8. Data-entry clerk
9. Human resources director
10. Service-desk manager
11. Service-desk attendant
12. Athletic director
13. Fitness director
14. Fitness or weight training instructor
15. Personal trainers
16. Group exercise director
17. Group exercise instructor
18. Junior aerobics instructor
19. Aerobics training coordinator
20. Junior programming director
21. Sports camp counselor
22. Aquatics director
23. Head lifeguard
24. Lifeguard
25. Swim instructor
26. Aqua fitness coordinator
27. Aqua fitness instructor
28. Children's programming director
29. Child care supervisor
30. Child care attendant
31. Martial arts instructor
32. Gymnastics director
33. Gymnastics instructor
34. Operations manager
35. Housekeeping supervisor
36. Locker-room attendant
37. Maintenance assistant
38. Building engineer
39. Assistant building engineer
40. Pool maintenance
41. Food and beverage manager
42. Snack bar attendant
43. Pro shop staff
44. Marketing director
45. Marketing assistant
46. Massage therapists
47. Membership representative
48. Member relations
49. Court sports director
50. Squash and racquetball pro
51. Head tennis pro
52. Tennis pro
53. Tennis desk attendant
54. Basketball coordinator
55. Basketball monitor
56. Manager on duty

Figure 6.1 Employee positions in a commercial health and fitness setting.

Grouping employees into an organizational structure that is easy to administer and classifies employees based on the goals of the organization is the next step. Various job categories may require different pay programs and practices.

For management purposes, group jobs so that tasks and responsibilities are appropriate for each category and the training and recruiting methods required to fill the jobs are similar. Once you complete this, you can develop many personnel practices, such as recruiting, training, employee communication, and payroll, to meet the requirements of the job.

In the health and fitness industry, there are at least five groups of employees to consider: upper management and supervisors, full-time staff (salaried), full-time staff (hourly wage), part-time staff (hourly wage), and outside contractors. Within each category there are subgroups that include employees from various divisions of the organization. For example, upper management includes the general manager, sales and marketing director, fitness director, aerobics director, and tennis director. Employee subgroups vary depending on the type and size of an organization. Figure 6.2 represents a sample employee list for a large multipurpose fitness center.

Developing a Compensation Program

A recommended approach for developing compensation programs follows. This is the traditional approach commonly used for problem solving in many businesses.

Employee Positions

Upper management

- Ownership group
- General manager
- Sales and marketing director
- Fitness director
- Group fitness director
- Tennis director

Full-time staff (salaried)

- Maintenance manager
- Front-desk manager
- Food and beverage manager
- Sales representative
- Controller or business office manager
- Manager on duty
- Assistant general manager

Full-time staff (hourly wages)

- Group fitness instructors
- Aquatics instructors
- Personal trainers
- Fitness center personnel
- Tennis instructors
- Racquetball instructors

- Service-desk attendants
- Bookkeeper
- Office staff
- Maintenance and cleaning
- Child care staff
- Food and beverage staff
- Pro shop staff
- Summer camp staff

Part-time staff (hourly wages)

- Aerobics instructors
- Aquatics instructors
- Personal trainers
- Fitness center personnel
- Tennis instructors
- Racquetball instructors
- Service-desk attendants
- Bookkeeper
- Office staff
- Maintenance and cleaning
- Child care staff
- Food and beverage staff
- Pro shop staff
- Summer camp staff

Figure 6.2 Employee positions grouped according to tasks and responsibilities.

Reprinted, by permission, from IHRSA, *2006 industry data survey* (Boston: IHRSA).

Identify Compensation Needs

Developing a compensation program begins with identifying needs. Some organizations might be in the start-up phase when they must install an initial pay program, and others may need a change in their compensation system due to problems with an existing system or new opportunities. Whatever the reason, identifying the needs is the most crucial aspect of compensation. Although there are many ways to identify needs, it is critical to have a reliable process that you can use to obtain the information you need.

THE BOTTOM LINE

Identifying compensation needs involves regular monitoring and observation, feedback from reliable sources, and obtaining information on current trends in the industry.

Some methods for determining specific compensation needs include the following:

- Observe the compensation experiences and problem areas that employees encounter in their work.
- Use opinion or focus polls with managers and employees.
- Perform personnel audits in which you question all aspects of personnel management, not just compensation.
- Use statistical analysis and personnel data to determine needs. Obtain benchmark surveys from industry organizations (IHRSA, IDEA). Consider using an information bank with job titles, responsibilities, and salary levels from similar settings to determine compensation rates.

Develop Goals and Objectives

Accomplishing these goals starts with setting specific objectives. Because much of personnel management is based on knowledge obtained from experiences, it is sometimes difficult to set specific objectives. Often objectives such as "Improve employee morale," "Provide greater internal consistency," or "Create a better quality of work environment" are used to quantify the desired objectives of an organization. Unfortunately, these nonspecific objectives are meaningless and can confuse rather than clarify a specific intent.

Set specific, quantifiable goals such as "Reduce the employee cost of health care by 25%" or "Delegate pay decisions to department heads or supervisors." Once you have identified goals, set up appropriate systems to evaluate cost and value.

Construct the Program

Based on the needs assessment and the stated goals and objectives, the next step is to construct the compensation program. Developing a formal compensation system in which everything is spelled out for every possible situation is highly unlikely. However, it is a good idea to establish standards in writing that serve to guide individual pay decisions. Such elements of a compensation program should contribute to better decision making, more consistency, and greater fairness.

A compensation program should never mean that the program itself makes the decisions and that the program becomes mechanical. Neither the program nor its procedures can be the decision-making process.

We mention here five standards to follow when developing a compensation program:

1. *Align compensation programs to fit the way you manage the business.* As with any business, health and fitness organizations are unique. Management styles, operating systems, and personnel concerns vary from setting to setting. A properly tailored compensation program reflects each of these factors and is developed with these values in mind.

2. *Make the program flexible.* A compensation program should adapt to a rapidly changing world. Develop the program so you don't have to reinvent the wheel if you make a change. Whether you incorporate wage scales, cost-of-living increases, pay for performance, or commission-based pay, each of these is subject to change at any time.

3. *Keep the program simple.* Consider all the supervisors and other managers who must support and administer the plan. It should make their job easier, not more difficult.

4. *Have a way to measure results.* There is no way of incorporating pay for performance if you can't measure performance. Use measures based on the goals of the organization. Possible measurements may include financial performance, division productivity, economic value, quality control, and customer service ranking.

5. *Don't make compensation a bad word.* Empower employees to understand the compensation process. If pay is to truly motivate employees to perform, then bring it into the open so that it can be understood. This doesn't mean sharing privileged pay information on employees. However, it does mean communicating and updating employees on the process.

Also consider two cornerstones of compensation management, surveying and job pricing. The data obtained from these processes are readily accessible, provide specific pay comparisons, and list current salary levels. Only through these methods can pay be sufficient to ensure competitiveness for the organization and fairness to its employees.

Compensation information is the basis for determining competitive pay and is vital for establishing fair pay. In response to the need for more and better compensation information, the health and fitness industry has invested a great deal of time and effort in developing survey information to improve compensation management. As a result, a variety of information is now available for managers in all settings to review and compare before establishing a compensation program.

When compared with more established businesses, the health and fitness industry is still in its infancy regarding salary data. Professional journals and industry organizations have primarily been responsible for salary surveys. The data obtained from these surveys can assist managers in establishing comparative benchmarks when recruiting and conducting performance evaluations. Keep in mind that pay variations exist between similar positions depending on the region, type, and size of facility and whether the organization is considered a low-revenue performer (25% less than average industry earnings) or a top performer (25% greater than average industry earnings). Table 6.1 illustrates these compensation differences among commercial health fitness facilities according to IHRSA survey data (2006).

A word of caution when using published salary information: It is essential that the data obtained from any survey be closely scrutinized before adjusting or setting wages and salaries. Managers need to know the size of the survey and how it was conducted, when, and by whom. Determine the sample size of the organizations participating in the survey. The goal is to find reputable and reliable surveys used by most health and fitness managers.

Perhaps the most common method for establishing wages and salaries is **job pricing.** This system starts by identifying all compensated positions, followed by a brief written description of each position (usually one paragraph). Next, prepare an organizational flow chart that illustrates position hierarchy and establishes a career path for employees to follow. Once you have completed this information, start pricing the jobs based on management's experience and salary information obtained from similar settings. Methods of obtaining compensation information include personal visits to other clubs, questionnaires, and telephone interviews with other managers.

Test the Program

After designing a compensation program, testing the program is the next step. A major component of testing is reviewing and questioning the legal and tax implications of the program. This process often requires working with an attorney and an accountant to make sure the organization is in compliance with the Fair Labor Standards Act.

During this time, you need input from all levels of employees. Take a what-if approach, questioning each aspect of the plan and deciding on any changes before implementing the program.

Implement the Program

Implementation means putting the program into operation and establishing the various procedures and reviews necessary to any new program. The

Table 6.1 **Compensation for Fitness Upper Management—Commercial Facilities**

| Staff member | Average | UPPER MANAGEMENT TAXABLE EARNINGS | | | |
		Top 25% (earn >)	Bottom 25% (earn <)	Individual facility	Chain
General manager	$75,886	$88,500	$54,350	$77,096	$68,740
Sales director	$50,053	$56,750	$35,913	$47,167	$56,482
Sales representative	$35,118	$41,569	$25,250	$35,374	$36,014
Fitness director	$47,587	$58,000	$36,919	$45,868	$50,659
Group exercise director	$29,190	$38,000	$16,276	$26,442	$32,724
Tennis director	$65,698	$85,000	$41,250	$66,056	$66,486

Data for table 6.1 adapted, by permission, from IHRSA, 2006, *Employee compensation and benefits survey results* (Boston: IHRSA).

ongoing application of the program illustrates if it is achieving the original goals established by management and employees. Of course, this phase never ends because implementation is dynamic, so expect regular changes and modifications. Finally, the nature of administrative and operational work involved in implementation will change, and the staffing required to perform the work must similarly change to meet new requirements.

Review and Revise the Program

Continual review of a compensation program will undoubtedly necessitate revisions or major changes. Causes for these revisions may be a change in operations, payroll regulations, financial status, or management. Managers will want to stay abreast of economic conditions affecting inflation. Each quarter, monitor changes in factors such as cost of living and consumer price index fluctuations. Annually review the state of the industry. Are pay rates for all positions staying constant or oscillating? Is the number of employees needed to operate various sizes of facilities staying the same or is a downsizing trend occurring? Is there still a high demand for health and fitness professionals? Is the overall growth of the industry continuing to reflect a positive change, or has growth slowed?

Consider all these factors when reviewing and revising compensation programs.

Making changes to an established compensation program is never easy, especially if the program has been successful and is understood by management and employees. However, waiting too long to make revisions may cause larger problems over time, so it is necessary to make regular revisions and act on them.

THE BOTTOM LINE

To remain innovative, you must update technology, stay in compliance with changing payroll laws, and adapt to the ever-changing needs of the organization.

You can adapt this process for developing compensation programs to fit any health and fitness setting. Although you can use this process as a basic management tool, the real challenge is to make the program reflect the personality of the business. Because fitness centers are unique and dynamic, clearly understanding the profile of the club, including short- and long-term goals and objectives, is essential.

Process for Developing Compensation Programs

1. Perform a needs analysis. Identify questions, problems, or opportunities by focusing on the following:
   - Hold discussions with department heads or supervisors.
   - Hold discussions with employees.
   - Examine reported issues, both member and staff related.
   - Perform personnel audits.
2. Develop objectives.
   - Set specific goals.
   - Consider impact on all phases of the operation.
   - Consider schedule format.
   - Determine if enough staff are available to meet these goals.
3. Construct the program.
   - Align the program to fit the way business is managed.
   - Make the program flexible to change.
   - Keep the program simple.
   - Have a way of measuring results.
   - Don't make compensation a bad word.

(continued)

(continued)

4. Test the program layout.
   - Consider the legal, tax, and accounting ramifications.
   - Play devil's advocate and consider what-if possibilities.
   - Determine whether it will stand the test of time.
   - Compare the program against alternatives.
5. Implement the program.
6. Evaluate the program's effectiveness.
7. Review the program.

Forms of Compensation

Employees in the health and fitness industry receive their pay in various ways. Each form of compensation reflects an organization's philosophy, managerial style, and commitment to its employees. Some elements of compensation include wages or salaries, overtime pay, commissions, bonuses or profit sharing, pay for time not worked, benefits, nonfinancial rewards, and compensatory time off.

The compensation elements mentioned in this section have the most practical value in compensation management. Managers should identify the specific elements of compensation that best fit their organization. Once identified, determine a value or cost for each item. Although this is sometimes difficult to do, it is the only way to fully understand and manage a compensation program.

Wages and Salaries

The term **wages** usually applies to payment for employee services rendered on an hourly or daily basis. Depending on the setting, this form of payment is generally received by front-desk attendants, maintenance personnel, weight-room trainers, and child care attendants. The term **salary** refers to compensation paid weekly, semimonthly, or monthly and describes the earnings usually paid to the owners, managers, and fitness, tennis, sales, and aerobics directors. Each form of compensation represents a fixed cost and the basis for administering other forms of compensation.

Overtime Pay

Service-desk attendants, weight-room personnel, child care workers, and most other nonsupervisory employees are eligible for overtime. By law, these employees must be paid time-and-a-half their regular base pay for each hour worked in excess of 40 during a week (this number will change from country to country and possibly region to region). You cannot combine or average work weeks beyond 1 week, and you cannot give compensatory time off (details follow) outside of a work week in lieu of overtime.

Most health and fitness organizations pay either time-and-a-half or double time for work on holidays or scheduled vacations. For those employees who occasionally work overtime, the additional pay they receive increases their overall rate of pay. The economics of overtime pay are important business considerations and need to be closely planned and scrutinized.

THE BOTTOM LINE

Regularly monitor employee overtime and instigate a procedure for obtaining overtime approval from supervisors. Without these safeguards in place, an annual payroll budget may erode quickly.

Commissions

Commission-based pay has become a popular method for compensating specialty employees in the industry. Sales personnel, massage therapists, personal trainers, tennis pros, and aquatics personnel are some of the employees who might receive remuneration from commissions. A straight commission plan pays employees a percentage of what they obtain in total sales. The rate of commission pay depends on industry standards and the estimated volume of sales generated. For example, a massage therapist could start at a commission rate of 60% to the therapist and 40% to the club. As the volume of massage sales increases, management could increase the commission to 70–30 to reward the massage therapist for an increased client base, allowing the therapist to earn more money and the club to receive additional revenue through increased sales.

Concerning sales staff, the IHRSA 2006 survey results (based on approximately 120 club responses) show that

- 45.5% of clubs give commissions based on a set fee per membership sold;

- 28.9% pay a commission as a percent of revenue generated, and the average commission in these situations is 9.6%; and

- 73.9% do not set a quota that must be reached before commissions can be earned.

Concerning personal trainers, the IHRSA 2006 survey shows that

- 46.2% of clubs pay a commission based on a percent of revenue generated, and 41.5% pay a commission based on a set fee per session;

- the average commission paid to those who earn a commission based on revenue is 49.3%;

- for those who pay a set fee, the average per session is $32; and

- 87.9% of clubs do not require that personal trainers meet a quota in order to qualify for a commission.

Although commission-based pay can motivate employees, commission-only plans may cause employees to sell more aggressively, sometimes generating unfavorable member reaction. Under this plan, an organization might find it more difficult to get commission-based personnel to perform other necessary duties.

Another plan gaining wide acceptance is the salary plus commission combination. Employees earn a basic salary to cover living expenses and they earn a smaller percentage of sales as a commission. This combination guarantees employees funds for paying current expenses and provides an extra incentive to sell their services.

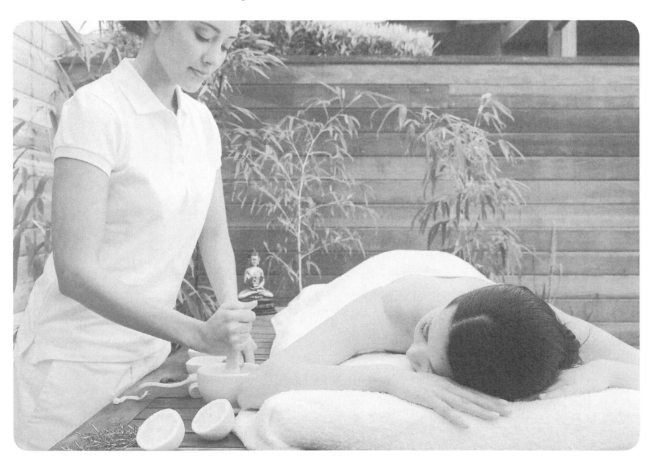

Specialty employees, such as massage therapists or sales personnel, are increasingly compensated through commission-based pay.

© Getty Images/Reggie Casagrande

Bonuses and Profit Sharing

Bonuses and profit sharing involve periodic lump-sum payments. The payments may be in the form of an annual or quarterly payment for meeting predetermined financial goals or a monthly bonus to sales personnel for reaching a preestablished new-member goal. Bonuses may also provide an incentive for such achievements as cost savings. For example, some clubs may structure the bonus plan entirely on quarterly net profits. With this approach, employees learn that they can have a positive impact on their quarterly bonuses if they are constantly watchful of all expenses associated with their division.

Industry data from the IHRSA 2006 survey show that

- 70% of clubs reported some form of a bonus plan;

- 66% of club management, 46% of sales staff, and 18% of other staff were eligible for the bonus plan;

- the main factor that was looked at when paying out a bonus was the overall performance of the club; and

- 59% of clubs reported paying out bonuses of more than $1,000.

For an employer, all such payments represent a variable cost. More important, many organizations believe that some type of bonus plan contributes significantly to improving overall operations and member services by providing financial motivation to employees. An example of a club-sponsored bonus program is explained in Ojai Valley Racquet Club Employee Profit-Sharing and Point System below.

Ojai Valley Racquet Club Employee Profit-Sharing and Point System

The Plan

Each quarter, on April 1, July 1, October 1, and January 1, the accounting department will compute the net profit (after all expenses) during the previous 3 months. We will designate 20% of that profit number for employee distribution as a cash bonus, no sooner than 30 days but no more than 45 days from the end of each quarter.

For the first three quarters of one's employment, we will pay 50% of this profit-sharing bonus to employees directly and hold back the other 50% to offset possible quarterly losses until computing the final annual profit at year-end. At this time we will pay the remainder of the 50% antiloss fund (net) to the eligible employees in addition to normal quarterly bonuses.

Who Is Eligible?

All hourly employees and some salaried personnel are eligible.

What Determines the Bonus?

1. Quarterly minireview results
2. Overall productivity with respect to others in the same department
3. The number of hours worked per week
4. Attitude toward each other
5. Length of employment
6. To what degree the department meets its expense budget

What's the Purpose of the Profit-Sharing Plan?

The purpose of the plan is to send each eligible employee an important message. The message is specifically spelled out in the amount of the employee's check (with respect to others in each department) and in the substance of the employee's quarterly minireview.

1. A check for a large percentage means you are meeting or exceeding your job requirements.
2. A check for a smaller percentage means that you are a valuable person but could use improvement in some areas.

3. A check for a small percentage means that your performance is not always what it should be.

4. No bonus means you should consider seeking employment elsewhere.

The overall objective of the plan is to help create a higher level of team effort and to tangibly reward those employees who are doing the best job for the club in their department.

What Are the Criteria for the Best Job?

1. Meeting expense budgets for the department as a whole (exceeding expense budget goals will result in a larger share of the total profit allocated to each department)

2. Meeting the needs of the members with regard to the function and purpose of each department

3. Supporting company policies, rules, and regulations and offering constructive criticism, in writing, to your supervisor when policies need changing

Point System

The profit-sharing plan is based on a point system. We have found that without the point system, the profit sharing becomes an entitlement rather than an incentive.

In the point system, each employee may receive both positive and negative points. Positive points include attending a club event, performing a special act for a member, suggesting an idea to improve the club, and any other positive acts to benefit the employee and the club. Negative points include tardiness, complaints, failure to attend a mandatory staff meeting, and any other acts that fail to meet the daily requirements of an employee.

Each item counts for a certain number of points, which are logged in each employee's workbook. We then total the points each quarter. Any negative net is used as a percentage, which is multiplied by the profit-sharing amount. For example, an employee who has −50 points receives 50% of the profit-sharing amount. Positive net is carried into the next quarter and eventually to the end of the year.

At the end of the year, the employee may exchange these positive points for vacation days or additional bonuses.

Performance-Based Pay

The logic behind **performance-based pay** is that improved performance should result in greater employee productivity, which in turn should result in improved business results. If this logic is correct, there is a financial return for improvement in employee performance. Managers must remember that pay increases for improved performance are considered investment spending. Few investment opportunities in the fitness setting yield a higher return for such a low risk. However, until the past decade this form of compensation was rarely discussed. Over the years, owners and managers have realized that by rewarding individual performance, the company and the employee both benefit. Performance pay creates a system of self-management. Employees not only perform their own tasks but also become watchful of the entire operations of the club. Over time, they understand that their productivity is linked to their success and income and to that of the company as well.

The disadvantages associated with pay-for-performance compensation are related to accountability. The measurements used for identifying performance improvement as it relates to increased business productivity are not precise and are rarely easy to assess from one day to the next. Supervisors must establish tangible goals that they can measure at least monthly. Possible goals could include an increase in monthly fitness revenue by 3%, decrease in monthly fitness expenses by 2%, or increase in the annual participation rate for fitness programs by 5%. Once managers determine goals, they must decide how each employee contributes to achieving these goals.

Another problem associated with pay-for-performance compensation is in the merit approach to productivity. Personal traits may be deemed as meriting a pay increase; however, they may have no impact on work effectiveness.

Administering performance pay involves establishing a performance rating system that identifies the methods of evaluation and how you will conduct the rating system. Once you complete the rating plan, determine how to link compensation to performance. Will you give compensation through salary increases, bonus payments, or a higher commission percentage? Will you reduce poor performers' pay if they do not achieve goals? After you have formalized this information, it is essential to communicate the plan to the employees, making sure they understand the process.

Pay for Time Not Worked

Pay for time not worked includes vacation time, holidays, sick-leave days, and special time off for such things as jury duty and military service. There is also pay for time not worked during working hours, such as scheduled rest breaks. Sick-leave days represent a form of self-insured sickness pay, providing employees with continued income in the event of a short-term illness. Vacation and holiday payments allow for a paid rest from work. For employees, payment received for these nonworked periods allows more time for families, recreation, and sometimes, most importantly, a needed break from the customer service business.

Benefits

Employee **benefits** provide protection against economic risks, including death, disability, and illness. Many of these are insured benefits, with the employer paying some or all of the insurance premium. For additional information on employee insurance, refer to chapter 16.

THE BOTTOM LINE

In some cases, employer-sponsored benefits provide coverage at a level the employee could not obtain as an individual.

Offering benefits to employees provides needed protection at a lower cost than would be available individually. Providing benefits can also assist in meeting the needs of the organization. For example, a retirement plan can help employees save for the future. Awarding a designated number of paid vacation days for each year worked can also show employees that management wants to reward them for their years of service. In today's market, providing a sound benefit package is necessary to attract and retain employees.

Each form of compensation can represent a significant portion of an employee's overall remuneration. However, usually only the financial elements of compensation are expressed in monetary terms; therefore, when you pay employees, all they see is the paycheck amount. They give little thought to the added benefits the employer pays for. Consequently, benefits are often viewed as soft costs. Employers should calculate a hard cost for such items as taxes (i.e., unemployment, workers' compensation, disability), health and life insurance, holiday and vacation pay, sick leave, retirement plans, bonuses, training and education, employee uniforms, and club membership. Only through this approach can employees see the total value of wages and benefits. Figure 6.3 provides a sample employee benefits worksheet that any organization can adapt to reflect an employee's complete compensation and benefits package.

In this model, an additional 32% was added to the base pay as a result of the benefits package. Understandably, most managers would view this figure as excessively high. However, a consideration when creating a similar model for employees is turnover. Often people do not stay long enough to earn all vacation pay, sick pay, or holiday pay. Others decide against taking health or life insurance. Consequently, depending upon turnover rates, a correction factor should be included to adequately represent payroll taxes and benefits.

A worksheet similar to figure 6.3 can also assist employees in understanding that if the organization incurs an increase in the cost of health care, employees might have to share some of the additional cost.

Nonfinancial Rewards

Although money is the driving force for most employees to work, there are some instances in which nonfinancial elements of remuneration are important and should be an integral part of a compensation program. In the health and fitness industry, working in a fitness environment is a perceived value to the employee. This value can relate to the social merits of helping people become physically fit or improving their self-image.

The job itself can be another area of great worth to the employee. Those entering the fitness field consider the opportunity to have a job that combines physical and social skills an added benefit. The opportunity to regularly use club facilities for personal workouts is also of value. Thus the work itself not only determines direct pay but also has psychological value.

Other forms of nonfinancial pay include club discounts, continuing education assistance, and in-house contests. It is the responsibility of an owner

ABC Athletic Club

Employee compensation and benefits worksheet
(assistant fitness manager, full-time)

	Hourly rate $10.00	Annual hours 2,080	Base annual earnings $20,800	
Taxes	BAE	Factor	Total	% of base
Federal unemployment	$20,800	0.008	$166	0.80%
State unemployment	$20,800	0.016	$333	1.60%
FICA (Social Security)	$20,800	0.0765	$1,591	7.65%
Worker's comp insurance	$20,800	0.024	$499	2.40%
Total			$2,589	12.45%

Medical insurance	Monthly	Annual	50% paid by employer	
Health Advantage HMO employee	N/A	N/A	N/A	
Health Source HMO employee	$128.00	$1,536.00	$768.00	
Total			$768.00	3.69%

Dental insurance
$14.64/staff/month at 12 months = $175.68
$7.32 paid by employer/month

at 12 months = $87.84			$87.84	0.42%
Paid holidays* Salaried (daily rate × 7)			$560.00	2.69%
Hourly employees (hourly rate × 2.5) (hourly rate × 1.5 × # of holidays)			$0.00	0.00%
Paid vacation* Salaried (hourly rate × 13 days)			$1,040.00	5.00%
Hourly employees (20+ h/wk) (hourly rate 3 average h/wk × 7-20 days)			$0.00	0.00%
Paid breaks* (hourly rate × 86.6)			$0.00	0.00%
Paid sick leave* (hourly rate × h taken) up to 32			$320.00	1.54%
Employee staff shirts ($8.00/shirt at 4 shirts/employee/yr)			$32.00	0.15%

(continued)

Figure 6.3 Employee compensation and benefits worksheet.

Training and educational courses* ($12,000/yr for qualified staff)		$1,000.00	4.81%
Total benefits (less benefits		$3,807.84	18.31%
included in	$2,920.00	salaried	14.04%
base earnings)	$0.00	hourly	0.00%
Net benefits	$887.84		4.27%
Bonus plan	$3,200.00		15.38%
Total compensation and benefits paid by employer		$27,477.44	132.10%

*Represents cost for nonproductive time.

Figure 6.3 *continued*

or manager to identify these areas for the organization and include them in the personnel manual as an added benefit.

Industry Pay Practices

Compensation for employees in the health and fitness industry is generally reflected as either an hourly wage or a salary (full- and part-time). A third category that also should be included is outside contractors. There are variations within each group depending on the setting, but you can group most employees under these three categories for the purpose of managing payroll.

Salaried Compensation

Salaried jobs are those in which the employee's input and decision making significantly affect the success of the business. Some salaried positions include the ownership group, general manager, sales and membership director and representatives, fitness director, aerobics director, tennis director, aquatics director, and others. Depending on the size of the organization, the salaried group can represent anywhere from 5% to 10% of the total number of employees and the average compensation can range from 15% to 20% of total revenue.

Organizations pay this group in three ways: salary, bonuses or profit sharing, and benefits. Managers usually compensate sales and membership personnel through a base salary, commission structure, or combination thereof. Performance pay has also become popular and is based on achieving preestablished goals set at the start of a fiscal year.

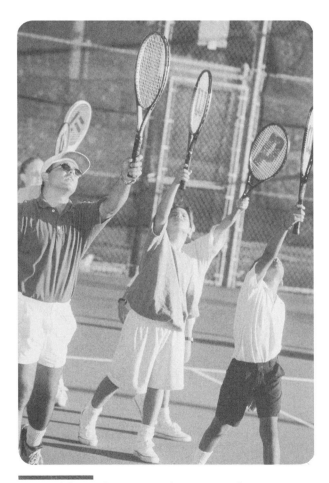

Some club employees—such as tennis director, aquatics director, and general manager—will be paid a salary that could include bonuses and benefits. Other employees are compensated with an hourly wage, and still others are considered outside contractors.

© Getty Images/Zigy Kaluzny

Hourly Wage Compensation

In the health and fitness industry, hourly wage employees serve in a number of positions. They can be front-line employees serving members, they can perform operational duties, or they can be in administration, assisting in the internal aspects of the business. Included in this group are service-desk personnel, weight-room instructors, child care staff, restaurant and pro shop employees, operations and housekeeping personnel, and clerical staff. Some of these positions require experience, certification, or education, whereas others require a short training period.

Although hourly wage positions have historically been the lowest paid, managers today are seeing the importance of fair compensation for those employees who provide face-to-face service to members. Currently, average pay for hourly wage employees ranges from minimum wage to $20 an hour, depending on the position. Hourly wage jobs pay a single rate or have step raises. In these jobs, the work is often learned quickly or in a predetermined time. Job duties can be set and the work standards achieved within a few months.

In these circumstances, when all employees must perform and produce the same, you should pay them at the same rate. It is only fair to have equal pay for equal work. Consider a wage progression scale for each position of this nature. Figure 6.4 provides a sample wage scale for evening housekeeping personnel.

Contractor Compensation

When developing and planning compensation, much discussion focuses on full- and part-time employees. However, a large percentage of workers in the health and fitness field are neither full- nor part-time employees but are instead **outside contractors.** Many are subcontracted (e.g., aerobics instructors, activity instructors, massage therapists, personal trainers). Some are hired for a specific time or task, and others are companies hired to provide a specific service (e.g., landscaping, legal matters, computers, sales, marketing). This form of compensation has been increasing in the industry and will continue to do so because of the advantages it provides.

ABC Athletic Club Wage Scale for Evening Housekeeping

Note: The following wage scale was established to provide supervisors with starting pay rates, incremental performance-review pay changes, and wage caps for each position in their division. This scale is based on average to good performance ranking for an employee's performance review. You can adjust the recommended pay rate accordingly if an employee exhibits either poor or excellent work habits. In some cases, starting pay rates are negotiable depending on a person's education, past experience, and level of certification.

Remember, ABC management must preapprove all starting wages and performance-review rate changes before you hire a person or perform an employee's performance review.

Wage scale (part-time/full-time)	
Length of service	Hourly pay
Starting wage	$8.15/h
30-day review	$8.50/h
90-day review	$9.00/h
1-year review	$9.25/h
2-year review	$9.50/h
3-year review	$9.75/h
4-year review	$11.00/h—maximum wage cap for position

Figure 6.4 Sample wage scale.

Subcontractors are generally paid per hour, per class session, or on commission. Usually, they are not covered by group benefit or retirement plans. Liability insurance is generally the responsibility of the contracting firm, which reduces employee risk. Personnel placement also becomes the responsibility of the contractor instead of the contracting company.

A disadvantage of using outside contractors is the lack of internal loyalty associated with being a part- or full-time employee. Contractors leave the premises once they have completed their class, client session, or task. Consequently, it becomes difficult to establish communication lines and to develop a sense of camaraderie or cohesiveness among coworkers. Because compensation amounts for outside contractors should be compatible with those paid to full-time employees, resentment could result if an employee were passed over for a position now being held by an outside contractor. Also, continually adhering to the tax statutes for what constitutes an employee–employer relationship is a difficult task for managers and supervisors. If the Internal Revenue Service (IRS) ever audits a club that is not adhering to these statutes, it can assess back-tax penalties.

Pay for outside vendors is based on a preestablished contract agreement for services rendered. This agreement has conditions that specify the terms of payment (monthly, quarterly, or annually).

THE BOTTOM LINE

Contracting with outside vendors has become popular because of the lower costs, better caliber of employee, lack of governmental paperwork, and lack of severance or union problems for the contracting business.

Most salaries and wages in the commercial health and fitness industry are expected to increase annually between 3% and 7%. Some positions, however, are expected to stay the same or even decrease, depending on an organization's profitability and regularly adjusted pay scales. A word of caution to managers of clubs that are experiencing continued revenue growth—do not develop a make-and-spend mentality. Reduced operating margins combined with the creation of new positions and continual pay increases can cause payroll expenses to slowly erode the economic growth of a club.

While providing regular wage and salary adjustments, many club operators also offer additional pay options and benefits. Managers may implement more creative pay for performance bonuses and commission structures to retain and motivate employees. In addition, organizations continue to increase their spending by using outside contractors.

KEY TERMS

benefits

commission-based pay

job pricing

outside contractors

performance-based pay

salaries

wages

RECOMMENDED READINGS

Berger, L.A., and D.R. Berger. 2000. *The compensation handbook*. New York: McGraw-Hill.

International Health, Racquet, and Sportsclub Association (IHRSA). 2006. *International employee compensation and benefits survey results*. Boston: IHRSA.

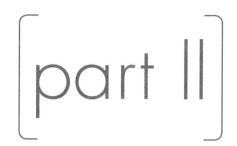

Member Recruitment, Retention, and Profitability

As a manager or club owner you need to be able to pay the bills. You also would probably like to get paid yourself. Part II presents an overview of the revenue-generating strategies you need to employ in your club. The adage "If you build it, they will come" has long been removed from the fitness industry. As competition has increased, the best club managers realize they need to take a strategic approach when it comes to marketing and selling their services, while also developing sound programs that motivate members to keep coming back.

In chapter 7, Casey Conrad discusses how to effectively market your facility for maximum traffic leads and traffic flow in your club. The best approach to marketing is a proactive one, where the plan is set in advance so that all staff members know what to expect and how to measure it. An unlimited number of marketing opportunities are available to the fitness industry, and we can get caught up in trying to evaluate them all. Follow Casey's guidelines, and you will be off to a great start.

Next, in chapter 8, Karen Woodard Chavez explains how to build an effective sales system by incorporating the front desk, phone calls, and the face-to-face sales process. Consumers have a multitude of choices in most markets. An effective sales person will effectively match the prospect's needs to the benefits the club has to offer.

The important topic of customer service is covered by Terry Eckmann in chapter 9. You will learn how to effectively communicate with members, by truly understanding what they want and then delivering it. Regardless of how strong your customer service skills are, there will always be a few unhappy people. Terry offers effective suggestions for dealing with disgruntled customers.

In chapter 10, Sandy Coffman tells you how to design programs that improve retention and keep members coming back for more. Sandy outlines a tried and true method for designing programs that will significantly improve any club's current level of programming.

Generating revenue outside of regular membership dues is no longer an option but is instead something that needs to happen in order for a club to be successful. In chapter 11, Cheryl Jones considers various ways club owners and managers can generate ancillary sources of revenue within their clubs. Cheryl offers some proven ways to make each of the most effective profit centers work for your facility.

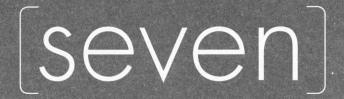

Marketing Your Facility

Casey Conrad

LEARNING OBJECTIVES

After studying this chapter, the reader will be able to

- understand what marketing is and its role in the success of a health and fitness club,
- appreciate the importance of the Parthenon (multipillar) approach to marketing promotion,
- understand the five pillars of marketing promotion, and
- apply the seven steps to creating a marketing piece that gets prospects to respond to advertising.

Tales From the Trenches

The name of the club and individuals in this story have been changed for privacy purposes.

I vividly remember my first day at the ABC Athletic Club because it only took me about an hour to uncover the primary reasons why membership sales had slipped so dramatically in the past 18 months. The club had been open just three and a half years. It had enjoyed a robust start, taking less than 12 months to reach 2,000 members, which is impressive for an 18,000-square foot (1,672-square meter) fitness-only club in a small midwestern town. However, after sustaining that number for 6 months, the club was experiencing a substantial net loss of memberships. When I walked through the doors, they were down to 1,600 members. That may not sound too bad, but those 400 members represented the majority of the club's net profit. Therefore, although the club wasn't losing money yet, it would start to do so very soon if it continued on its current path.

Although there were a few other smaller fitness facilities in the area, the loss wasn't due to either a new competitor opening their doors or an existing competitor lowering prices. It also wasn't because of the physical appearance of the club, as it was still new and featured all the latest and greatest equipment on the market. Furthermore, the club was kept clean, and the staff were as consistent as one would find in most clubs. Simply stated, what had happened was that the newness of the club and the initial promotional hype had both faded, and the club operator was not marketing the club in a way that would maintain a consistent flow of new prospects.

I discovered this by asking one very simple question: "May I see your marketing plan?" John Knapp, the owner, looked at me and said, "Do you mean the ads we have been running?" That one answer told me that John Knapp and the ABC Athletic Club were guilty of one of the most common business mistakes club operators make—failing to have a clear, concise, month-by-month marketing plan that outlines exactly how the club is going to drive prospect traffic through the doors, resulting in consistent membership sales.

Without a written marketing plan that I could look at, I was forced to do a marketing audit of the ABC Athletic Club by asking John a series of questions. Exactly what type of advertising was the club doing—newspaper, radio, television, direct mail, flyers? For each type, how often did they use those mediums in the course of a year, what exactly did the ad say and offer, what type of response rates did they get, and what was the ultimate success rate for membership sales? Did the club have any type of referral programs? If so, were they done at the point of sale with new members or were they for all members? What were the incentives being offered, and what percentage of new members each month came from referrals? How did the club follow up with prospects who had toured but did not enroll? Did the club have any type of materials that went out to members who had ended their contracts? Did the club do any type of marketing with other businesses in the area? For example, did they distribute guest passes, flyers, or brochures, or use lead boxes (small entry boxes that get people to submit their information to receive something for free or a chance to win something)? In addition, did the club work with any corporations or small businesses in the area to try to reach their employees? What about philanthropic efforts in the community?

As I continued to ask the questions, my clarity on the biggest problem facing the club increased in direct proportion to John's level of frustration at himself for not realizing sooner that his lack of marketing diversity and his lack of a substantive plan were literally killing the business he had worked so hard to build—a business he both wanted and needed to succeed for him and his young family.

John was motivated to learn and excellent at following directions. With some long hours spent extracting information from contracts, sales forms, and the club's computer software, he was able to go back and compile a substantial number of reports that would help to assess the marketing efforts that had been used. Such information as how many calls came in from an ad, how many appointments showed, and how many members were enrolled; how many referrals were obtained each month a campaign was run compared to those months where there was none; what the breakdown was each month of all sales sources; and how many letters were going out to nonmembers or former members and what the conversion rate was of those joining. Although it was a long and tedious process to collect this and other data, the information was critical to evaluating past performance and helping to make intelligent future marketing decisions.

Once all the information had been collected and analyzed it was time to help John put together a 12-month marketing plan that would outline every single marketing activity he would do in the course of a year. With the data from the past three and a half years, a budget, and a full understanding of the skills and time available to John and his key staff, we began the process, first by deciding which marketing activities would be done each month. Once that stage was completed, we could go back and determine specific campaigns based on the time of the year as well as outlining the offer that was intended to be used. Of course, we knew that if changes needed to be made because of performance issues, new knowledge, or feedback, it was possible. However, having the detailed plan established a clear course of action with a destination in mind that could be measured.

Over the next several weeks, the first 6 months of the plan were outlined, with the involvement of myself, John, and the sales manager, Michael. What both John and Michael quickly realized was that in addition to the comfort of not having to throw together an ad or come up with an idea at the last minute, having a plan on paper allowed for a synergistic relationship between all marketing efforts. This, they realized, would ultimately lead to greater effectiveness and ultimate honing of their annual marketing plan.

After 2 months of operating the business with a marketing plan, I returned to work with John and Michael on the second 6 months. Allowing some time to pass would mean that their understanding of their own plan would be better and the knowledge they gained would make outlining the second 6 months much easier. This proved to be true, but more important were the results the ABC Athletic Club was realizing. Their multifaceted marketing plan had resulted in a 146% increase in club traffic over 2 months. This meant 25% more sales, which meant they weren't at a negative net growth anymore. Both men were confident that the following month would actually see greater results and positive growth. In addition, the club was now tracking the results of each and every marketing effort. This was allowing for objective evaluation of how the club's marketing dollars were being spent.

Twelve months later, I checked back in with John. He had completed 1 full year of using a marketing plan and was reaping the benefits. His membership had grown back to over 1,800 members, with a consistent positive membership growth of 20-30 members per month. He and Michael had taken the year 1 marketing plan and made some changes and additions for year 2. The process was quite easy and both felt good knowing that the decisions were based on qualitative data, not just what they thought sounded good at the time. It took some time, resources, and energy to complete, but as John told me, "Having a marketing plan in place is making the day-to-day operation of this business easier and more effective. I only wish someone had told me about it before I opened my doors!"

Traditional marketing has taught that there are four *P*s: product, or what the business is selling; place, meaning the location where the product (or service) is sold; price, meaning the cost of the product; and promotion, which refers to everything businesses do to get their products into the hands of the consumer. Newer textbooks have added a fifth *P* to the marketing mix—person, or the target market that a product is trying to reach.

All five of the marketing *P*s have an impact on one another and must be seen as interdependent when making marketing decisions. For instance, if the target market (person) is baby boomers, the club will probably have more recumbent bikes than upright bikes (product). Likewise, if a new operator has two potentially good locations (place), the location that is more convenient to or has more surrounding stores that are attractive to baby boomers will have the advantage.

As you can see, product, place, price, promotion, and person all influence the creation and ongoing development of every health and fitness club. However, once the club doors are open, only one *P*—promotion—will stay high in the club operator's daily priorities.

Marketing can be defined as all functions involved in moving products from producer to consumer. The key word in that sentence is *all*, because successfully driving prospects to a club requires a variety of marketing efforts (promotion). The famous line from the movie *Field of Dreams*, "If you build it, they will come," does not apply to the building of a health club. Regardless of how great the equipment, services, and staff are, if not enough prospects come in, the club won't stay in business.

As a result, although *marketing* traditionally refers to all the *P*s of marketing, this chapter is going to use the term to refer to any and all types of promotional marketing. Unfortunately, managers get so caught up in the day-to-day running of the facility that marketing often gets forgotten or put off until the last minute. Michael Gerber, author of *The E-Myth* (1986), calls this the "doin' it, doin' it, doin' it" syndrome. Even when a club has a marketing agenda, the daily demands of operating the club often result in last-minute marketing decisions, copy creation, approval, and ad production. Ultimately, this can mean poor quality and response rates.

A well-thought-out promotional marketing plan is the key to success. By taking the time to create an annual marketing plan, your club will be positioned to gain maximum exposure, increase response rates and sales, and refine its marketing efforts year after year.

This chapter is going to walk you through the elements of creating an effective **marketing plan.** It will first discuss the marketing Parthenon, or the five categories of marketing efforts every club must use to achieve success. Several examples within each of these categories will be outlined. Next, it will provide a step-by-step guide for designing any marketing piece for maximum response rate. Finally, it will outline a 12-month marketing-grid template, allowing you to put your new skills and strategies into effect.

Marketing Categories and the Parthenon Effect

An effective marketing plan comprises five different marketing pillars, or categories: external marketing, internal marketing, guerrilla marketing, community outreach, and corporate outreach. Having a mix of all five areas accomplishes two important things. First, it allows you the deepest penetration into your community, gaining **top-of-mind awareness (TOMA).** TOMA refers to when a business or its product or service has reached a high level of consumer awareness. Where some products or services look to gaining national awareness, for most club operators, having a high level of TOMA within a single community is the ultimate goal. Experience has shown that TOMA increases exponentially with the number of marketing efforts happening concurrently in any one marketplace. Second, including all five marketing categories will provide you with greater security. The reason for this has to do with the **Parthenon effect** (see figure 7.1).

The Parthenon is a classic Greek temple where the roof is supported by many pillars. The fewer the pillars, the more susceptible the roof is to falling. For example, if the building only had two pillars, the roof would fall if something happened to the first pillar. With three or more pillars you have greater stability, even if one of them fails.

The same concept holds true with club marketing. The more pillars a club uses, the stronger its marketing effort will be. If a club uses only one type of marketing and that strategy fails to work, the club will have no sales—it put all of its eggs into one basket, so to speak. If, however, a club has many different types of marketing efforts happening concurrently, even if one or two of them don't seem to work, prospects will still be driven through the club doors because of the other efforts.

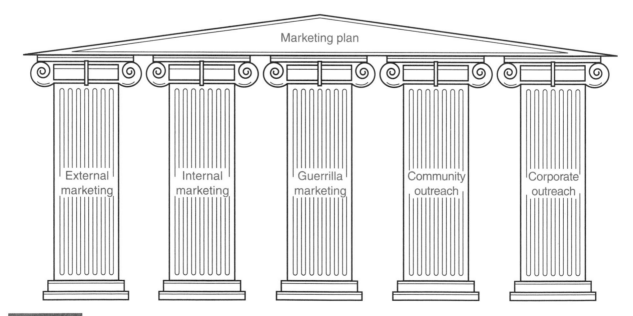

Figure 7.1 The Parthenon effect and the five pillars necessary for an effective club marketing plan.

Knowing the importance of the Parthenon effect, let's take a deeper look at each pillar in order to fully understand its role and possible marketing ideas within each.

External Marketing

External marketing refers to any traditional marketing effort that reaches a large number of people simultaneously. This type of marketing includes such mediums as newspaper, television, radio, and large direct mailings. As you might suspect, external marketing is almost always more expensive than other marketing efforts. Unless unique circumstances exist (for example, if a facility has been the only club in town for many years), external marketing is necessary for success because it is typically the only form of marketing that can reach large numbers of people immediately, allowing the club to create the all-important TOMA.

That said, it is imperative to take a careful and realistic approach with external marketing so as to not spend the entire marketing budget on external marketing, thus relying on one pillar and putting the club at risk. Although that advice may sound easy enough, when you look at the cost of delivering a simple postcard to a resident household, it is easy to see how quickly the money is spent. For example, a common postcard mailing will cost around 35 cents per piece with a minimum order of 5,000 to 10,000, which means that one single mailing will range from $1,750 to $3,500. If a club tries to go with smaller quantities, the cost goes up. The point is that it's easy to spend lots of money on external marketing. Let's take a look now at the most common external marketing options for clubs.

Newspaper Ads and Inserts

Newspapers are the most logical form of external advertising for single-club operators because they reach a good portion of the local market. In smaller towns with a local newspaper, ads are usually reasonably priced. However, in large metropolitan areas, the price can be outrageous, even cost prohibitive.

There are two different marketing options with newspapers: display ads and inserts. A **display ad** is placed within the pages of the newspaper. With any newspaper ad, it is important to follow three rules for choosing placement. The first is the section of paper. If the paper has different sections (e.g., business, general, health), try to put the ad in the section that will be most visible to your prospects.

If the club is for women only, for example, don't put the ad in the sports section; instead, go with the lifestyle section.

The second element for choosing newspaper ad placement is physical location on the page. Depending upon the size of the ad, where it goes on the page can make a big difference. For instance, if the ad is smaller than a quarter of a page, you don't want it to go in between two other ads unless you change the border of your ad to contrast with the other two ads; otherwise the ad will blend in and get lost. (Note that you rarely are given this kind of information before the ad runs.) It would be better for the ad to go on the edges of the paper where the eye has a better chance of seeing it. Although you technically have no control over the placement of an ad, you can greatly increase your chances of obtaining the best possible placement by establishing a strong relationship with both your advertising representative and the editorial assistant at the paper. Approach them in a friendly manner and emphasize that because these ads represent a huge portion of your marketing budget, you are curious as to how to get the ideal placement for optimal readership and response rate. When you get a favorable spot, make sure you stop by with a guest pass or a gift certificate for a small service at the club, along with a thank-you note. If this is inappropriate for your organization, a simple thank-you note will go a long way. In the event that you get poor placement (and usually a poor response rate), follow up with a phone call. Politely express your concern that the placement negatively affected your response rate and ask if there is any way to get better placement next time. Being nice all the time is the key. Experience shows that a positive relationship will lead to much better placement.

The final element for ad placement is the actual page number in the newspaper. Obviously, good placement in the pages is desirous; think of how few people finish reading the entire paper. If you have any control over it, the earlier you can place the ad in the paper or the section, the better the chances are of it being read.

In addition to newspaper display ads, a common form of club marketing is **newspaper inserts,** or flyers. Flyers are typically sheets of paper that have a local business ad photocopied or printed on them. Although they can often be more expensive than a newspaper ad of the same size, they have several advantages. First, because these pages literally fall out of the paper when the reader opens it, they have a much greater chance of being read. Second, bright colors can be used, which further increases the chances of the ad being seen. Finally, because the insert is a single sheet, readers will be more apt to hold onto it, whereas the newspaper is often thrown away—even when the reader meant to keep a coupon or article.

The important thing is to test both newspaper mediums and figure out which one gives a greater **response rate.** This would involve running the exact same ad as both a display ad and an insert and tracking the response and enrollment rate from each source. This concept will be discussed in greater detail later when reviewing the concepts of benchmarking, tracking, and analyzing marketing efforts. For now, suffice it to say that the ultimate judge and jury of any marketing efforts is the consumers' response. Clubs may find that for one type of promotion inserts are ideal but for others display ads are better suited. The key is to test, track, and retest.

Radio

Radio is another potential external marketing medium that, although it can cost more than the newspaper, is usually more viable than television for smaller clubs. But before a club operator gets caught up in the exhilaration of hearing the club advertised across the airways, a careful consideration of the pros and cons should be considered.

In determining if radio is the right advertising medium for a club, the first thing to consider is the **marketplace size.** For a single-club operator in a large metropolitan area, or a little fish in a big pond, the use of radio may be a poor investment. However, if the club has multiple locations in one area, radio advertising can be cost effective.

Another consideration is the **radio-to-marketplace ratio.** That is, how many radio stations are in the area? If the number of stations is high, the listener population is more spread out, making it potentially more difficult to reach the numbers necessary to justify the investment. The converse holds true as well. You can pinpoint this type of information through listener profiles as well as through the quarterly marketplace report of the station.

If you can justify radio advertising in your marketplace, the next task is purchasing spots. A **spot** is a single running of a radio ad. Options and costs for radio advertising are as varied as health club memberships. Basically, the cost of spots is based on rating points, the time the spots will be aired, and the length of the ad.

The number of listeners a station has in the area determines rating points, and the higher the number of listeners, the greater the expense. *Airtime* refers to when an ad will run. Obviously, a spot during peak hours costs more than an off-peak slot. Another option is purchasing run-of-the-station packages, which means that you have no control over when the ads will be aired. Finally, costs increase with the length of the ad, which is usually 15, 30, or 60 seconds.

With almost all radio advertising, you will usually be asked to buy a set package based on the total

Newspaper Advertising Facts and Tips

- Frequency is more important than the size of the ad. Therefore, if you have $2,000 a month to spend on newspaper advertising, you are much better off running smaller $500 ads each week of the month versus buying one $2,000 ad.

- Before signing any contract, try to have an article written up on the club in exchange for purchasing advertising. The representatives will likely tell you that they have no influence with this, but their manager can have influence with the editor if they know it can result in a long-term contract for the paper. This is particularly true with regards to the opening of a new club since it is a worthy topic for the business section of even the smallest newspaper.

- Newspapers typically either charge by the inch or use a **rate-keeper program.** By the inch, you will contract for a certain minimum number of inches per year and the rate goes down as the total contracted number of inches goes up. With a rate-keeper program, the advertiser must place an ad each week but without any type of size requirement. The rate typically isn't as good (because you could conceivably run the smallest available ad every week), but it is more economical than buying a la carte.

- When discussing insert prices with the representative, find out if printing is inclusive or exclusive. Also note that there is an additional charge for color paper or inks.

number of spots you wish to run. Don't be afraid to negotiate. Of course, negotiating price based on quantity is one thing, but there are other options to explore. For instance, you can negotiate price based on the time of year. What many people don't know is that the prime selling month for clubs is the worst month for radio stations because most retailers spend much of their radio budget on holiday offers. Not only should you be able to get a better price break in January, but if you have bought a package that runs over several months, you can negotiate to have the spots weighted to air more frequently in the first few weeks of January.

Once you have negotiated your package, it is time to put the ad together. For many operators this can be the most frustrating task, and they turn to the radio station for assistance. Although stations are often eager to help (sometimes as a way to close the deal), using their help can be potentially dangerous. Radio stations are in the entertainment business; hence they usually create entertaining ads. Clubs, however, don't need an entertaining radio ad—they need an ad that gets listeners to take some form of action. In advertising this is referred to as a *direct-response ad.* Therefore, whether it is to call, stop by and visit the club, or actually enroll, every ad must ask the listener to take some action. These response strategies will be discussed later in this chapter.

Using radio correctly and creatively can add another dimension to promotional efforts for selling club memberships. Make sure you take the time to do your homework, design a good direct-response ad, and use your negotiating skills to produce a package that gets you the exposure needed to make it a profitable investment.

Television

In years past it was unlikely that a small club would be able to afford any type of television advertising. However, with the advent of cable television and hundreds of national, regional, and local stations, television is a possible medium that can have substantial benefits for those who have the budget. First, if the ad is done correctly, television lends a huge degree of credibility—more than any other medium. Second, it can reach a large number of people in a relatively short period of time, possibly boosting sales quickly. Third, because of the large number of stations, ads can now be directed at a more defined market audience. Finally, some research concludes that television advertising has a more lasting effect on consumers because it involves seeing and hearing and can create an emotional response in viewers more easily than print advertising. Of course, all the benefits of television must be balanced against the reality that any advertising spot is costly to produce, is costly to change, and, like radio, requires a level of frequency that will require a substantial investment—especially if the club is in a large marketplace.

First, you must determine if television will fit into your budget, which means you need price lists. Unless you have had previous experience with buying television ads, it is recommended that you hire a local **media buyer** who can assist you with the entire process. The good news is that the buyer does not get paid unless you proceed with a purchase. After you provide target market information and an estimated budget, the buyer will provide a list of appropriate stations based on demographics and ratings. Usually the buyer will also provide viewer data, allowing you to analyze which stations will most likely reach the consumers you want.

Most clubs look at local cable stations or possibly specialty networks, like the Food Network or Discovery Channel, that air on a regional level. These types of spots can be purchased anywhere from $5 to $35 per run depending upon both the station and the time being aired. If you have the budget you can spend a lot more per spot, but most small clubs won't be considering local network spots during Oprah that cost $500 for one 30-second spot!

Similar to radio, media buyers can put together package options, bringing down pricing or adding free spots that typically run during off times and are given by stations as an incentive to buy. The good news is that media buyers know what they are doing and can negotiate small and large packages to fit a wide variety of budgets. That said, television is similar to radio; frequency is imperative. Therefore, you are better off running more spots in a shorter period of time than trying to stretch them out over months. Again, your media buyer will assist you in making good decisions.

The next aspect of television advertising is putting together the actual ad. It will be impossible for even the most amazing makers of home videos to produce their own ad. Poorly produced ads scream mom-and-pop business, defeating the credibility that comes with television advertising. Therefore, you will want to hire a professional to produce the ad. Although this, too, is dependent upon your marketplace and media buyer, you should plan on spending between $2,000 and $5,000 for a 30-second ad. If you are buying a package of spots from one local cable station, you can typically get the spot for cheaper, and if it is the right time of year and you are spending enough, sometimes you can get it thrown into the deal for free. This is where a media buyer becomes invaluable to the process. Of course, the complexity or simplicity of the ad will influence the price, as will the choice of music and whether you use professional actors. All of this must be negotiated and put in writing before you begin production. You do not want to think you agreed to one thing only to get into production and have the producers tell you it will be another $1,000 to get what you want.

Although many people are unaware of it, **stock video footage** can be repurposed for commercials as a way of keeping costs down. These video clips are available for purchase, allowing you to use the video and simply create your own voice-over. Two sites that offer these types of services are www.thoughtequity.com and www.spotrunner.com.

One final word on ad production is remembering to factor in a **trailer.** The trailer is typically the last 5 seconds of a 30-second ad that are left blank. This space is where the advertiser will place the call to action. For small clubs, the trailer is imperative, allowing you to run the same commercial for many months or years but being able to change the offer as frequently as is needed. Changing the trailer still costs money, but it is much cheaper than having to produce an entire ad.

Television can add a powerful punch to your marketing efforts, but can also be a budget drain if not done correctly. Be certain to use a media buyer and talk with other small businesses in the area before making any commitments.

Yellow Pages

For many club operators, the Yellow Pages are a sought-after external marketing vehicle. (And if you aren't seeking it, a salesperson will seek you!) For years, the Yellow Pages would have been the first place where a prospect's fingers would do the walking, so to speak, to find a club. Yellow Pages, however, can be an expensive form of advertising and many club operators are reporting that the response from this medium has dropped so dramatically that they are radically reducing the size of their ad and in many cases going to simply a single-line listing, which every club operator should have as a minimum.

If a club is going to make the investment to have a larger display ad, it is important to ensure it is a good one. Like newspaper advertising, Yellow Pages representatives offer to have their office lay out the ad as part of the investment. This can be a problem, however, because the result is that every ad often

looks the same and the reader is not drawn to any particular ad except by size or by alphabetical listing. Therefore, when designing a Yellow Pages ad, it will be important to follow the design standards for creating an ad that gets a response, which will be covered later in this chapter.

Finally, unlike the other marketing pieces that a club operator will create, a Yellow Pages ad must stand the test of time because it cannot be changed for 1 full year and, if done improperly, will torture a club operator each month when making the monthly payment!

Direct Mail

Direct mail refers to any type of mass mailing (5,000 or more pieces) sent to prospects within a demographic area. The mailing can be in the form of a letter, card, or postcard and is typically done through some sort of mailing house or direct-mail company that coordinates everything from the creation of the piece to the buying of the list to the mailing itself.

One of the most popular forms of direct mail in the club business is postcards. The reason for this is twofold. First, postcards are the least expensive form of direct mail; in the United States, they range anywhere from 35 to 40 cents per piece. Letters are next, ranging anywhere from 50 to 80 cents, followed by cards, which can cost as much as $1 each depending upon how fancy the card stock and printing are.

Aside from the offer to the consumer, perhaps the most important aspect of any direct-mail campaign is the list of names and addresses of those who will receive the piece. A well-selected list can result in a high level of response, whereas a poorly selected list can result in a huge expense without any financial return. There are four ways a club operator can maximize the selected list.

1. If the club has an existing database of members, a direct-mail company can take the list and back-run it to tell the club exactly where its members reside. This is done by having the club send the mailing company a file of their membership list by street name and zip code only. This ensures that the list is not being spammed. The company will then generate a report that shows a map of the area by street and where the club's membership base is coming from. From there, two approaches can be taken: Either market to the nonmember households in the neighborhoods where existing members live or try to market to areas where the club isn't currently pulling from.

2. When a club is new and doesn't have a membership base to analyze and strategize from, the operator can create an **isochrone map.** The isochrone is the area surrounding a club where residents are most likely to buy a membership at the club. It is typically referred to by a certain radius around the club. Using a street directory of the area, the club operator should determine the isochrone of the club. Once those boundaries have been established, the operator, along with a willing and able passenger, should slowly and systematically drive the streets surrounding the club. As they drive through the neighborhoods, a visual assessment of the area will be the determining factor as to whether the street (or portion thereof) is highlighted in green as a neighborhood that seems prospective, in yellow as a questionable neighborhood, or in pink as an undesirable neighborhood. With that information, a direct-mail company can work with an operator and choose streets for list selection. Certainly this process is time consuming, but if a club does not have any data to make reasonable decisions with yet and the club manager wants to try to make a somewhat educated guess as to the list, this is a reasonable approach.

3. Managers can use categories to narrow down their list selection. Of course, distance from club, age and gender of prospect, and household income are the most basic filters. List companies, however, have an amazing amount of information on people, and for a price you can buy a very specific list. For example, if an operator were opening an exclusive, high-end club, a list could be bought that selects only those people within a certain distance of the club who have a certain household income, own a gold or platinum American Express credit card, belong to a country club, and are married. So long as the proper criteria are selected, the more specific the list, the greater the chances are for a higher response rate.

4. Perhaps the least attractive and least effective way to select a list is by using a specific zip code. Unfortunately, if a club operator doesn't know better, this shotgun approach to direct mail often gets recommended. Given the cost of putting together even an inexpensive postcard and the reality that a .5% response rate is considered good, this approach should be avoided at all costs.

Finally, in addition to needing a good offer and using a good list, the last element of direct mail is the concept of testing. Before spending thousands of dollars on a huge mailing, it is highly recommended that you do a small test sample of around 500 pieces. Even if the test isn't done in full color, so long as the layout and other elements are consistent with what the final piece will look like (and how it will be delivered), testing a piece can save you lots of money, time, and frustration.

Tips for Direct Mail

- *Don't make the piece too complicated.* This typically happens when the club tries to put too much information onto the piece. A good rule of thumb is to have no more than 60% coverage on any side of a direct-mail piece.

- *Make the piece look important.* With postcards, this can be done with proper color selection or graphics. With letter campaigns, it can be accomplished through paper selection, embossing of envelopes, or using stamps instead of a postage machine.

- *Make the piece unique.* Perhaps you can use a scratch-and-win technology or shrink-wrap a refrigerator magnet to the postcard.

- *Make the piece personal.* Certainly using first and last names will help, but another idea is to use return address stickers or a hand stamp to make it seem less like junk mail.

- *Make the size stand out so that the piece doesn't get thrown in with other junk mail.* There is no doubt that bigger postcards are less apt to get lost in all the other mail.

- *Use hand addressing with smaller mailings.* Some marketers believe that the open rate of hand-addressed envelopes is more than twice as high as labels or printing.

Coupon Packets

Another popular form of advertising for smaller clubs is the coupon mailer. These are envelopes of coupons that go into everyone's mailbox on a monthly or quarterly basis. Typically these mailings are coordinated by mailing houses or people who own franchised coupon-mailer businesses. The coupons are geared toward home owners, with offers for things like oil changes, carpet cleaning, yard work, and house cleaning. Most mailing houses ensure that there are no competing businesses within any single coupon pack. Many clubs have tried coupon mailers because they are inexpensive and potentially reach many households. The jury is out as to the effectiveness of this medium, however; some club operators swear by them and others swear at them. If you use this form of marketing, just make sure you follow the steps to creating a direct-mail piece that works, as outlined later in this chapter.

Internal Marketing

Although many people think internal marketing refers only to those things that are done inside a club, that is not the case. **Internal marketing** actually refers to a variety of activities and promotions that originate from within the club and are done on a smaller scale than most external marketing. This does not mean, however, that internal marketing is less effective. Much to the contrary, it is often internal marketing activities that bring in the largest percentage of new members to a club. Let's review the most important types of internal marketing.

Point-of-Sale Referrals

Referrals are the most powerful and plentiful source of new members in the fitness industry. Between 60% and 70% of all fitness sales come directly from referrals. As a result, it is vital that you have a strong referral promotion at the point of sale that gives the new member an incentive to tell others about the club. This means having a program where new members are given special guest passes to share with their friends. In order to make this referral program strong, three components are necessary: value, scarcity, and urgency.

Value is exactly what it sounds like—customers perceiving that the program has value for them. Creating value with a point-of-sale program can be accomplished in several ways. For one, the passes should have a time frame that is longer than passes used in other promotions. Therefore, if a club has 1-week guest passes printed on the back of every employee's business cards, the point-of-sale referral passes need to last longer, like 10 days or 2 weeks. A second way to create value is by designing attractive passes using heavy stock and full-color printing. A third way is to make sure a dollar value is printed on each pass, letting the customer know what the pass is actually worth. A final way to create value is to offer new members some sort of incentive if their referrals join.

The second component necessary for a strong point-of-sale referral program is scarcity. **Scarcity** means that there is a limit on the offer. Limiting the availability of an item—creating scarcity—helps to increase its value by using the principles of supply and demand. The easiest way to tap into this concept is by limiting the number of special passes a new member receives.

The third component is **urgency.** Urgency is what makes a customer take action sooner rather than later. The power of urgency is why every coupon has an expiration date and every offer is available for a limited time. Point-of-sale referrals can use the power of urgency two ways. First, if you inform new members that the passes are part of the enrollment process, there is a greater likelihood of obtaining names at that moment. Second, even if new members don't register for the guest passes at the point of sale, a 30- or 60-day expiration date can be placed on the offer. Doing this provides the salesperson with a follow-up opportunity and gives the members a second chance at the passes, perhaps at a time when they feel more comfortable giving referrals.

With an understanding of the concepts behind point-of-sale referrals, let's discuss how the program will actually be implemented. Obviously, a system needs to be followed whereby a new member is always given a presentation about the referral program and then asked to provide names. In clubs, typically one of two different approaches is followed. The first approach is to include a section of the membership agreement that explains the program and has spaces for the member to put the names of referrals. The second approach, and perhaps the more successful approach, is to have a new-member referral form that is separate from the agreement (see New-Member Guest Privileges on page 129 for an example). A separate, attractive form has a greater perceived value to the customer. In addition, if names are not obtained at the point of sale, the form serves as a useful follow-up tool for the salesperson. The only potential downside is that without the program being included on the membership agreement, a salesperson who is uncomfortable asking for referrals can more easily skip the referral presentation without being held accountable by management. This is costly for both the club and the salesperson.

New-Member Guest Privileges

As a member of the club, you are entitled to bring guests to the facility for a standard daily rate of $_____ per visit. At the time of your enrollment, however, you are given the opportunity to register for five free guest passes allowing five different friends of yours, local residents 18 years or older, to use the facility free of charge for (time of pass). Each of these passes is a $_____ value, bringing the total value to $_____. Please fill out the form below with the names and contact numbers of those people you would like to receive the special passes and we will register them today.

This is one way we like to say, "Welcome to the club!"

Member name: _____

Date: _____ Membership #: _____

Home #: _____ Work #: _____

Who Comes to Mind?

- Family
- Neighbors
- Close friends
- Coworkers
- People with whom you socialize
- Friends who currently work out

Guest's name	Contact #
1. _____	_____
2. _____	_____
3. _____	_____
4. _____	_____
5. _____	_____

❑ I have been fully informed of my new-member guest privileges and I do not wish to take advantage of these passes at this time. I also know that these passes are good for 60 days from the date of my enrollment and that I can redeem them at any time during their validation dates.

_____
Member signature   Date

From M. Bates, 2008, *Health Fitness Management*, 2nd ed. (Champaign, IL: Human Kinetics).

Existing Member Referrals

Although a club must tap into the power of point-of-sale referrals, it should also constantly provide existing members with incentives to refer their friends. Therefore, at least three times per year a club should run in-club referral programs where the club offers its members something special if they refer a friend who enrolls at the club.

Of course, the same components that make a successful point-of-sale referral program should be incorporated into existing-member referral programs—value, scarcity, and urgency. As for creating value, one of the keys to successful referral campaigns is having interesting incentives and gifts. This could be something as simple as a sweatshirt with the club logo embroidered on it, or it could be something more sophisticated like a weekend for two to a nice hotel or resort in the area. There are many companies that sell vacation vouchers specifically for promotional purposes. With a minimum purchase, club operators can offer weekend getaways or 4-day vacation packages valued in the hundreds of dollars that only cost the club $10 to $40. Regardless of the gift or incentive you offer, scarcity can be generated by advertising that there is a limited number of the special gifts, and urgency is simple to create by having a well-documented deadline for the promotion.

Finally, in order for any in-club referral campaign to be successful, promotion throughout the club is absolutely necessary. The club must tell members about the promotion on a number of levels, including signs in the club, verbal discussions, letters, and even e-mails. It is amazing how many times people need to hear, see, or experience something before they take action.

In-House Specials

Of course, one simple and cost-effective method of internal marketing is to offer members some sort of special that doesn't go out to the public through external marketing. For instance, clubs could send a personal letter to members telling them that for the month of December the club will waive the enrollment fee to anyone they directly refer so long as they use the gift certificate provided to them in the mailing. Finally, an in-house advertised special doesn't even have to be done through a mailing but rather can simply be advertised throughout the club with posters, banners, signs, and employee discussions.

Missed-Guest Mailers

Even clubs that enjoy an excellent closing ratio on tours given will have a large number of guests who don't enroll. The biggest mistake that most clubs make is not marketing to these **missed guests** once they have left the club. This happens because it is time consuming and difficult for the club to organize the effort. According to the most recent industry statistics, however, someone who has had an experience with a health club is 300% more likely to buy a membership than someone who has never visited a facility! Combine this fact with the small cost of marketing to missed guests, and it only makes sense to organize the effort.

The first step in organizing missed-guest mailers is data entry; that is, ensuring that the sales team (or administration staff) is entering into the club database the names, addresses, phone numbers, e-mail addresses, and primary areas of interests for each guest. In addition, using some sort of coding system that identifies the primary reason for the guest not enrolling will be important for future marketing efforts. Think about it—if the club were going to run an 8-week Women on Weights program, it would be much more effective to send out a mailing to female guests who visited the club within the past 6 months, who wish to tone and firm, and who gave time or money as their primary reason for not joining rather than simply mailing to all the women on the list. Only by identifying what fields need to be tracked and systematically entering the information into a database can this type of efficient, targeted marketing occur.

Alumni Mailers

Similar to missed guests, another overlooked, inexpensive marketing opportunity is marketing to former members, also referred to as **alumni members.** Certainly, these people didn't renew their membership (or even cancelled), but they are fitness minded and might be ready to come back. They are certainly more likely to join a health club than someone who has never worked out at a club before. Of course, the same principles of data entry apply to alumni mailers as they do to missed guests.

Guerrilla Marketing

Guerrilla marketing refers to any type of marketing effort that is typically done by the club staff at the grassroots level. Generally speaking, these efforts are less expensive ways to advertise. However, don't equate lower cost with lower response. Some grassroots marketing is the most powerful and least expensive form of marketing because it reaches people at a more personal level.

The key to any guerrilla marketing effort is organization and consistency. First, organize efforts that are going to be the most effective for the type of client you're trying to reach. For example, if you operate a women's-only business, finding other businesses, venues, and activities frequented by female clients will reap the greatest rewards. Therefore, working with local hair and nail salons or women's clothing stores is one type of ideal guerrilla marketing opportunity. As is the case with any marketing, trial and error is the only thing that will tell clubs what will and won't work in their marketplace.

Second, get the entire staff on board to ensure that the guerrilla marketing is consistently being done month after month. Regardless of what guerrilla marketing efforts are implemented, they are an important part of the marketing Parthenon and allow clubs to reach many prospects at low or no cost. Let's look at the most common forms of guerrilla marketing for clubs.

Lead Boxes

Lead boxes are small boxes placed throughout the community. Typically the boxes have some sort of advertisement on them, enticing consumers to fill out an informational slip that either gives them some sort of free trial membership or enters them to win a short-term membership to the club. Club salespeople contact local businesses and work out an arrangement whereby the lead box can be placed in a strategic location where customers will see it. In return for allowing the club to place the lead box in the business, typically some sort of reciprocation is given to the business. This could be anything from a month-to-month membership, services at the club, or the opportunity to market the products and services of the business to the club members.

Marketing products and services are often the most popular form of reciprocation with small, owner-operated businesses because owners of these businesses don't usually have a lot of extra time and would prefer help in growing their profits. Each week the appropriate salesperson visits the business, picks up any slips that have been entered, and calls the prospects and either informs them they were the winner or offers them a free trial membership. Although some club operators are negative about lead boxes, others obtain so much success with lead boxes that they are their primary form of marketing. Think about it—even if the location is terrible and not many people fill out the informational slip, the lead box itself is an inexpensive, miniature billboard promoting the club.

There are hundreds of businesses in any community that provide club salespeople with endless opportunities for placement, but experience has proven that if you want customers to fill out the informational slip, some businesses are better suited for lead boxes than others. Choosing a business where customers have to wait a short period of time is ideal because it gives them enough time to fill out the slip. Although not an exhaustive list by any means, some of the more successful locations include the following:

Hair salons	Tanning salons
Nail salons	Restaurant waiting areas
Day spas	Maternity shops
Women's clothing stores	Doctors' office waiting areas
Quick car service waiting areas	

Take-One Displays

Similar to lead boxes, take-one displays are placed on countertops of local businesses. The display consists of trifold brochures placed in a brochure holder for people to take. The advantage of take-one displays is that most businesses will allow this type of outreach in their lobby or on their countertops, whereas some will not allow lead boxes. The disadvantage is that take-one displays do not capture the name and phone number of prospects. However, if the option is a take-one placement or nothing, it is a great marketing tool. Further, even though they do not capture names, take-one displays can be a powerful type of marketing to create TOMA.

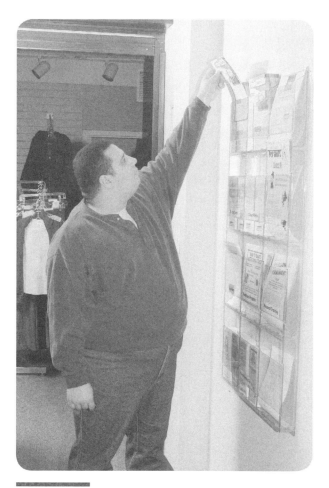

An inexpensive take-one display is a guerrilla marketing tactic that contributes to a club's top-of-mind awareness (TOMA).

Business Cards for Employees

Although the idea of having business cards for employees certainly isn't new, the reality is that all too often club managers do not provide their employees with business cards unless they are directly in sales. This is a big mistake because studies have proven that when people have business cards, not only are they more likely to network, they feel a greater sense of ownership and pride in their place of work. Therefore, all employees working 20 or more hours per week should have printed business cards with their name on them. (Don't use generic cards with a place for them to write their name in—such cards look unprofessional.) Employees should be trained and encouraged to pass these cards out to as many people as possible, and nonsalespeople should be given a reward if one of their business cards comes back to the club and the person joins. Given the small costs of printing a standard business card, this is a great way to get your club's name out.

Joint Marketing Promotions With Local Businesses

There will be many instances where club employees engage in a conversation with a local business but for some reason the business cannot or will not allow a lead box or a take-one display to be placed in the facility. This does not mean, however, that the business won't be interested in forming some sort of **joint marketing promotion** with the club, whereby both businesses benefit from allowing one another to share customers. There are many ways to develop such a relationship. For example, both businesses could print coupons for each other and distribute them to their respective customers. Another example would be if each business set up a table in one another's business for one day a month; the club could do fitness testing for the customers of the partner business and set up an informational table in the lobby. The same types of businesses that were identified in the section on lead boxes would work well for joint marketing, but since time to fill out a slip is not an issue, many more options exist. Some of these would include the following:

Car washes	Bridal shops
Beauty salons of any sort	Children's furnishing shops
Massage therapists	Car dealerships
Bagel shops	Health food stores
Bike shops	Fast-food locations
Sneaker stores	Home equipment stores
Day care centers	

Direct Referral Programs

Unlike internal marketing referral programs that are designed to generate member referrals, the direct referral program is where clubs establish a strong enough relationship with other professionals that those professionals are willing to directly refer their clients to the club. There are two ways that direct referrals can be given. First, special passes can be created that the professional gives to clients or patients. Like take-one displays, the downside to this type of referral is that the prospect may or may not take action and call the club. The other way, which requires a much stronger relationship between the professional and client as well as the professional and club, is where the client's name is actually given to the club, which then contacts the client. Although direct referral programs are much more difficult to establish and sometimes take years to develop, once established they can create a solid referral base that brings new members into the club at a low cost. Several types of professionals who are open to direct referral programs and have a large clientele to draw from are as follows:

Doctors of any type	Cellular service salespeople
Hair and nail salon employees	Insurance salespeople
Real estate agents	Home equipment salespeople
Car salespeople	

The guerrilla marketing activities mentioned here are only a few of the many efforts that can be established. As you might suspect, guerrilla marketing is only limited by your imagination and work ethic. A wonderful source for hundreds of guerrilla marketing activities is a book called *Guerrilla Marketing* by Jay Conrad Levinson (1990). This author has published dozens of guerrilla marketing books, but this is the original book and the best one to start with. If you like the basic premise and wish to get even more guerrilla marketing ideas, review the other books.

Community Outreach

Community outreach is any type of activity that focuses on community-building activities. Although it is called *community outreach,* this pillar is not directed toward getting an immediate response from prospects. Rather, community outreach is more about creating goodwill in the hearts and minds of those who live in the area. It is designed to make people feel good about your company while also creating brand awareness, not immediate sales. Still, community outreach is important. When someone reads an article about your club or a press release on fitness that mentions your club, they will be much more apt to read it and believe it compared with advertising that was paid for. Further, when community members attend an event that the club has sponsored or provided an auction item for, it will build credibility. Of course, the challenge is organizing such activities and events, since they take a lot of time. Following is a discussion of popular community outreach activities for clubs.

Press Releases

One of the most powerful ways to positively influence someone's decision to begin a regular exercise program is through education. When people clearly know how an exercise program is going to affect them and their lives, they will be more likely to join. By sending out regular press releases on the benefits of regular exercise, you can establish a great relationship with the media. They will begin to see you as an expert and will contact you for quotes and photos during key times of the year.

When writing a press release, follow two basic rules:

1. Do not try to sell anything! The press will simply throw it out.

2. Concisely answer the standard questions:

- Who: Who is the release about (both you and the end consumer)?
- What: What is the relevant, factual, interesting information to tell?
- Why: Why should people care about this information?
- Where: Where is the activity?
- How: How can the reader get more information?

When sending out press releases, remember that the newspaper is not obligated to print them. You may send out releases for multiple months without the slightest bit of interest from an editor. As discouraging as this can be, it is imperative to be consistent with your releases, earning the respect and trust of writers and editors. Eventually the day will arrive when there is either a slow news month or a writer is in a pinch for a story, opening the door to using your materials. Once a relationship is established, assuming you have provided good material and are pleasant to work with, you may become a regular source for the paper or television.

In addition to press releases on the benefits of exercise, it is important to let the community know what your center is doing. For instance, if your center is running or participating in a philanthropic effort, let the media know. Follow the same format as you did for writing the other press releases. Figure 7.2 is a sample press release that tells the community about the participation of a health club in a communitywide health campaign.

Speaking Opportunities

A powerful way to gain community exposure is through speaking engagements. In every town, small or large, there are numerous groups that meet monthly and are always looking for speakers. Some groups meet for breakfast, some for lunch, and others for dinner. Some engagements will be for 10 minutes, and others will want you to speak for an entire hour. Start with smaller presentations and work your way up to longer lectures, gaining confidence and a following along the way. In addi-

tion, depending upon how much exposure you are in need of, you can choose your engagements by the type of group. For instance, some groups, like the National Association of Women Business Advocates (NAWBA), are predominantly women, and other groups, like the Lions Club, traditionally have more male members. Of course, depending upon the composition of the groups' members and the time available to make changes, you can adjust your presentation accordingly.

At the end of every presentation, be sure to announce to the audience that you are available to speak to other organizations and if they know of someone you should contact, you would appreciate the referral. With time you can create a public image as the health and fitness expert in your community. This type of image can create other community and marketing opportunities for you and your facility.

Contributions to Community Efforts

A great community outreach program is to do various fund-raising activities. For instance, there are always walkathons and other outdoor events that members and staff can participate in. These fund-raising activities are already organized and sponsored by other people. Simply get your members and staff to go out and support the event. To maximize your exposure at such events, ask everyone to wear a club T-shirt. For those with a small budget, it is always fun to have a special T-shirt made for the event, giving them out only to those who participate. One word of advice, however, is pass them out at the event, not beforehand—it improves the participation rate!

A philanthropic effort is anything that your center does that contributes to a cause. In ways it is similar to fund-raising, but it's usually done at the club level, not organized by someone else. For instance, every year the Salvation Army asks people to donate unwanted coats in order to prepare for the upcoming colder weather. Your club can run a coat drive and get members to bring in their older coats. Even better, coordinate the coat drive with a marketing campaign and give new members a discount on their enrollment fee (or some time free) if they bring in a coat for the cause.

Another way to support the community is by sponsoring a local sport team. Regardless of what team you support (e.g., soccer, softball, Little League), having your name on the shirts of a couple dozen kids or adults is wonderful exposure. When friends and family members see the shirt, they may not know who your company is, but when they later see an ad the connection is made, winning the hearts and minds of community consumers.

NEWS

FOR IMMEDIATE RELEASE

Contact: Healthy Inspirations
[Name]
[Phone]
[E-mail]

GO RED FOR WOMEN MOBILIZES WOMEN TO JOIN THE FIGHT AGAINST HEART DISEASE

Healthy Inspirations [City] Supports the Campaign to Promote Women's Health

[City, State]—February 2007—Thousands of Americans will help women fight heart disease this February when they participate in the third year of the American Heart Association's **Go Red for Women** initiative.

Go Red for Women began in February 2004 to raise awareness that heart disease is the number one killer of women. Nearly twice as many women die each year of heart disease and stroke than all forms of cancer combined, including breast cancer. Perhaps more importantly, new research has determined that obesity alone increases the risk of heart disease. As obesity in the United States continues to rise, so will heart disease. The grassroots campaign has since grown into a vibrant national movement as more women, men, celebrities, health care providers, and politicians embrace and elevate the cause of women and heart disease. The campaign provides women with information on healthy eating, exercise, and risk-factor reduction, such as smoking cessation, weight maintenance, blood pressure control, and blood cholesterol management.

To reduce the risk of heart disease, the AHA recommends that women visit their health care provider to assess their health risks. Women are also encouraged to commit to a healthy lifestyle of exercise, proper nutrition, and not smoking. For more healthy heart tips, recipes, or a schedule of Go Red for Women activities, call 888-MY-HEART (888-694-3278) or visit www.goredforwomen.org.

During the month of February, Healthy Inspirations in [City] supports Go Red for Women by offering complimentary body composition evaluations for women. The evaluations examine body-fat percentage, fat-free mass percentage, hydration level, and resulting risk factors. The assessments, which will be given throughout the month, will help women understand their personal health and how to make healthy lifestyle changes to decrease the risk of developing heart disease. To schedule an appointment, contact Healthy Inspirations at [phone].

About Healthy Inspirations

Healthy Inspirations is a women's weight loss and healthy lifestyle center focusing on long-term weight loss. With over 70 locations worldwide, Healthy Inspirations provides nutrition programs, exercise, relaxation therapy, and personal coaching and support for its members. The Healthy Inspirations in [City] is located at [address]. For more information on Healthy Inspirations, visit www.healthyinspirations.us or call [phone].

Figure 7.2 Sample press release about the involvement of a club in a health campaign.

Corporate Outreach

Corporate outreach is exactly what it sounds like—any activity that reaches out to the employees of a company with the hopes of getting them to enroll. Corporate outreach is different than corporate sales, which is when a company actually subsidizes a portion of employees' health club membership. With the former, the club is trying to directly influence the employee to personally buy a membership.

Many single-owner clubs struggle with corporate outreach for two primary reasons: a lack of available time for visiting companies, and a lack of comfort

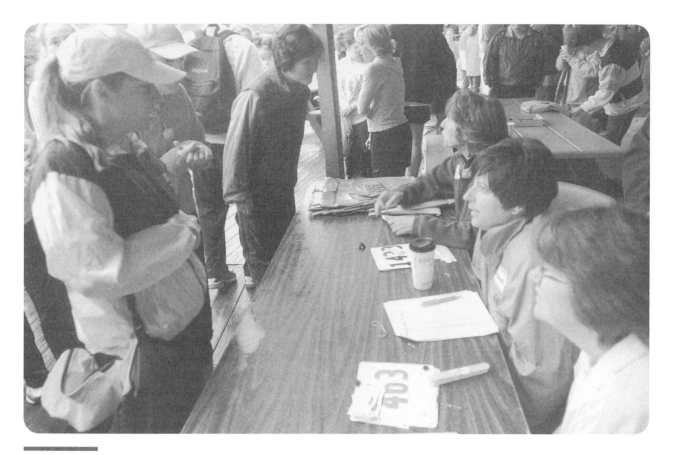

Fund-raising activities such as walkathons and other outdoor events provide an opportunity for club staff and members to support worthwhile causes and at the same time promote the club to the general public.

in contacting a human resources manager to discuss a marketing relationship. However, corporate outreach doesn't have to be complicated or take a lot of time. There are many low-cost, creative ways to work with local companies. The most obvious, of course, is using your current membership base to identify both potential companies and the key contact person. Like all sales, calling someone through a referral is always easier than **cold calling** a stranger. Using your membership database (if you obtain employment information on your contracts) or your sales team, you can quickly build a list of potential prospects.

If for some reason this list-building tactic doesn't work, try a corporate business-card drop at your front desk. Simply place a fish bowl at the front desk and have members drop their business card in to win dinner or some other prize that you have obtained or purchased. From those cards, you can have the sales team contact the member at work and find out the corporate contact name or perhaps names of coworkers who might like some club information. Once you get the name of a corporate contact, send that person a letter and then follow up to try to get some sort of exposure at the company,

such as paycheck stuffers, e-mail broadcasts, health fairs, and company fitness classes.

• *Paycheck stuffers.* One way to get exposure in a company is to make an arrangement with the human resources department to put a letter or flyer into the paychecks. This ensures that every employee is getting the information. Even with companies that use electronic payroll services, employees often receive a check stub or a printed receipt verifying the deposit on payday. Therefore, attaching the promotional piece to the preprinted check stub or receipt is still an option.

• *E-mail broadcasts.* In today's day and age, electronic mediums are a wonderful tool. Often businesses have e-mail servers that can deliver e-mail to every employee at the push of a button. When this is available, try to take advantage of it!

• *Health fairs.* If you are really organized and have the equipment and the staff to do it, one way to get into businesses is by offering to do an on-site health fair. This is where you set up a table and perhaps offer body composition and blood pressure screening in exchange for being able to pass out information on your club.

• *Company fitness classes.* If your club has the staff and a company is open to the idea, another great way to reach corporations is by offering group fitness classes on-site. If staff is plentiful and the demand is present, a schedule of three sessions per week can be offered. However, even if staff is limited, many corporations will allow you to offer a yoga or mind/body class once a week.

Balance Among the Five Pillars

To create an effective marketing program, clubs must embrace the Parthenon concept and use all five pillars in their efforts. In summary, external marketing includes the more traditional, higher-profile mediums. Internal marketing refers to letter and referral campaigns done through the club's members and lists. Guerrilla marketing entails a variety of grassroots activities that can be done by employees at no or low cost. Community outreach refers to any activity or effort that promotes goodwill for the club. And finally, corporate outreach is any effort targeted at a local company with the hopes of gaining exposure and members directly from employees. Table 7.1 summarizes the advantages and disadvantages of each marketing option.

When creating a marketing plan, a manager must ask the question, "Does the marketing plan have a good balance among all five pillars?" The key lies in ensuring all pillars are used each month

Table 7.1 Advantages and Disadvantages of External Marketing Options

Marketing option	Advantages	Disadvantages
EXTERNAL MARKETING		
Newspaper ads and inserts	Reaches a lot of people.	Expensive.
Radio	Reaches a lot of people. Can change ad quickly.	Expensive. Can be too broad and hence ineffective.
Television	Creates tremendous credibility with consumers.	Expensive. Unless ad is done correctly, it can look cheap.
Yellow Pages	First place many new home owners will look.	Expensive. Fewer and fewer people are using the Yellow Pages.
Direct mail	Goes directly into prospects' mailbox. Can be targeted a number of ways.	If using a mail house, must run 5,000-10,000 at once, hence expensive for smaller operators. Can get lost in the masses of junk mail.
Coupons	Reaches a lot of people at a low cost.	Many other items are in coupon pack, so may not get seen.
INTERNAL MARKETING		
Point-of-sale referrals	Easy to obtain from new members. Low cost.	None.
Exiting-member referrals	Low cost. Members naturally refer anyway.	Requires planning and implementation.
In-house advertised specials	No cost. Up-sells and cross-sells to existing members are easy.	Must promote in creative ways or else members become blind to in-club signage.
Missed-guest mailers	Low cost. Someone who has been into your club is more likely to join.	Must manage the database. Phone follow-up needed to maximize response rate.
Alumni mailer	Low cost. Former members are more likely to join.	Must manage the database. Phone follow-up needed to maximize response rate.

GUERRILLA MARKETING		
Lead boxes	Low cost. Proactive source of leads.	Quality of lead can be low. Must manage placement and follow-up of boxes.
✳ Take-one displays	Low cost. Can get into places where you may not typically reach prospects.	Not capturing names. Must manage placement and follow-up of displays.
✳ Business cards	Low cost. Makes employees feel important.	Must justify cost when employee turnover is high. Must teach employees how to proactively pass them out.
Joint marketing promotions	Low or no cost. Reaches similar-minded customers.	Time factor in establishing relationship and putting together materials.
Direct referral program	Low or no cost. Reaches similar-minded customers. Lead is typically high quality, high conversion.	Takes months to establish rapport and trust with the referrer.
COMMUNITY OUTREACH		
Press releases	No cost. Potential for free press.	Time needed to put together release. Must manage database of media contacts.
Speaking opportunities	No cost. Reaches many prospects within the community.	Difficulty in finding staff member who is comfortable with speaking and eloquent. Often engagements happen early in the morning or after business hours.
Philanthropic efforts	Creates goodwill within community. Usually low cost to participate.	Time consuming. No immediate sales generated, hence difficult to justify.
CORPORATE OUTREACH		
Paycheck stuffers	Low or no cost. Viewership almost certain.	Time consuming to establish such a relationship.
E-mail broadcasts	No cost. High open rate.	Time consuming to establish such a relationship. Cannot promote memberships.
Health fairs	Directly work with employees. Proactively acquire names.	Time consuming. Sometimes low turnout at corporation.
✳ Company fitness classes	Establishes good relationships with employees. Fun environment.	Must pay instructor. Must deal with substitutes. May have low turnout.

with the appropriate balance that creates the greatest number of new prospects. Certainly, the more marketing efforts a club does simultaneously, the greater the synergistic effect of creating TOMA, which ultimately means more prospects walking through the club doors.

Although every club has different needs that will be determined only through trial and error, the following is a good rule of thumb to start with:

- One external marketing campaign per month (if newspaper is primary medium, this means a minimum of one ad per week but the same campaign for the entire month)

- Three internal marketing activities per month (these should be scheduled so that at least one of the activities is running at any given time during the month)

- Four guerrilla marketing activities per month (again, these four activities should span the entire month)

- One community marketing activity per month

- One corporate outreach activity per month

Figure 7.3 provides an example of a marketing grid that reflects balance among all five pillars.

Marketing Grid

Month	External marketing	Internal marketing	Guerrilla marketing	Community outreach	Corporate outreach
January	Newspaper ad run twice a week for the first 2 weeks, then once a week for the rest of the month ("Merry Fitness, Happy New Rear" ad) 50% off enrollment fee	POS referral: free T-shirt with five names and phone numbers Existing member referral: $50 gas card when friend enrolls Alumni mailer: come back at old rate	10 lead boxes 10 "take-ones" Flyer exchange with four local businesses	Weight loss press release	Paycheck stuffer with MetLife
February	Newspaper ad once a week Two-for-one enrollment fee Free heart-healthy booklet as secondary offer	POS referral: 1-week passes Existing member referral: fleece vest Missed guest offer: 2-week trial for $29	10 lead boxes 10 "take-ones" Flyer exchange with four local businesses	Heart Month press release Blood drive at club	Health fairs at two local companies
March	Newspaper ad once a week First 10 pounds free	POS referral: 1-week passes Existing member referral: $50 Visa card Alumni mailer: 1-month trial with PT $99	10 lead boxes 10 "take-ones" Fitness Testing Month at local health food store	Osteoporosis Month press release	Health fairs at two local companies
April	Newspaper ad once a week	POS referral: 1-week passes Existing member referral Missed Guest mailer: 1-month trial with PT $99	10 lead boxes 10 "take-ones" Guest pass distribution at dry cleaners	World Health Day press release	Paycheck stuffers with four local banks Weight loss competition among the four banks

Figure 7.3 Part of a 12-month marketing grid that lists marketing activities in each of the five pillars.

Steps to Creating an Effective Marketing Piece

Whether it be a newspaper ad, a direct-mail piece, or an inexpensive flyer that employees will pass out around town, creating a marketing piece that gets the greatest number of responses is the goal of every business. Most ads are ineffective simply because the writer was not familiar with the basic elements necessary for effectiveness. Even when writing a letter to a missed guest or a prospect, the same principles apply. Let's review the eight steps to creating an effective marketing piece.

1. *Know your target market.* Ask yourself what your **target market** is—who you are trying to reach (e.g., exercisers, past exercisers, nonexercisers, seniors, moms, executives). Next, ask yourself what these people's concerns are, and finally, what solution your product or service offers them.

2. *Create the headline.* The **headline** is the first thing that is read in the marketing piece. This is true whether it is a letter, postcard, or billboard. Many businesses make the mistake of putting their logo or company name at the top of a letter or direct-mail piece. This is a classic mistake, and it is costly because the logo or name becomes the headline and therefore is ineffective. The headline must grab the reader's attention. The headline is said to be 80% of an ad's effectiveness; it must scream a benefit or promise that is important to the reader. If possible, it should be emotional, and it should use the word *you*. Have it answer the question, "What's in it for me?" The headline should include power words like the following:

- New
- Free
- Announcing
- Simple
- Powerful
- How to
- Amazing
- Easy
- Effective
- Exciting
- Crucial
- Last chance

3. *Clearly state the benefits.* This part of your piece is the **body copy,** and it should focus on the specific benefits the person is going to get from your product.

- This is not about feature dumping; that is, it is best not to list everything a club has to offer since many of the items may not appeal to all readers and they may assume that a club with so many features is too expensive.
- People don't care about 42 pieces of equipment, they care about saving time! Along the same lines as feature dumping, too many ads simply state a feature rather than focusing on the benefit that feature has to the reader.
- Benefits should be stated emotionally, such as "Keep you motivated," "Help you avoid boredom," and so on.
- If using a letter, break up the body copy with subheadlines. **Subheadlines** are key words and phrases used to signify a new paragraph and typically are either centered with spaces before and after or are underlined. If you are using these concepts correctly, paragraphs should be no more than four or five sentences before a subhead occurs that regrabs the reader's attention.
- If you are going to educate the customer, make sure the information isn't too technical. Keep it simple! For example, if the strength training equipment has a certain type of technology, instead of getting into all the details of the cams or levers, it would be better to simply say, "Cutting-edge technology allows you to maximize your workout without fear of injury."
- One way to write effective body copy is to tape yourself talking to someone about the benefits.

4. *Make the offer.* The **offer** simply tells the reader exactly what you are offering (e.g., free visit, short-term trial, brochure). Outline to readers exactly what they need to do to take advantage of the offer (e.g., pick up the phone, call today, redeem coupon). A secondary offer is an invitation for readers to take action, even though that action doesn't require them to buy. It is a way to get them to respond so you can put them on your mailing list and target marketing to them. The secondary offer should be something that is free and has a high perceived value to the population you are trying to reach, such as the following:

- Low-fat cookbook
- Report on how to exercise at home
- Exercise audio and workbook program
- Brochure on the benefits of exercise

5. *Give them a guarantee.* A **guarantee** of some sort makes your offer more enticing to the reader. Guarantees take the risk off the buyer and place it on the seller, making it easier for the buyer to justify the purchase. People who respond to a guarantee are usually ones who wouldn't have bought otherwise. There are many different types of guarantees:

- Price guarantee
- Refund guarantee
- Service guarantee
- Results guarantee
- Reference guarantee

Make the guarantee as specific as possible. Clearly establish the exact criteria that must be met in order for the guarantee to take effect. Of course, don't make the guarantee if you can't deliver!

6. *Call to action.* The **call to action** is a way to motivate readers to take action now. A call to action usually comes in two ways:

- A bonus or incentive
- A deadline that needs to be met

With some offers you can take a **tiered approach** to the call to action. For example, an ad could give multiple incentives if readers call or enroll before a certain date. After that date an incentive remains, but it is diminished. For exam-ple, if they enroll before a certain date they might receive $100 off, a free nutritional assessment, and a starter kit for getting fit. If they enroll after that date but before the end of the month, they still get the nutritional assessment and the starter kit. The greater incentive is designed to get the reader to call sooner rather than later.

7. *Make it better than risk free.* If you want to really motivate people to take action, make your offer better than risk free. Do this by giving them something for taking action, even if they decide not to buy the product or service. Continuing with the example for the call to action, the club could make the offer that even if readers decide after 2 weeks that the membership isn't for them, they can keep the starter kit as a way of saying thank-you for trying out the club. If you can tie this bonus into something educational, you have a real winner! For example, if you made one of the gifts in the call to action an audio and workbook exercise program valued at $29.95, it serves a dual purpose: It has a high perceived value, and it hopefully will help influence the reader to remain a member.

8. *Add a postscript.* If you are writing a direct-mail letter, always use the postscript. The **postscript** (P.S.) is one of the most-read sections of a letter, second only to the headline. Use the postscript to restate your most important benefit to the customer, the incentive, and the deadline.

KEY TERMS

alumni members
body copy
call to action
cold calling
community outreach
corporate outreach
display ad
external marketing
guarantee
guerrilla marketing
headline
internal marketing
isochrone map
joint marketing promotion
marketing plan
marketplace size
media buyer
missed guests

newspaper insert
offer
Parthenon effect
postscript
radio-to-marketplace ratio
rate-keeper program
response rate
scarcity
spots
stock video footage
subheadlines
target market
tiered approach
top-of-mind awareness (TOMA)
trailer
urgency
value

REFERENCES AND RECOMMENDED READINGS

Gerber, M. 1986. *The E-Myth*. New York: HarperCollins.

Gerber, M. 1995. *E-Myth revisited*. New York: HarperCollins.

Levinson, J.C. 1990. *Guerrilla marketing*. New York: Penguin.

Ries, A., and J. Trout. 1993. *The 22 immutable laws of marketing*. New York: HarperCollins.

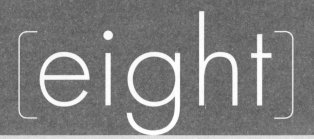
[eight]

Increasing Sales

Karen Woodard Chavez

LEARNING OBJECTIVES

After studying this chapter, the reader will be able to

- recognize the importance of the relationship between membership representatives and service-desk staff,

- be successful when using the phone to sell memberships,

- understand how to create urgency during the tour, and

- appreciate the importance of properly preparing yourself to sell.

Tales From the Trenches

Ian's new club was scheduled to open in 2 months, and the market research, design concepts, financing, and hiring were all coming together nicely. There was no doubt in his mind that he was going to have the nicest club in the area. He had spent a great deal of money on the design and was sure that people would notice this and appreciate it right away.

As he was discussing the presales planning with his staff, it sounded like his staff had all the information about the club that they would need in order to presell memberships. Although he had an aggressive presales budget, he was confident that the club would sell itself.

After the first couple weeks of presales, Ian was reviewing the sales numbers and was surprised to see that out of the 80 people who had come in for information, only 20 had actually bought a membership. He asked the staff why this was and they gave answers ranging from, "They wanted to think about it," to "It's too expensive." He quickly scheduled a meeting to review the features of the club and asked his sales force to push people a little harder. A week later sales had gone up slightly but nowhere as high as he had forecasted they should be.

Ian began to panic and wondered if he was taking the right approach. A couple of colleagues suggested talking to a consultant, which he thought might be a good idea. He had no idea where to start, so he contacted IHRSA, an organization that serves the industry by offering educational opportunities and other services. IHRSA gave Ian a list of consultants, and he made his decision based on the consultants' Web sites and brief conversations with a few of them over the phone.

The consultant Ian hired was able to come to the club within 1 week of the initial phone call. Once the consultant had a chance to meet with Ian and his staff, she then watched how the sales staff performed during the actual sales process. It quickly became apparent to the consultant what the problems were, and she prepared a report and an action plan for correcting the problem. The consultant's analysis included these points:

- Sales personnel were not spending enough time developing rapport with the clients. People will not buy from someone they do not feel comfortable with.

- Sales personnel were too focused on the features of the club and did not spend enough time on the benefits to the individual. People won't buy something unless they understand exactly how it will benefit them.

- Sales personnel were not comfortable overcoming objections. Whenever potential clients said they wanted to think about it or it was too much money, the salespeople simply let them walk away.

The consultant offered the following solutions to these problems:

- Train all staff on how to build trust and rapport with their clients.
- Train all staff on focusing on the benefits of the membership and what the client will get from those benefits.
- Train all staff on how to overcome objections and help them understand that objections are normally a request for more information.
- Make sure that all sales personnel understand all of the previous points so that they do not feel they are pressuring people into buying.

Ian read the analysis and plan for improvement and agreed to hire the consultant to do this training and to also train someone on his staff to carry on the training after the consultant left.

Within 2 weeks of the consultant completing the staff training, Ian saw an immediate impact on the closing percentage. Before the training, his staff members were closing memberships 25% to 35% of the time. They were now closing memberships 50% of the time and Ian was confident that this would increase to over 60% within the next couple of months.

By the time the club had opened Ian was slightly behind his initial projection, but he was confident he would quickly get back on track. More importantly, he now understood the importantce of a thorough sales training program. His initial mentality was, "if you build it they will come." The reality was that his market offered many clubs to choose from and well-trained salespeople would make the difference between the club being successful or failing.

This chapter details several functions in the selling process. Before those functions are addressed, however, it is critical to clarify two elements:

1. *Strong sales skills are critical to the success of any venture.* Club operators often fall into the trap of believing that a beautiful facility will ensure their success. However, the market is very competitive and only the best will thrive. Most people do not like to exercise, so getting our services to consumers is not about simply giving a tour and wowing them with our facility and equipment. It is about understanding the reasons they would say *yes* or *no* to exercise and creating a compelling reason to say *yes*.

2. *Strong sales skills are not about technique or manipulation.* Strong selling skills are simply about two things—being the leader and having good communication skills. As you will read in this chapter, this includes listening, asking the right questions, providing the right solutions, and creating comfort in the decision.

This chapter will cover three essential elements of selling:

- Fostering the partnership between the reception desk and membership department
- Turning telephone calls into appointments
- Maximizing the face-to-face selling process

We will not address lead generation or prospecting since they have already been covered in the marketing chapter. However, note that the ability to generate your own leads rather than relying on the advertising campaigns of the club will be critical to your success.

Fostering the Partnership Between the Service Desk and Membership Department

This section focuses on how clubs lose business due to a lack of partnership between the service-desk staff and the membership staff—an area over which we have direct control.

In a **partnership,** two or more parties contribute to a joint interest in addition to sharing the risks and profits. You've got a solid partnership between the **service desk** and membership department if you see the following qualities among service-desk staff:

- Having a clear understanding of their role as it relates to membership sales

- Giving accurate information
- Understanding exactly how much information to give
- Giving consistently positive and friendly greetings
- Creating a good first impression for **membership representatives**

Conversely, energy needs to be put into creating or strengthening the partnership if you're seeing the following:

- Incomplete guest cards
- Inconsistent greetings
- Inconsistent verbiage
- Inability to take control
- Lack of knowledge
- Poor attitude toward membership representatives

Tools to Strengthen the Partnership

Fortunately, there are several tools you can implement to strengthen the sense of partnership among your staff. Here we discuss communication, incentives, and relationship support.

Communication

Communication is vital to a strong partnership. Follow these guidelines to improve communication between the service desk and membership department.

- Choose a liaison from the service desk to attend certain membership meetings and elect a liaison from membership to attend service-desk meetings.

- Issue a weekly update for the two departments that includes updates on promotions, such as where advertisements may be running, upcoming membership events to be familiar with, upcoming projects the department may need help with—anything they need to know that will make them feel a part of the process rather than the last to know.

- Keep an appointment sheet at the front desk. As membership representatives come in for the day, they will write their appointments on the sheet with any special notes the desk needs to know. This tells the service-desk staff who is coming in for the day so they can give a more familiar greeting when the

prospective member comes in, which is a professional and proactive way for the service desk to create a positive first impression on the prospective member.

Incentives

Incentives are one of the best ways to create a direct relationship between behavior and results; that's why so many clubs pay commissions as a large part of the compensation package for membership representatives. Clearly, it would not benefit the club to have a large part of service-desk compensation be commissions; however, some sort of incentive helps the service desk start paying more attention to the membership sales process and what it takes to make it successful.

THE BOTTOM LINE

Since service-desk staff members are partners in membership sales, they should get some kind of perk when the club reaches its membership sales goals.

The following are some tools your club can use as incentives:

- Split a small percentage of total membership commissions with the service-desk staff. The split can be based upon the percentage of total hours worked by each staff member. For example, if the service-desk bonus for membership hitting or exceeding the goal is a pool of $500, a staff member who worked 20% of the hours gets a 20% bonus, or $100.
- Dinners, movie tickets, and club services are also valuable incentives.
- Don't get stuck on giving an incentive based on the end result. The process has to work well in order to end successfully. Consider rewarding aspects of the process that are crucial at the service desk (i.e., greetings, phone verbiage, how they receive prospective members, guest cards being completed accurately, looking for people whose memberships are expiring).
- Make sure all staff who are eligible for an incentive are aware of it and know how to get it. We often assume that staff members have all the information they need to do their jobs well when this is not always the case.

Relationship Support

The most important thing we can do to support the partnership is to make sure that service-desk staff get the appropriate training from the beginning. Often they are trained by the service-desk manager, operations manager, or owner and the emphasis is on answering phones, receiving members and guests, scheduling, and so on, with little attention paid to the importance of the membership process and how to affect it positively. Have the membership sales director incorporate membership training into your program, which will build a better relationship with the service desk from the beginning.

Additionally, when service-desk employees do something well, let them know they did a good job and thank them. Even if they need to improve on something, let them know they did it 90% right and tell them how they can make it 100% right, making sure to model the behavior for them.

Guest Cards and the Service Desk

The **guest card** is one of the first points of contact with a prospective member and thus is a strong sales tool for the membership representative. Although most clubs have a guest card, they don't maximize its benefits. If designed and used correctly, it can be one of the best tools for building rapport, gathering needs and motivation information, and setting the sales process up for success.

Characteristics of a Well-Designed Guest Card

Well-designed guest cards have the following characteristics:

- The most user-friendly cards are 8.25 by 5.5 inches (21 by 14 centimeters) or smaller.
- They include space for the basics: name, address, occupation, past club experiences, interests, and needs.
- They provide space for both evening and daytime phone numbers as well as e-mail addresses.
- They provide space for referral information in the section on how they heard about the club. This is by far the best area for building rapport early with the guest. It allows the marketing representative to develop commonality with the guest by saying early in the conversation, "I see that Susan Crawford referred you to the club—she's been a member here for years. How do you two know each other?"

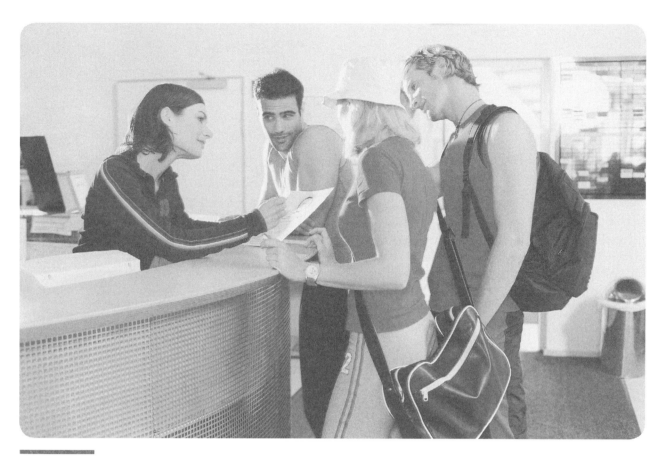

The service-desk staff are an integral component to the membership process. The relationship between the service desk and the membership department should be considered a partnership.
© Getty Images/Altrendo Images

- Because guests may try the equipment during the tour of the club, a liability waiver is included. It should not include a full health history questionnaire, however; most guests are coming in to tour the club and it is unnecessary at that point.

Effective Use of the Guest Card

Too often when a guest approaches the service desk and inquires about membership information, the service-desk staff member responds in a somewhat apologetic tone, "Sure. Would you mind filling this information out first?" Instead, when a guest inquires about membership information, we want to train the service-desk staff to respond with, "I'd be happy to tell you about membership! I'm going to have you take a second to complete this information and I'll get a membership representative to answer all your questions." When the staff member takes the position of *directing* the guest rather than *asking* the guest, the guest is less likely to buck the process and we are more

likely to get complete information. The service-desk staff also should be trained on the purpose of the guest card so they can explain it to a questioning guest.

Turning Calls Into Appointments

Mastering phone skills is a critical link in sales success. It is often what transforms a prospective member into a full-fledged member. Certainly, we need to master face-to-face sales skills as well, but without phone skills, we can end up throwing marketing dollars away or pushing qualified prospects into the arms of our competitors.

To master phone skills, this section will cover the following:

- Why we are at a disadvantage on the phone
- Mistakes to avoid
- Setting yourself up for success

Disadvantage Factor

First contact with a prospective member on the phone versus first in the club can present a few disadvantages. Here's why:

1. *No visual cues.* The exchange is entirely based on tone and verbal skills. They cannot see you, your warmth, the beauty of the club, or the energy of the members. For most people, visual cues are a large component in how they process information. Without them, it's difficult to build rapport.

2. *No environmental control.* When you are speaking with someone on the phone, you have no environmental control. For example, if you call prospective members at work, they may be dealing with countless distractions while speaking with you; thus, their environment may make it difficult for them to focus on their discussion with you. You don't know exactly what is going on, but you sense they are not entirely with you. Sometimes we take this personally (which is wrong), and sometimes we recognize it right away and do the right thing, which is schedule time for them to come into the club.

Six Mistakes to Avoid

Let's review some of the mistakes that cause us to sound as if we are selling the club over the phone. After listing some of the mistakes, we'll provide simple, proven solutions.

Mistake 1: Asking for the Appointment Too Soon

As you read this, you may be thinking, "Wait a minute—isn't the purpose of the phone call to schedule an appointment?" That's correct, but the point is that getting the appointment and getting the prospective member to show up for it are a strategic process. For example, the vice president of sales for one of the largest club chains in the United States revealed that the organization has a measly 30% show ratio for telephone appointments—70% of appointments don't show. He explained that this happens because they train their membership representatives to go for the appointment within the first 45 seconds of the phone conversation.

If you are pushing hard for the appointment on the phone, one of two things will happen—either callers will hang up or they will agree to an appointment because they don't know how to say no to you. However, even if they agree to an appointment, the odds are unlikely that they will actually show up.

Mistake 2: Asking for the Caller's Name and Phone Number Too Early

It is crucial to get the caller's name and phone number, but if we do it too early, it will feel pushy. How many times have you answered a telephone inquiry with a cheerful voice, asked for the caller's name, and then felt the caller's voice drop to a flat, defensive note? How about when you've asked for a phone number and the caller didn't want to give it to you or made up a number instead? When you ask too soon, it tends to destroy rapport. This connection with the prospect is critical, and it must be earned.

Mistake 3: Laundry Listing the Club

When you laundry list the club, you are listing all of its features and programs. The phone rings, and the ensuing conversation sounds like this:

Membership representative: "Hello, this is Membership."

Caller: "Hi, I'd like some information about what you offer. Do you have yoga?"

Membership representative: "Oh yeah, we've got a great yoga program. We also offer several other classes like stretching, dance, sculpting, step, high impact, low impact, spinning—all the stuff you'd expect, plus we have a pool, eight tennis courts, full-court basketball, sand volleyball, free weights, techno gym machines, and a full cardio area with 10 treadmills, 6 recumbent bikes, 6 upright bikes, rowing machines . . ."

We think that if we tell the caller enough about our facility, it will sound as though we have a lot to offer and thus build value in the caller's mind. The problems with this reasoning are as follows:

1. Most callers have something specific in mind that made them call. Part of our job is to find out what that is and build desire around it. In laundry listing, we completely ignore that basic tenet of selling and blast them with general information rather than telling them what they want to know.

2. Many callers will have no idea what spinning classes or recumbent bikes are, so when we use these kinds of terms, we merely add confusion and discomfort rather than build rapport.

Mistake 4: Price Quoting

This is one of the most controversial sales issues in the industry. The way we handle it separates the successful appointment setters from the unsuccessful.

The predictable opening statement on 90% of incoming calls is "Hi, I'd like some information about your rates." Most membership representatives believe that because rates were the first details requested from the caller, they must be the most important concern. The reality is that most callers are not sure what questions they should ask and price happens to be the easiest one for them—not always the most important one. Instead of either detailing the membership prices or defending why you can't give prices, acknowledge what they are looking for (which results in the caller being less defensive), determine their true concerns, and then give the appropriate information and schedule an appointment. If necessary, you can give a range of prices, as we'll discuss later.

Mistake 5: Lack of Preparation

Lack of preparation on the phone refers to the following:

- Not having a goal for the number of appointments you want to get from calls
- Not knowing how many calls you need to make in order to schedule your desired number
- Not having a system for tracking call data
- Not taking notes on calls
- Not scheduling specific times to ensure that calls are made daily
- Not using a guideline for calls

Lack of preparation is a costly mistake that can set the stage for failure. We will address the solutions to this problem in the section Setting the Stage for Your Success.

Mistake 6: Lack of Calling Frequency

This is one of the most costly call mistakes, and it is also the one that happens the most. Even the best salespeople cannot hit or exceed their goals if they are not talking to enough people. Often membership sales staff sit down to make calls, get in touch with some of their leads, and schedule a few appointments, but the ones they don't get in touch with during that call time get moved to the next day rather than called again the same day. Lack of frequency in calling slows the appointment-setting process, which ultimately creates more work for you and less financial reward.

Setting the Stage for Your Success

As we've seen, there are many potential pitfalls when it comes to phone skills. Fortunately, there are some simple, proven ways to avoid them. Here we'll look at ways to prepare yourself for success with incoming, follow-up, and confirmation calls.

Incoming Calls

When it comes to **incoming calls,** the good news is that they called us—they're interested. Let's look at the following continuum (figure 8.1), with 0% to the left, which equals *cold*, and 100% to the right, which equals *sold*.

Statistics show that when people call a business to ask questions, they are more than 50% sold on buying the product or service. In other words, when they call, they already have made up their mind that they're going to buy—they just don't know who they're going to buy from. So with incoming calls we have the opportunity to move them to 70% or 80% sold, which usually results in an appointment. When we have an appointment with people who are already 80% sold, all we have to do is move them 20% to 100%! Therefore, it is critical to set ourselves up for success from the beginning. Here are 10 phone success tips you can implement immediately.

Phone Success Tip 1: Set Goals for Phone Calls   Goals should include the total number of calls you're going to make, appointments you will get from those calls before you stop, new-prospect calls, and current-member calls for referrals. To know these things, you need to know your bigger picture—how many memberships you want to sell, how many appointments you need in order to sell those memberships, and how many phone calls you need to make to prospective members in order to schedule those appointments.

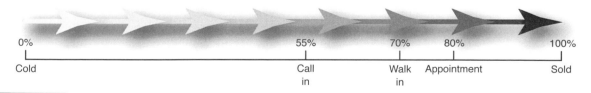

Figure 8.1 The cold-to-sold continuum.

Phone Success Tip 2: Be Prepared and Organized

Goals are a huge aspect of preparation for phone calls. Other elements include the following:

- Being in the right mind-set
- Having and consistently using a data-entry and tracking system (either manual or automated)
- Taking notes during the conversation so you can be more familiar with them when they arrive for their appointment or more organized when making follow-up calls
- Using a call guideline or script

Phone Success Tip 3: Use a Script

The response to phone scripts goes two ways. Some membership representatives cringe because they see scripts as being awkward and forced, and others get excited because they know that a good script is a great guideline for sales success when used correctly. If you fall into the cringe category, think about it this way: Any TV commercial, movie, or Broadway stage production usually comes across as very natural. However, the whole production is scripted. The reason it comes across so flawlessly is because it is practiced to the point that it becomes second nature. Granted, both sides are scripted, which is vastly different from what happens when you are on the phone with a caller, but there are some similarities. The biggest similarity is that once you have practiced your script to the point that it becomes second nature, you can become conversational and focus more on listening versus what you should be saying next. You become more present, which allows you to respond in a more effective and creative way.

You should use a script that provides the ability to acknowledge, assess, and ask for the appointment. Take a look at the script in Turning Calls Into Appointments on page 151 for an example.

Phone Success Tip 4: Use a Unique Selling Position

Your **unique selling position** is what makes you different and better than the competition, and when you use it correctly, it is what makes prospective members realize that your club is the club for them. A unique selling position can be based on programs, services, facilities, staff, equipment, or philosophy. In order for it to work, it has to be relevant and desired by the prospective member.

Phone Success Tip 5: Maintain Control

Maintaining control does not mean dominating the conversation. Instead, make sure that you are directing the conversation by asking questions. Your phone conversation should be a mix of 70% asking questions or listening and 30% giving information. The essence of professional selling is professional questioning, whether it is face to face or on the phone. That is one of the reasons why a script works so well—it gives you the questions to maintain control and direction. Think about what you want to accomplish and formulate your questions to do so.

Phone Success Tip 6: Exude Energy

Having energy doesn't mean we should gush on the phone or wildly exaggerate when speaking. Simply speak more clearly and slowly, enunciate more, smile when you speak, stand when you speak, look at yourself in a mirror when you speak, and add affection to your voice.

Phone Success Tip 7: Set the Appointment

You're probably thinking that setting the appointment is obvious; it should be, but it is not. Some clubs don't feel it is important to set appointments; they see it as too high pressure. Those clubs usually say something like, "I'll be here from 2 until 10 this week, so just stop by when you can." Here is why that approach doesn't work:

1. It shows the caller that you don't have much going on and that your time is not valuable.
2. It puts you in the position of providing terrible service if callers show up and you and all the other membership representatives are busy giving tours. Now they have to wait, which might drive them to go to your competitor down the street who can help them now.
3. By not scheduling appointments, you can't manage your time effectively—you never know when you will be really busy or not busy enough.

Remember, the entire goal of the phone call is to schedule the appointment. By doing so, you can provide better service, manage your time more effectively, and increase your ability to close sales.

Phone Success Tip 8: Get the Caller's Phone Number

Getting the caller's phone number is critical for your ability to follow up and reschedule in the event something prevents the appointment from happening. As mentioned earlier, if we ask for the caller's name and phone number too early in the call, we more than likely won't get it because in the caller's mind, there is no good reason for us to have it. However, if we request this information toward the end of the call after we have built some rapport and have set an appointment, then it makes sense for them to give it. The best approach is to simply say, "Raul, in case any of my previous meetings are running late, how can I contact you?" Raul would give his number

Turning Calls Into Appointments

Greeting

"Hello, this is Membership, how can I help you?"

Acknowledge Needs and Qualify

"Sure, I'll be happy to give you some information. Do you have a pen and paper so you can jot a few things down?"

"Will this membership be for you or will someone else be joining you?"

"I'm sorry, I didn't introduce myself. My name is (give your full name). And you are . . . ?"

"Have you been to the club?"

"What would you like to do in the club?"

"What time of day will you be taking classes (lifting weights, exercising)?"

"(Caller's name), what you'll find makes us different from other clubs is _____ and _____. Does that sound like it might fit with what you are looking for?"

"(Caller's name), from what you've explained to me, the membership options that would suit you best range from _____ to _____ per month. Does that fit with what you had in mind?"

Schedule the Appointment

"The next logical step is for you to come into the club, have a workout on us, get a feel for the club, and see if it's a match. If you like it, then we can sit down and go over your options."

"Is this afternoon good for you or is tomorrow better?"

"I've got some time available at ___ a.m. or ____ p.m. Which works best for you?"

"OK, (caller's name), I've got you down for _____ on _____. Do you need directions to the club? In case anything comes up, your daytime number is _____ and your evening number is _____? There we go then. I'll look forward to seeing you on _____ at _____."

"Oh, by the way, if there is someone you'd like to bring with you to the club—a friend, family member, or coworker—I'd be happy to host them as my guest as well."

"OK, we'll see you on _____ at _____. Bye."

Let the caller hang up first.

and you would ask if it is a home or office number. If it his office number, you would say "Great! And your evening number is . . . ?"

Phone Success Tip 9: Invite the Caller to Bring a Friend This tip can double your sales leads if you do it correctly. After you have set the appointment, invite the caller to bring a guest. It sounds like this:

"OK, Laine, I'm looking forward to seeing you at the club tomorrow evening at 6:30 for a spin class and to see the club. I think you're really going to enjoy it. And by the way, if there's someone you'd like to bring with you—a friend, family member, or coworker—please feel free to invite them. They'll be my guest."

It is critical that you make this offer after the appointment is set, not before. If you offer before scheduling the appointment, it will delay the scheduling because they will have to think of people to invite and then check with them and get back with you. In the process, they may lose their steam and you may lose the appointment altogether.

Phone Success Tip 10: Make the Visit an Event The best and simplest way to make the visit an event as opposed to just a tour is to schedule the caller to come in for a complimentary class, training session, assessment, or workout in addition to seeing the club. Make this event the focal point. This also gives prospects the opportunity to try before they buy and build their desire for belonging to your club.

Follow-Up Calls

Now it's time to approach follow-up calls and leaving messages. **Follow-up calls** are calls you make to a prospective member who has either seen or visited the club but has not joined yet. The purpose of the call is to schedule an appointment to come back into the club.

When to Make the Follow-Up Call   If you have given a club tour and the prospective member did not join, when do you follow up? The range of answers to that question is usually from 3 to 7 days. Every once in a while, someone will answer correctly, "Within 24 hours."

If you're calling a residence, call no earlier than 9:00 a.m. during the week and 10:00 a.m. on the weekends unless you have permission to call earlier, and call no later than 8:00 p.m. in the evening unless you have permission to call later. You may also want to check your state laws with regard to time frames for telephone sales.

How Often to Call   If you have given a tour, the person did not join, and you follow up with a phone call, how many times do you call before you stop? A good philosophy is to call until the prospective member says either yes or no. That may be 15 calls, but if done right, you will get your answer. You should never stop calling just because you think the person might not be interested.

THE BOTTOM LINE

Most membership representatives cringe at the thought of calling a prospective member several times. But by giving up too soon, they miss the success that is just out of reach.

The three-round call system will allow you to make enough calls and achieve higher phone success, and here is how it works:

• *Round 1*—When you come into the club in the morning, sit down to call all your leads. You will get in touch with some, but for those you don't get in touch with, do not leave a message because you will call them back in the afternoon.

• *Round 2*—In the early afternoon, sit down again to make more calls. Call the leads you were not able to reach in the morning. Again, you will get in touch with some and won't be able to speak with others. For those leads you are unable to speak with, do not leave a message because you will attempt to call them again in the evening.

• *Round 3*—In the evening, sit down for a third time to call all the leads you have been unable to speak with today. For those you are still unable to speak with, leave a message.

What to Say on a Follow-Up Call   There are several formats for leaving messages or speaking live to prospective members. One of the most effective tools if you have toured with someone is the great news call. It sounds like this:

> "Hi, Cory! This is Karen Woodard with the ABC Club. I've got some great news for you based on our conversation the other day. Give me a call as soon as you can at 303-444-5555. In fact, if you can call by 6 p.m. on Tuesday, even better! I think you're really going to like this."

This format can be used for leaving messages or speaking live. The benefit is that you start with a positive. At all costs, avoid starting a conversation with a negative.

> "Hi, Cory, this is Karen Woodard with the ABC Club and I'm just calling to see if you've had a chance to speak with your partner about joining."

When you make this kind of call, there is no reason for the prospective member to call you back.

When making the great news call, the following three elements must be included:

1. The news needs to be relevant and desirable to prospective members. It can be promotional, program related, service related, and so on.

2. The phone call needs to be delivered with energy and urgency in your voice. Additionally, mention a time and day to call you by.

3. If you have to leave a message, do not give the great news away in the message. The prospect has to call you back to get it; otherwise, it defeats the purpose.

A critical element to remember when leaving messages is this: Don't spill your candy in the lobby! In other words, don't leave long, drawn-out messages that give the prospective member no reason to call back. If you have placed between five and seven calls and left messages with no response, then you need to make the reality-check call. This usually prompts a response either way and provides clarity on how to proceed with the prospective member.

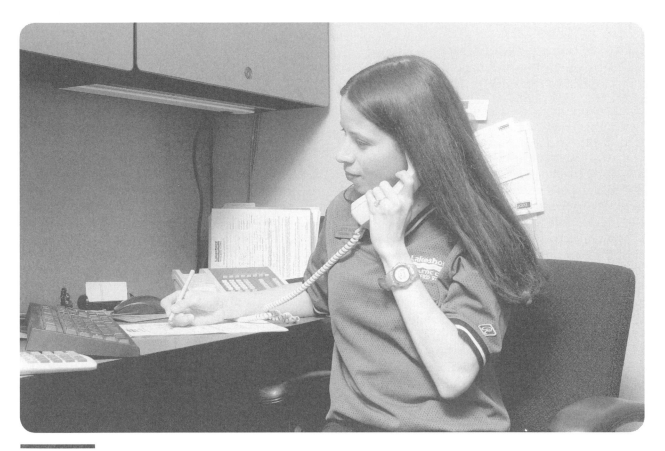

The mastering of phone skills is directly related to sales success. Feeling comfortable when talking on the phone can go a long way in turning a prospective member into a full-fledged member.

"Hi, Cory! This is Karen Woodard with the ABC Club. I've left a few messages and haven't heard back from you so I don't know if you are not getting the messages or if this is something that you're not interested in at this time. Please call me and let me know either way. If you tell me you're not interested, then I won't leave updates for you and I won't be offended. Thanks for your courtesy, Cory!"

Confirmation Calls

Confirmation calls are a follow-up to an appointment. When you schedule appointments with callers, more than likely you write them down and make them a priority because they are directly related to your personal, professional, and financial success. Callers, on the other hand, may not place the same importance on the appointment because it is related only to their fitness; thus, they may forget about it and not show up. The best way to decrease the chances of this happening is to confirm every appointment you make. For example, if it is

Monday evening and you schedule an appointment with a caller for Wednesday afternoon, call her on Tuesday evening to confirm. By confirming your appointments, you will display professionalism and courtesy as well as increase your show ratio for appointments.

Maximizing the Face-to-Face Selling Process

This section will give you the tools to maximize the face-to-face selling process as well as create a more comfortable buying environment for both the buyer and yourself. Traditionally, the goal of the sales process has been to close the sale. However, if we view that as the only goal, we will slow the entire process down. Instead, view it as what it is—a process that has multiple steps:

1. Building trust and rapport
2. Performing a needs assessment and asking qualifying questions

3. Building desire on the tour

4. Presenting the price

If you don't do each one in order, you can't get to the next goal. If you have not built rapport, you won't be able to get the best information during the needs assessment. If you don't get specific information during the needs assessment and qualification, you won't be able to build desire on the tour. If you don't build desire on the tour, it will be more difficult to close the sale. This often leads to a lot of follow-up work, which slows the process down and makes more work for you. The message here is to focus on each step to make it easier to get to the close for both you and the prospective member.

The best membership representatives take the time to do the rapport building, needs assessment, and qualifying questions before the tour. Then they use the tour to build desire, create differentiation, use trial closes, handle objections, and close on the tour. The weakest membership representatives start the tour, then perhaps do the needs assessment, maybe ask some qualifying questions and do some trial closes, handle objections after the tour, and maybe close the sale after the tour.

How can you possibly build desire and show prospective members what they want if you don't know what that is? Strong membership representatives invest time before the tour so that they know how to build desire for prospective members. The close becomes a matter of flow. That is why it is important to spend 3 to 5 minutes with the prospective member before showing them the club. During that short time, you'll be able to customize the tour to the needs of the prospective member.

Ideally, this should take place in the lobby away from the service desk and out of the line of traffic. If you have a sitting area or a café somewhere in the lobby, it will work beautifully. Be sure to find a place where you can sit for a few minutes rather than standing. You want to create comfort. Don't take prospective members into a sales office both before and after the tour; most prospective members have had an experience with the office before and don't like it.

Now that we have taken a look at the big picture, let's break it down into the elements that make it successful.

Building Trust and Rapport

All successful sales philosophies have one element in common—building a good relationship with the prospective member. When buyers feel they have a relationship with you, there will be less tension, defense, and fear of exploitation (see figure 8.2). Instead, there will be trust, rapport, and more sales!

Building trust and rapport doesn't really start with you; it starts with the service desk and is continued forward with you. This is why it is imperative that the membership sales department and the service desk have a solid working relationship, as discussed in Fostering the Partnership Between the Service Desk and Membership Department on page 145. Here is where we take it to the next level: building the relationship between yourself and prospective members once the service desk has passed them on to you.

The Introduction

A strong introduction is simple and includes a few key elements:

1. Use the prospective member's name.

2. Extend your hand first to shake—be the leader.

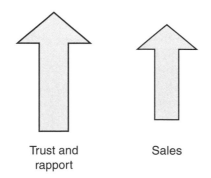

Trust and rapport   Sales

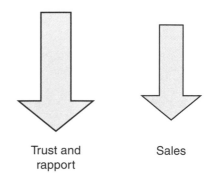

Trust and rapport   Sales

Figure 8.2   The relationship between trust and rapport and sales.

Preparing Yourself to Make the Sale

The time we spend mentally preparing ourselves for success in the sales process is critical. What we do to prepare ourselves before our professional day begins has an exponential impact on not only that day but also each day thereafter and therefore our career. We are constantly bombarded by other people's actions, thoughts, and words, most of which may not be positive. In addition, our own self-talk creates our reality. If our self-talk is not constructive, supportive, and forward moving, then we end up moving backward with respect to our own image. Therefore, we must continuously prepare ourselves to be the best.

Let's take a look at some tools to achieve this. One is the cold-to-sold continuum, which was introduced on page 149. This continuum applies just as much to the seller as it does to the buyer. The only difference is that sellers need to be at 100% sold every moment of every day. The following tips will help you stay focused:

- Love selling—it is a choice. Don't accept a sales position because you don't mind selling. Truly excellent membership representatives love the sales process.

- Know your big picture in life. Think about what you want for yourself over the next year, 5 years, and 10 years and break it down into five categories: personal, physical, financial, spiritual, and relationships. Write out your goals for these areas and stay on track with them.

- Keep visual reminders of your life goals. Magazines, catalogues, and photos are good resources for visual images that reinforce what you want. When you find the image that fits what you are working toward, cut it out and paste it into a book and review the book regularly.

- Know your sales goals and stay on track with them. Know what your monthly goals break down to on a daily basis, and never let yourself get more than 2 days behind before you catch up. It is a lot easier to make smaller corrections than it is to make a big one.

- Read industry publications. Stay abreast of what others in the industry are doing in order to confirm your good work and get new ideas.

- Read sales books and listen to sales tapes. There is an abundance of industry-specific and nonindustry sales material that will rocket your performance ahead.

- Listen to motivational tapes. Motivational tapes help us to break out of a rut and see things in an entirely new light.

- Role-play with your coworkers. Most membership representatives hate role-play, but it shortens their learning curve and speeds them to higher sales results. Take 20 minutes once per week and role-play whatever aspect of the sales process you want to improve.

- Have weekly sales meetings, which can be a huge motivational tool when done correctly. When you attend, be prepared to participate and learn.

- Proactively seek help with your sales performance. Don't wait for the sales director to inform you that you are not performing to the expected level. "I need your help" will be music to your sales director's ears and hasten your success.

- Use the club. It seems obvious, but when we are regular club users, we can fall into the habit of doing the same thing over and over again. Try everything in your club. Use all the equipment, take all the classes, swim in the pool, have a massage—the variety will help you to sell those areas even better.

- Brainstorm on urgency. Be clear about all the reasons a prospective member should join today versus come back. By creating urgency in the sales process (having prospective members join the first visit), we build momentum.

- Eat well and get rest. In selling you have to be 100% on all the time. Make sure you are taking breaks throughout the day and eating. It's hard to stay motivated when you are starving and exhausted.

- Commit to your own success. Promise yourself that you will do whatever is ethically and legally possible to be successful in your position. Commitment doesn't guarantee success, but lack of commitment guarantees you'll fall far short of your potential.

- Motivation is like bathing—if you don't do it every day, you could stink. If you don't motivate yourself every day, your sales could stink.

Since you usually get what you expect in life, expect the best for yourself.

3. Introduce your full name as a matter of professionalism.

4. If the person doesn't have an appointment, state your position and offer to answer any questions.

5. Avoid asking, "How are you today?" It is a nervous filler question that is irrelevant to the scenario, especially if it is the first time you are meeting this person.

6. End the introduction with a question that is relevant to the process—take the lead.

By starting the process with a strong, simple introduction, you set the stage for your professionalism and credibility. This is critical in the process of building rapport. Have you heard that people decide in the first 7 seconds whether or not they like you? It is unfortunate and true. Think about your own experience. We often make a quick decision based upon appearance, initial action, or conversation. In sales, this can be deadly. In addition to your introduction, the following factors can affect how the prospective member perceives you:

Breath	Voice tone and
Oral hygiene	volume
Physical hygiene	Eye contact
Physical appearance	Nonverbal skills
Choice of clothing	Facial expression
Vocabulary	Energy
Presentation skills	

All of these factors have a major impact on our relationship with the prospective member, but the last one is especially important. The energy factor is how you relate to prospective members based on their energy. Think of a scale with 0% being asleep and 100% being bouncing off the walls.

Most prospective members fall between 30% and 50% when they come into the club for their first meeting with you. To maximize the rapport-building process, you want to match their energy and be just a hair above it. Therefore, if the prospective member comes in at 35%, you want to be at 40%. If you were at 100%, the prospective member would be trying to figure out if you were for real. Take a few seconds to read prospective members' nonverbal communication (e.g., facial expression, posture, fidgeting, curiosity) in order to gauge their energy level before you approach them.

THE BOTTOM LINE

Meet people where they are rather than expecting them to come to your energy level right away. The trust will start to build and they will move in your direction.

Once you have introduced yourself, the process has begun. From this point on, you want to have your process in place. However, remember that it is not mechanical or interrogational; it is conversational. This means you are going to need to be an expert listener. As you ask questions, listen and respond based on the answers. Don't simply ask the questions on your list regardless of what the prospective member has just said. Certainly, you want to have questions that will allow you to move through the process, but the key is to remain conversational.

Open the conversation to further build rapport rather than just going right into the needs assessment. For example, use the guest card and the information the prospective member has given you. Make sure you are using vocabulary that is relevant to the prospective member from a cultural perspective and technical level. If the person is wearing something of note—a piece of jewelry, a shirt from your alma mater, something unique or recognizable—comment on it and develop a conversation about it if the conversation is there. Most important of all, you must be present and listen to the prospective member.

Keys to Effective Listening

Most of us believe we are effective listeners, but research indicates that most of the time we listen at about 25% of our potential, which means that we ignore, distort, misunderstand, or forget 75% of what we hear. Lazy listening ends up costing a great deal in lost sales, misunderstandings between members and staff, and miscommunication among staff members.

We seem to think that if we tell prospective members a bunch of stuff, then they'll want to join. But how do you know what they want you to tell them if you are constantly talking and not listening? To be effective, you should be speaking about 30% of the time and listening 70% of the time. Listen to your coworkers when they give tours and have them listen to you to see what the reality of that equation is.

There is no doubt that being a great listener is a challenge. You must hear information from the speaker, give it meaning, determine how you feel about it, and respond, all in a matter of seconds. That's a lot of processing! Fortunately, the following steps will help you do just that:

1. *Hear.* When conversing, let the other person speak with no interruptions from you. Leave a moment of silence to ensure the person is done for the time being. This may be difficult for those of us who are not so comfortable with silence.

2. *Interpret.* After you hear what has been said, it's time to interpret the message. Interpretation includes not just the words but also the tone, nonverbal cues, and our own filters. Filters include our perceptions, memories, biases, expectations, attention span, feelings, needs, and so on.

3. *Evaluate.* Here is where we may start speaking. Ask questions and analyze the information without jumping to conclusions.

4. *Respond.* After we hear, interpret, and evaluate, we can confidently make thoughtful responses that reassure the speaker that the message was heard, understood, and evaluated properly.

Effective listening requires all of these steps, but too often we shortcut the process by going directly from hearing to responding. Some factors that cause this include the following:

- Our own filters
- Fatigue
- Lack of focus
- Mental overload
- Being harried
- Sales styles
- Distractions
- Lack of training

Fortunately, we can become better listeners in a relatively short amount of time. Here are some guidelines to assist you with this process:

- Take notes.
- Slow your mind.
- Slow your mouth.
- Control distractions.
- Control your emotional buttons.
- Repeat important points.
- Show interest.

- Pay attention to nonverbal cues.
- Be a whole-body listener.
- Ask open-ended questions.

To put these into action, catch yourself in the act of not listening. Then, substitute the bad habit with one of the new habits from this list. If you start consciously practicing better listening skills, you'll find the results are worth it. If you have only been listening 30% of the time and make the switch to listening 70% of the time, that is a 130% increase in effectiveness. A 130% increase in effectiveness would have a phenomenal impact on your sales production. As a bonus, if you take that 130% increase in listening effectiveness and extend it beyond your professional life into your personal life, your relationships will reach new heights.

Emotional Connection in the Sales Process

When prospective members don't join the club on the first visit, most membership representatives believe it is for one of the following reasons:

- They lack motivation.
- They are not the true decision maker at home.
- They are unable to make an exercise program work in their schedule.
- They aren't financially qualified.
- They have to get in shape before joining the club.

Indeed, some of these reasons may be the cause of prospects not joining. All are external reasons, which would indicate that the reason they didn't become a member appears to have nothing to do with the membership representative.

There is, however, another side to this picture—the internal aspect that offers other reasons prospects don't buy on the first visit:

- We don't prepare properly.
- We don't ask the right questions.
- We don't create and sustain trust.
- We don't create value.
- We present the buying question too soon.

This section will focus not on technique, but complementing your professional sales skills with an emotional connection that inspires the prospect to join today. The goals in creating an emotional connection are facilitating the buying process, building trust, keeping the new member as a long-term member, and creating a referral stream. As you read on, keep this thought in mind: You can earn a commission using a sales technique, but you can earn a fortune building relationships.

Trust Busters   What makes prospective members not trust us? Following are several trust busters:

- Preconceived notions the prospective member has about the industry as well as salespeople in general
- Preconceived notions on our part about the prospective member
- Inappropriate appearance (i.e., if we are dressed unprofessionally)
- Inappropriate demeanor (i.e., vocabulary that is too technical, abrasive, or negative; keeping prospects waiting; not following through on what you say you're going to do; faking answers you don't know)
- Needing to make a sale rather than simply wanting to get the prospect involved in the best program

Selling styles can also be trust busters. Table 8.1 compares three trust-busting styles with trust-building styles. Review them and see where your sales style falls.

Trust Musts   Now that we have identified what will bust the trust, let's focus on the trust musts that create an emotional connection. Trust musts include the following:

- Listening to understand, not to reply
- Analyzing needs to avoid forcing a fit with the club
- Maintaining warm, focused eye contact
- Showing respect for prospects
- Talking to them on their level
- Repeating points that are important to them without sounding like a parrot
- Having passion for what you do
- Maintaining composure at all times, especially when they express objections
- Offering guarantees that you can support (e.g., satisfaction guarantees, program guarantees, pricing)

Now that we have removed trust busters and checked our trust musts, we're on the way to creating an emotional connection in the selling process. The following tips will get you the rest of the way there:

1. Know prospective members' true motivation (not just their interests and needs) and use this knowledge throughout the tour to build desire. For example, when they tell you what their goals are, your next question could be, "It sounds as though you're very clear about your goals. What's your motivation for getting there?"

2. Use feeling questions throughout your introduction and club presentation.

   An example would be, "Tell me what it's like for you when you feel your absolute best. When was the last time you felt that way?"

3. Help them to visualize their results and being a part of the club.

4. Genuinely agree with them when appropriate.

5. Build urgency based on their motivation, the programs, and promotions throughout the tour.

6. To create a stronger bond and a more immediate feeling of belonging, introduce staff and members who are relevant to the prospective member's needs.

7. Have a genuine interest in prospective members' success in achieving their health and fitness goals. When you are only looking for your own immediate gratification (i.e., commission), that success is short lived. When you have a hand in someone else's success, that connection can last a lifetime.

Certainly, there are many ways to sell memberships. Choose the style that provides the least resistance and the highest return, which is typically based on the professional sales skills of preparing, professional questioning, creating value, building rapport, building trust, creating emotional connection, and asking for the sale. Examining your style for these qualities will assist you in mastering emotional connection.

Performing a Needs Assessment and Asking Qualifying Questions

Now that we have established trust, honed our listening skills, and started building an emotional connection, we can move forward with the **needs assessment** and qualifying questions, two critical elements in the sales process that often end up being rushed or missed altogether. These two elements allow you to investigate

Table 8.1 Comparison of Sales Techniques

Trust busters	Trust builders
Focus on closing: Disregards any rapport building, needs assessment, qualifying, or customization and puts a lot of energy into the tail end with the close. Feels like a hard sell.	*Focus on building rapport:* By focusing on the front end with more rapport, needs assessment, qualifying, and customization, the focus becomes needs and solution based. Feels genuine to the buyer.
Pitch products: Becomes canned and focuses primarily on features. Often irrelevant to the buyer. A fast answer is ready for everything.	*Listen and learn:* Allows you to zero in on the details the buyer wants most. Customized to the buyer.
Overcome objections: Doesn't give the prospect a chance to express emotions or real concerns. Can become adversarial. Often involves outdated closing techniques.	*Resolve concerns:* Invites the buyer to open up. Your response becomes more investigative or consulting versus simply responding with an answer (e.g., "Can you tell me more about that?"). Tendency is to reach a natural conclusion and mutual commitment that joining is the right fit for the buyer.

what will and will not allow prospective members to join the club today. In addition, they provide information that allows you to do the following:

1. Build desire on the tour.
2. Create urgency.
3. Understand the prospective member's concerns before they become objections.
4. Handle objections while on the tour.

Needs Questions

Needs questions will tell you why the prospective member is interested in joining. They cover interests, needs, and motivation and should be asked before the tour in order to be the most useful. Usually the conversation goes something like this:

Membership representative: "Bob, what would you like to do at the club?"

Bob: "Well, I'd like to play some basketball, maybe swim a bit, and lift weights."

At this point, the membership representative has discovered what Bob is interested in but has not yet uncovered Bob's needs. To do that, the conversation should progress as follows:

Membership representative: "Well, Bob, we certainly can provide excellent programs and equipment for you in those areas. Tell me, what is it that you want to accomplish with basketball, swimming, and weights?"

Bob: "I'd like to work on my coordination, my heart, and my strength."

The membership representative has now discovered Bob's true needs. Read on as the representative uncovers the motivation:

Membership representative: "It looks like you have some pretty clear goals in mind. Kudos to you, because most people aren't quite so clear about their goals. Do you mind if I ask what is motivating you to have those goals?"

Bob: "Well, I used to play basketball in high school and we have our 20th reunion coming up. During the reunion there's a basketball tournament and it's been a while since I've played."

Too often, we go only as far as the interests or activities that the prospective member wants and mistake those for needs. We need to continue to probe for the needs and motivation. The motivation is imperative since it is the force that causes any of us to act on something. Furthermore, it allows you to build urgency for the prospect without appearing pushy because you are using their motivation instead of yours for them to join.

THE BOTTOM LINE

If we use prospective members' motivation for them to join, the process becomes much more genuine and more powerful; when we use our motivation, it comes across as pushy.

Read on to see how their motivation can help create urgency:

Membership representative: "Oh, your 20th reunion. So you want to play well, feel good, and look good. How much time do we have to accomplish your goals?"

Bob: "The reunion is in 3 months."

Membership representative: "No worries, Bob. Your timing is great. If we start now, we can make it happen."

Qualifying Questions

At this point, the membership representative has enough information to know what will make Bob say *yes*, but not enough information to understand what will make Bob say *no*. Now is where the **qualifying questions** come in to uncover any concerns before they become objections after the tour. You never want to find yourself giving a great tour with energy and rapport and then losing your momentum because a bunch of objections are thrown at you later. By asking qualifying questions before the tour, you can uncover problems and have more time to work through them while you are on the tour.

Qualifying questions uncover the five major areas of concern before they are expressed as objections.

- Eagerness and motivation to join
  - Question: "When are you planning on making your decision to start a fitness program?" or "When are you wanting to start your membership?"
  - Concern expressed: "I want to think about it," "I'm shopping around," or "I'm not sure I can commit."
- Decision-making ability
  - Question: "Is there anyone else who will need information on this decision?"
  - Concern expressed: "I need to talk with my spouse (doctor, insurance company, employer)."
- Time availability
  - Question: "How many days a week are you planning on using the club?" and "What time of day works best in your schedule?"
  - Concern expressed: "I don't think I can make time in my schedule," or "I'm too busy."

- Financial ability
  - Question: "Our membership rates range from _____ to _____. Does that fit with what you have in mind?"
  - Concern expressed: "I can't afford it," or "It costs too much."
- Other limitations
  - Question: "Assuming you feel that the club works for you, is there anything that would hold you back from joining today?"
  - Concern expressed: "I don't live here yet," "I am recovering from an injury," "I have to get in shape before I join," and so on.

These qualifying questions will help you to uncover any concerns that may exist. When you uncover the concerns, they should not always be handled at that moment. This is still before the tour, which means it is fairly early in the sales relationship and you don't want it to feel adversarial. Concerns or objections are best handled on the tour.

Building Desire on the Tour

The purpose of the club tour is twofold: to create differentiation between your club and the other facilities in town and to build desire for the prospective member to purchase membership. This section will cover some of the most effective ways to build desire. Too often, we become tour guides, giving tours that are informative but not very exciting for prospective members. When we build desire, we are taking the information they have already given us and using it to build anticipation for them to become members.

Some foundational elements need to exist before you can build desire on the tour. These elements include the pretour work:

1. Building rapport and commonality
2. A strong needs assessment to understand the experience level, needs, and motivation of prospective members so that you understand what would make them want to join your club
3. A complete qualification process to understand what might make them hesitate to join your club

Once this foundation has been laid, you have the platform to build desire. Now let's look at some of the tools you can use to accomplish this goal:

- Show genuine excitement and enthusiasm for how the club will work for prospective members. Vary the tone in your voice and use other nonverbal skills such as animation of the face, smiling, raising the eyebrows, and so on.

- Customize the tour by taking prospective members to what they want to see first. This is their tour, so show them what they want to see, not what you want to show them. Avoid doing the same cookie-cutter tour every time.

- Know their motivation and verbalize it frequently on the tour. Using their motivation to join is much more powerful than using your motivation.

- Introduce prospective members to other staff throughout the tour. The purpose of this is to create as many bonds as early in the process as possible so they feel that they are a part of the club already. Of course, your staff should be warm and welcoming. Be careful when introducing a prospective member to current members, however—this can backfire unless you know the member well.

Create Urgency

Probably one of the most important ways to build desire is to create urgency. When we create urgency, we are reminding prospective members why they should join today. This element is either missing or is done incorrectly on the vast majority of tours. When it is done incorrectly, it feels like pressure, and when it is not done at all, it delays the sales process and can even lose the sale to another facility. There are three ways to create urgency: promotions and price, programs, and personal motivation.

The health and fitness industry has historically used promotions and price to create urgency, but it is not the most effective method because it is based on our motivation rather than the buyer's. It sounds like this: "If you decide to join today, we can waive your enrollment fee (add an extra month, enter you into our drawing . . .)."

Program urgency is very effective and is based on a specific starting time of a program, league, class format, and so on. If they miss the opportunity to sign up now, it would delay involvement for another 6 to 8 weeks or however long the program lasts. It sounds

Pretour Power Questions

Review the following list of pretour power questions, which will allow you to uncover needs, motivations, and qualifications. Incorporate these into your presentation to maximize your success:

- How did you hear about us?
- How much time do we have today?
- Most people join the club for one of four reasons: medical or rehab, sport performance, appearance or fitness, or social reasons. Which of these would you say is your main motivation?
- Tell me more about that.
- When was the last time you felt really good about your fitness level? What's changed?
- Would you like to go back to that same level or somewhere in between?
- Will this membership be for yourself or will someone else be involved?
- What is your time frame for making a decision?
- Picture yourself as a member 6 months down the road. Ideally, what would be different with your fitness?
- Where are you in your decision-making process?
- Tell me about your past club experiences. What did you like most at your last club? What did you like least?
- What recreational activities are you planning on incorporating into your fitness program?
- How often will you be using the club?
- What would you like to see first?
- What would you see today that would tell you this is the club for you?
- Is there anything that would hold you back from getting started today?

like this: "Tyrone, you mentioned that you wanted to start playing tennis again and need some help. Well, your timing is perfect—our beginning player clinic starts this Tuesday and we have a space available. Let's get you in there!" Program urgency is only effective if it speaks to the needs or motivation of the buyer. If your club has not offered leagues or session programs in the past, this may be a good opportunity to start offering them.

Personal motivation is the third way to create urgency and is also very effective. It is based on why prospective members told you they need the club. It is a gentle and encouraging reminder for them to not delay their results any longer. Here is what it sounds like: "Shanti, I am so glad you're here. I was thinking about what you said earlier about wanting to lose some body fat, pick up some speed, and get stronger before the summer biking season. This is the perfect time for you to start. If you start now, you'll be seeing results within a few weeks. After all, tomorrow's results start today!" Note that when you discover buyers' needs, always find out if there is a time frame with which they want to accomplish their goal. This will be a huge tool to create urgency based on their terms.

To be the most effective at creating urgency, use a combination of all three methods and use them all throughout the tour, not just at the end. If we create urgency throughout the tour, it feels more encouraging and builds excitement for the buyer.

Create Differentiation From Our Competitors

Do not read this section if you have the only club in your community, have absolutely no competition in your market, and close 100% of your sales on the first visit. If this is not the case, however, then this is the section for you! The focus of this section is how you can create differentiation in your market and in the buyer's mind on the tour.

We attempt to create differentiation in our marketing messages but often forget to do so on the tour. We sell our club, but we don't sell how our club is different from the competitors. In creating differentiation, you establish in the potential members' mind that this is the club for them, so it is paramount to your ability to confirm the sale. The best tools to accomplish this include

- establishing and using your unique selling position,
- knowing what your onlies are, and
- knowing your competition.

Let's discuss each of the three tools and how to incorporate them into your sales presentation.

Establishing and Using Your Unique Selling Position   Your unique selling position refers to the characteristics that favorably differentiate you from your competitors. It is an honest benefit statement that caters to the specific needs of the prospective member. It is based on six elements: programs, services, staff, equipment, facilities, and philosophy. Within these six categories, you need to determine what your club does or has that is different. Most facilities base their unique selling position on features rather than on philosophy, which can be dangerous because your competitors can duplicate anything you do that is feature oriented. They cannot, however, duplicate your philosophy and thus the delivery of that philosophy. Your philosophy is typically focused on who and how you serve. Take some time to develop and simply articulate the philosophy that makes your club different. Once this has been articulated, the entire staff should understand it and be able to deliver it both verbally and in their actions.

How you will integrate this unique selling position into your tours and conversations is simple. It sounds like this:

> "Brian, you mentioned earlier that you're concerned about not coming to the club regularly and getting the value from your membership. What you will find makes us different from the other clubs in town is that on a monthly basis, we print a report of all members who have not been in the club during the previous month. We then contact those members to determine how they can best use their memberships. What that means to you is that we don't let you slip through the cracks and waste your membership. Does that sound like it would benefit you?"

Knowing What Your Onlies Are   Onlies are similar to the unique selling position. An only is something that is exclusive to your facility, tends to be more feature oriented than benefit oriented, and is specific to the needs of the buyer. If onlies are not related to the buyer's needs, they are irrelevant. They can be mentioned in the following way:

> "Alison, you mentioned you spend the majority of your time with free weights—you'll be interested to know that we are the only club in the city whose dumbbells go in 2.5-pound (1-kilogram) increments instead of 5-pound (2.25-kilogram) increments."

Know Your Competition The only way you can develop and use a unique selling position or onlies is if you know your competition. Go to all of your competitors every 2 to 3 months and research what they offer in terms of programs, service, staff, equipment, facility, and philosophy. It is critical to stay abreast of your position in the market based on the position of your competition. The best way to approach this is honestly rather than sneakily. You are visiting the competition to determine their strengths and weaknesses in the areas of onlies, not for a sales tour. Before going to your competitor, phone the club manager or owner with the following:

> "Hi, Jorge, this is (your name) with (your club) and I'm calling because we would like to come over and see your club. I'd like to have you show me around and schedule some time for you to come over and see our club as well. When would be a good time for both?"

By being honest and upfront, you minimize the defensiveness of the competitor and maximize the results of your visit and the relationship.

Once you have scheduled the appointment, take the analysis form (Competition Analysis on page 164) with you and peruse it in the car before you go into the facility. By reviewing it beforehand, you'll have a more specific idea of what to look for. Do not take this form with you into the club, however.

By using the tools of a unique selling position, onlies, and knowing your competition, you will not only be able to sell your club but sell how your club is different from the competitors and ensure that buyers need not look further. When we create differentiation, we expedite the sales process in a gentle and educated way.

Ask Trial Close Questions

Trial close questions are a terrific tool for membership representatives to test the waters and monitor the interest level of the prospective member. The purpose of the trial close is to

- affirm the buyer's enthusiasm,
- uncover any remaining concerns,
- handle those concerns, and
- give you the perfect opportunity to ask the prospective member to join.

All of these points are critical in the sales process. However, most membership representatives don't ask any trial close questions at all.

Therefore, when they ask prospective members to join, they have no idea what they might be dealing with in terms of enthusiasm level or concerns. By asking trial close questions, you end up expediting the sales process because you know exactly what the prospective member is thinking and feeling at the time and dealing with it immediately.

Depending on the size of your club, you can ask 5 to 9 questions. It is important that you vary the questions so you don't sound like a parrot repeating the same thing over and over again. Additionally, when you ask trial close questions, you want the delivery to be conversational, not confrontational. Thus, you will need to practice asking the questions so you are comfortable enough to deliver them conversationally.

The best times to ask trial closes so they come across naturally include the following:

- As you show a part of the club: "Sara, this is our yoga studio. How does it feel to you?"

- As you leave a part of the club: "Raj, does it look like our free-weight room has what it takes for you to get the workout you want?"

- Hallways or transition areas: "Denise, from what you've seen in the club so far, does it feel like the club will work for you?"

As you can see, trial close questions can be open-ended or closed-ended questions. Can you see how the three sample questions would reveal the prospective member's level of enthusiasm or concern and give you an opportunity to handle those concerns? Additionally, they give you an opportunity to ask the prospective member to join if the time is right. For more examples, peruse the following list of trial close questions:

- "Is the club what you expected?"
- "Where do you think you'll be spending most of your time in the club?"
- "How does the club feel to you?"
- "On a scale of 1 to 10, where is the club for you?"
- "Does it look like we'll be able to meet your needs?"
- "Do we have what you're looking for?"
- "Is this the kind of class that would work for you?"
- "So, do you think you'll join?"

Competition Analysis

Evaluator _____ Date _____ Time _____

Club name _____ Phone _____

Address _____

Price structure	Enrollment	Monthly dues	Annual dues
Individual			
Couple			
Family			

Facilities

Group exercise rooms # _____   Approximate ft^2 (m^2) _____

Floor type _____   Classes/wk _____

(Attach schedule)

Free weights (selection rating 1 2 3 4 5 6 7 8 9 10) Size S M L XL

Selectorized machines: Type _____ # _____

Separate women's area _____ Size S M L XL Type of equipment _____

Circuit training area _____ # of stations _____ Type of equipment _____

Classes/wk _____

Cardio area equipment type and # of each _____

_____

_____

Spinning studio size _____ # of bikes_____ Classes/wk _____

Aquatic facilities: Indoor lanes # _____   Outdoor lanes # _____

Racquetball _____ # of courts _____ Charges _____

Squash _____ # of courts _____ Charges _____

Tennis _____ # of courts _____ Charges _____

Basketball _____ # of courts _____ Charges _____

Volleyball _____ # of courts _____ Charges _____

Track _____ Laps for 1 mile (1.5 kilometers) _____

Child care _____ Hours available _____ Charge/child/h_____

Tanning _____ # of beds _____ Charge _____

Massage _____ # of rooms _____ Charge _____

Fitness testing services _____ Charge _____

Personal training _____ Charge _____

Pro shop _____ Type of products _____

Beverage bar_____ Beer, wine, juice, smoothies _____

Restaurant/snack shop description _____

Spa facilities description _____

Sauna _____ Men's _____ Women's _____ Coed _____

Steam _____ Men's _____ Women's _____ Coed _____

Whirlpool _____ Men's _____ Women's _____ Coed _____

Locker-room size _____ Amenities _____ Condition _____

Other facilities not listed _____

Major points of differentiation from the market _____

Rating	Very poor				Average				Excellent	
Outside appearance	1	2	3	4	5	6	7	8	9	10
Cleanliness	1	2	3	4	5	6	7	8	9	10
Smell	1	2	3	4	5	6	7	8	9	10
Atmosphere	1	2	3	4	5	6	7	8	9	10
Attitude of staff	1	2	3	4	5	6	7	8	9	10
Attitude of members	1	2	3	4	5	6	7	8	9	10

From M. Bates, 2008, *Health Fitness Management*, 2nd ed. (Champaign, IL: Human Kinetics).

Rating (continued)	Very poor				Average				Excellent	
Energy of club	1	2	3	4	5	6	7	8	9	10
Equipment condition	1	2	3	4	5	6	7	8	9	10
Location	1	2	3	4	5	6	7	8	9	10
Visibility	1	2	3	4	5	6	7	8	9	10
Parking	1	2	3	4	5	6	7	8	9	10
Club condition	1	2	3	4	5	6	7	8	9	10
Greeting/good-bye	1	2	3	4	5	6	7	8	9	10

From M. Bates, 2008, *Health Fitness Management*, 2nd ed. (Champaign, IL: Human Kinetics).

Of equal importance to asking the trial close questions is your response to the answers. When you ask a trial close question, listen for one of three types of answers: very enthusiastic, lukewarm, or negative.

If you hear an enthusiastic answer, terrific! This is a green light for both you and the prospective member. If you hear a lukewarm or apathetic answer, don't let it go—probe it. For example, if you know Sara is looking for a great yoga program and you ask, "Sara, how does the yoga studio feel to you?" and Sara responds unenthusiastically with, "Uh, it's nice," don't just let it go. Probe it by asking further but with a soft delivery, "I thought you would be more excited about our yoga studio. Tell me what you're thinking." Trial closes help you to move forward—don't allow yourself to stumble by not probing when you get an answer that is less than enthusiastic or even negative.

When you ask the appropriate number of trial close questions throughout your tour and probe the answers to understand how the prospective member feels, you will know when it is time to invite that person to join. Trial closes allow you to get to this step smoothly, professionally, and confidently.

Handle Concerns or Objections on the Tour

The majority of membership representatives handle objections in two ways: at the end of the tour or not at all. Neither of these choices is optimal, the second choice for obvious reasons and the first choice because it is predictable and tends to build pressure for both the buyer and the seller.

Typically we fall into this habit simply because we have not done our due diligence and therefore do not have the tools to know what the concerns are. There is also a part of us that does not want to hear *no*.

As a more effective alternative, enhance your sales skills by handling objections while on the tour instead of waiting until the end of the tour. The benefits of handling objections on the tour include increased comfort, less pressure, a more conversational style, and a lighter energy, which all add up to a more conducive buying scenario. Picture this: You are walking through the club with the prospective member, who has a concern about whether she can fit club use into her schedule. At that point, a conversation such as the following may be appropriate:

Membership representative: "Maria, I was thinking about what you said earlier about being able to get into the club as much as you want. It strikes me that with how much you like this area, it will motivate you to come into the club. What are your thoughts on that?"

Maria: "You're right, I do love it. But I'm still a bit concerned that I'll join and not come in enough to get my money's worth."

Membership representative: "Hm, I can see what you're saying. It sounds as though it is a value concern for you. Is there anything else that might hold you back from feeling that the club would work for you?"

Maria: "No, that's it."

Membership representative: "OK. Would it be all right if we took a few minutes to see how this could work for you?"

Maria: "Yeah, I would really appreciate that."

Membership representative: "Super—I'm glad you're willing. Let's start with small steps. We want you to be successful and feel good about your decision with the club. Let's figure out where we can find an hour twice a week in your schedule. When do you typically have the least amount of activity or demand on your time?"

Maria: "That's a hard one. I'm always on the go. I have meetings in the evenings and my lunches are usually scheduled as well. I'm all over the place."

Membership representative: "It does sound like you're busy. Maria, let's go for two mornings a week before work. Come in by 6 a.m. and we can make sure you get your spin class in and have a strength workout before we get you to your office by 8 a.m. How does that work for you?"

Maria: "Six a.m.? I can't commit to that twice a week!"

Membership representative: "OK. Let's do one day during the week at 6 a.m. and then a weekend day of your choice for a more leisurely pace. How does that sound for starters?"

Maria: "Oh, I like that. I can do that."

Membership representative: "Excellent. I know that you'll be happy with that decision."

In this conversation, the membership representative handled the concern in a matter of 1 to 2 minutes in a conversational way as she and Maria were in an area that was particularly appealing to Maria. The conversation could occur as you are standing in such an area or perhaps walking and talking. This allows you to skip the pressure of sitting down after the tour to go over concerns or handle objections.

In addition, the membership representative proactively brought up the concern rather than waiting for Maria to bring it up at the end. This style eliminates pressure because the element of surprise is removed since you are simply discussing a point in a conversation that was brought up earlier.

Thus, to handle objections on the tour successfully, there are a few things you will need to do:

- *Qualify before the tour.* Qualifying questions differ from needs assessment questions in that needs questions tell you why the prospective member wants to join the club. Qualifying questions tell you what might hold the prospective member back from joining today. The sooner you have this information, the more time you will have to work through the concerns on the tour. Therefore, ask these questions before the tour.

- *Use 5 to 9 trial close questions on the tour.* Remember that these questions assist you in accomplishing four things: affirming enthusiasm, uncovering remaining concerns, handling objections on the tour, and assessing the buyer's position.

- *Use the seven steps for handling concerns.* This method is outlined here:

1. Listen to the concern with no interruptions.

2. Paraphrase the concern so you know you understand what was said and the prospective member knows you understand.

3. Isolate the concern (determine that what was expressed is the only concern or that there may be more).

4. Question the concern, which simply means asking if it is appropriate to find a solution.

5. Provide a solution. Here is where you will continue to probe and ultimately come to a solution that works for both the prospective member and the club. The solution may be right on the tip of your tongue or you may need to be a little more creative. Take your time here—it is not a race to see who can speak first or fastest.

6. Confirm that the solution you offered works for the prospective member.

7. Make the offer to join once the solution has been confirmed.

By handling the prospective member's concerns on the tour, you change the entire dynamic of the sales process, resulting in a more comfortable buying scenario, which typically results in more buying. When buyers trust the seller, they are more likely to purchase. Handling objections on the tour makes you more trustworthy and professional, and it differentiates you from your competitors and produces more first-time closes than handling objections at the end of the tour.

To incorporate this style into your sales presentation, practice the simple steps described in this section: qualify before the tour, bring the concerns up while on the tour, ask trial close questions to probe, and use the seven steps for handling concerns. Give yourself 30 days to become proficient with this style and you will experience a noticeable difference in your sales results.

Presenting the Price

You've just done a fabulous job with a prospective member. You built rapport to a point where you both felt comfortable, the trust was high, you qualified him, and he's a hot prospect. You masterfully did the needs assessment and you know the club can meet his needs. On the tour you escalated his desire even higher. You tested the waters with trial closes and he's ready to sign up. You sit down to do the price presentation with him, however, and the energy changes, he decides he needs to think about it for a while, and he leaves without joining today.

What happened here? Aside from not handling the objection, it could have something to do with how the prices were presented. This section will focus on how you can present prices in a more masterful way and thus improve your first-time closing rate.

Seven Steps for Presenting the Price

A smooth and confident price presentation can make or break the close. Presenting the prices is not the close; the close should take place far before you go over the price details. If you wait until the price presentation, you make price the focus of the close and put yourself at a disadvantage. When presenting prices, follow these seven steps:

1. *Get out of your own head.* Oftentimes we apologize for our prices because we either don't think the club is worth what we are asking or because we might not be able to afford to be a member at the club. This attitude comes across and poisons the way we sell.

2. *Financially qualify the prospective member within the first 3 to 5 minutes.* You should ask your qualifying questions before the tour to uncover concerns before they become objections. A good

choice to uncover any financial concerns would be, "Malcolm, what price range are you considering for membership?" He will respond in one of two ways: He will say, "I'm not sure, how much does it cost?" or he will tell you what he has in mind.

If he is unsure of what he can spend, begin with, "Malcolm, our memberships at the ABC Club start at $45 per month and go to $75 per month. Does that fit with what you have in mind?" If it does, he's qualified and you can continue with your other qualifying and needs analysis questions. If at any point before you go on tour he starts to ask detailed questions about the different memberships in the range you just gave, simply respond with, "Since it looks like our range fits with your range, let's wait to go over those details until after you've seen the club—it'll make a lot more sense then."

If he responds with a number that works with the pricing structure, then your response should be along the lines of, "Excellent! We have several programs that will work for you." If he responds with a number that does not work with your pricing structure, you should respond with, "Our memberships at ABC Club start at $45 per month and go to $75 per month. Are you firm at $35 or can you stretch a bit?" If he can stretch, you'll know he has just qualified himself financially and price will not be an issue.

If the pricing does not fit with what he had in mind and if he cannot stretch, then you may want to respond with, "Malcolm, I can understand that the membership price may not work for you, so we have two options at this point. If you don't feel as though you want to take the time to see the club, I understand; however, know that I would love to show you the club." By doing this, you are gracefully giving him an option to leave without feeling embarrassed and you are still letting him know that you want him to see the club. If he leaves, that's OK—he wasn't financially qualified.

3. *Relax—they've already said yes.* Since you've already verified that pricing isn't an issue, if you aren't confident in presenting the pricing, prospective members will get a mixed message. Continue to support their decision with positive language and genuine enthusiasm. The more comfortable you are with the numbers and membership options, the easier this becomes. Additionally, slow down when you speak. Being able to relax during the price presentation simply takes practice, so frequently role-play price presentation.

4. *Have a professionally printed price sheet with options.* List no more than four options on a price sheet so it doesn't get confusing for the prospect. If there are too many options, it's too much to think about and make an immediate decision. Simplify your pricing structure and printed presentation to encourage an easier decision-making process. On the other hand, clubs that offer only one option end up shooting themselves in the foot. You always want to offer a choice so that a choice can be made; otherwise, the only choice is whether the membership does or does not work.

5. *Always start with your most expensive membership and address it as your most popular membership.* If that membership doesn't work, you can always go down to the next option, but if you start in the low or middle range, you've limited your options. Additionally, if you start at a low or middle price, it may appear that you are tacking on extra fees for additional services. When you start high and from the perspective that this is the best membership package, you will sell more of them and if you need to go down it will be received more positively.

6. *Break the information down into smaller pieces and test the waters as you go along.* Sometimes the numbers can get confusing, so make sure you cut through the fog by breaking it down and not getting too far ahead. A big mistake membership representatives make is to present all the options all at once, speaking too quickly and leaving the prospective member confused.

7. *Close each option before you move to the next one.* How many times have you presented a price, the prospective member asks about a price lower on the sheet, you proceed to discuss that price, and the prospect responds with "OK, now what is this other price?" The problem with this is that you haven't gotten any feedback on what you presented originally—you don't know whether it will or will not work for the prospect. The best way to get this feedback is to say, "I'd be happy to tell you more about that membership. Before I do, though, tell me what your thoughts are on this price we've just gone over."

That's it—the seven steps to making your price presentation a detail and not the point. Let's take a look at the whole format put together:

"Malcolm, I'm excited you've decided to join the club today. I know you'll get what you want and more from your membership, so

let's see which one works best for you. We have a few options, and the one I'm going to recommend first is our full-service membership. It's our most popular membership because it's our best value and here's why: It includes everything you've seen in the club today plus towel service, and you get privilege pricing on tanning, massage, and pro-shop items. Can you see why this is our best value?"

"Now, there are two ways you can take care of your membership—you can choose the annual program or the monthly dues program. Which would you like to hear about first?"

"All right, the way the monthly dues program works is all we need to start your membership today is your enrollment fee of $125 and the monthly dues of $55. How does that work for you? Great, then let's go ahead and finish up the details."

That's all the price presentation needs to be. If Malcolm wanted to know more about the annual plan, you would have found out exactly what his thoughts were on the monthly dues, handled anything that needed to be handled, and then proceeded to close him on the annual plan. By creating this flow, you will make price a detail and not the point, and you will notice a significant increase in your first-time closing skills.

Closing the Sale on the Tour

As mentioned, most membership representatives wait until the end of the tour to close the sale, and some never even ask prospective members for their business. One study from *Sales and Marketing* magazine (1999) shows that 73% of sales reps across all industries do not ask for the sale at all. The upside is that there is an abundance of business for the membership representatives who are willing to ask for the prospective members' business.

What causes this common but costly delay? There are numerous justifications, but we will focus on the primary three.

1. *Rigid training*—Many clubs are locked into a traditional, inflexible style of training that does not allow for any spontaneity or playful creativity. Membership representatives who do too much talking and not enough listening further characterize this style.

After-Sales Service and Follow-Up

Not only have you just sold a membership, you've also gained a new long-term relationship that will be pleasurable and profitable. Often, clubs believe that all we need to do is get the member. Believe it or not, that's the easy part. Now we need to keep the member. This is what we call *retention*. The opposite of retention is *attrition*, which refers to the members we lose each year.

Attrition is one of the biggest problems facing most clubs at this time. Here is the irony: The cost of getting a new member is much higher than the cost of keeping current members. The reality of the situation is that new members are an asset that needs to be taken care of by you and the rest of the club staff. Here's a list of things you can do to make sure new members are happy with their decision and remain with the club for years to come.

1. As soon as prospective members become members, schedule their fitness assessment within 24 hours if possible. Get them in the habit right away if they are not already practicing fitness enthusiasts.

2. Get them involved with other things as well, such as a class, lesson, or social function.

3. Introduce them to as many staff members as possible so they feel a part of the club immediately.

4. Send a personal, handwritten thank-you note the day they join.

5. Call them a week later to check in and make sure they are comfortable and enjoying the club. The reception you get from this call will likely be positive. However, if there is a problem, be prepared to deal with it immediately rather than pass the buck to someone else. How expediently and gracefully you handle potential problems here will determine the propensity for longevity.

6. Call them on the first day of the month to talk about the club's referral program.

7. Call them every 2 months from the date they joined. It is crucial to maintain this relationship with your members. That way, if they have any problems, they know who to come to for resolution. In addition, they will bring their friends to you as referrals.

These seven tools are no-cost ways for you to have a positive impact on member retention and increase your referral base.

---

2. *Fear of offending*—Some membership representatives feel that asking prospective members for their business will somehow offend them. However, prospective members are actually expecting us to ask for their business and if we don't, we are sending a mixed message that perhaps their business is not that important to us.

3. *Philosophy or style*—Clubs that practice this philosophy are missing the boat. Clubs are something that people want to feel a part of. Prospective members want to be invited to join and feel that they are important.

The benefits to shifting the closing from the end of the tour to during the tour include the following:

• Relieves pressure from the buyer and the seller.

• Presentation is more conversational and thus spontaneous and natural.

• Creates more differentiation between your club and your competitors.

• Expedites the sales process.

When you ask prospective members to join and they say yes, be prepared to respond with, "That's excellent—would you like to see the rest of the club, or would you prefer to get your membership taken care of and see the club at a later time?" That may seem shocking, but what we fail to realize is that more often than not, prospective members come into the club ready to buy.

By asking the prospective member to join on the tour, you will close more sales in general. Closing on the tour reflects a delivery of confidence, professionalism, and comfort that is a refreshing departure from the canned sales styles of the past.

KEY TERMS

confirmation calls

follow-up calls

guest card

incoming calls

membership representative

needs assessment

partnership

qualifying questions

prospective member

service desk

unique selling position

REFERENCES AND RECOMMENDED READINGS

Woodard, K.D. 2000. Selling Power: 120 Ways to Sell More Club Memberships. *Sales and Marketing Magazine.* Boulder, CO.

Ury, W. 2007. *The Power of a Positive No.* New York: Bantam Books.

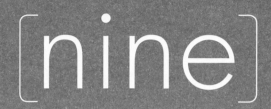

Focusing on Customer Service

Terry Eckmann

After studying this chapter, the reader will be able to

- recognize the importance of customer service,
- understand avenues of training to enhance customer service,
- explain essential communication skills for exceptional service,
- discuss emotional intelligence and self-management in customer service, and
- monitor the success of customer service.

Tales From the Trenches

Owning and operating a business sounds exciting. You can be your own boss, with no one to answer to but yourself. Sounds good in theory, but in practice owning your own business means that every person who walks through the door is your boss. Every customer is the key to determining whether or not you stay in business. It is essential as a business owner or manager to make customer service the highest priority. The team members you employ must also share the philosophy that the customer is always first. We can always learn more about how to provide quality customer service. When the student is ready, the teacher will surface.

One such customer service teacher was Susan. Susan was a front-desk manager who taught her associates new things about customer service every day. She didn't actually tell them specific tips, strategies, or techniques to provide exceptional customer service; instead she served as the customer service queen in action. She had the ability to turn some of the most difficult situations into situations with a positive outcome. Her secret? She listened. She would always seek first to understand and then she worked with the client to find an acceptable solution. What she sometimes learned was that the customer was angry and frustrated about many other things and was dumping all that emotional baggage on the first person who was in a position to listen.

One day a customer was angry because the lap swim times had been changed due to a time conflict. Susan listened as the woman screamed that she'd had it with this place and was never coming back again. When the customer seemed to have said all she was going to say, Susan said, "I am so sorry that we have inconvenienced you today. Time is such a luxury and it sounds like you really had to work to fit this into your schedule. What can we do to make this up to you?" The woman stormed out. Several minutes later she came back in the door and said, "I'm really sorry. I behaved badly and I appreciate you taking the time to listen to me vent." She went on to tell Susan about some personal problems she was struggling with at the time. She continued to be a loyal customer for many years to come.

Another key to good customer service was shared by one of Susan's older adult clients. When she would come back from spending the winter in Florida, she would share stories about all the group fitness classes she attended. She would talk about the music, the choreography, the variety of class options, and the people she met in the classes. One spring, however, she returned and had nothing to say about her group fitness classes. When asked if she was able to participate in exercise classes on her winter vacation, she said, "Yes, and I didn't like them." It turns out that the music was similar, the class options were much the same, and even the choreography in her favorite low-impact classes was similar. She said, "I just really didn't like those classes at all. You know, I went to class three times a week for an entire month and the instructor never even asked me my name." Knowing and using names is a key factor in providing exceptional customer service!

Customer service is essential for success in the fitness industry. Fitness professionals will be successful if they provide exceptional customer service, and the fitness organization will be successful if its foundation is exceptional customer service. This is because the fitness industry sells services. A product is tangible; it takes up shelf space, has a shelf life, and can be inventoried, depreciated, and taxed. A service, on the other hand, doesn't exist until a person requests or requires it. A **service** is defined as an action that one takes in order to help another person achieve a goal or objective. A **customer** is any person who requests or requires these services. Customers include every person inside and outside the organization we must interact with to perform our job correctly. **Customer satisfaction** occurs when a product or service meets or exceeds a customer's expectations.

This chapter provides an overview of customer service. Topics include the importance of customer service, the two categories of customers, what the customer wants, training staff to provide exceptional service, communicating with customers, dealing with difficult customers, and monitoring the effects of customer service.

Recognizing the Importance of Customer Service

We live in a rapidly changing world, and fitness clubs continue to be challenged by a roller-coaster economy, new competition, changing demographics, and shifts in the fitness industry. Club members are continually affected by instability at work and in personal lives. These challenges make exceptional customer service in the fitness industry an important practice every minute of every day. The goal of customer service is to create a friendly, comfortable, clean, and well-maintained environment that will retain current members and regularly draw new members. **Exceptional customer service** is exceeding the customer's expectations by going the extra mile and adding that special touch. Serving members must be the number one priority.

THE BOTTOM LINE

Successful organizations anticipate, meet, and exceed customer needs.

According to LeBoeuf (2000), the majority of customers quit doing business with a company because of indifference toward the customer by an employee. The following statistics on reasons why customers quit doing business with a company support the importance of customer service and the impact a single employee may have on customer retention.

- 1% die
- 3% move away
- 5% develop other relationships
- 9% leave for competitive reasons
- 14% are dissatisfied with the product
- 68% quit because of an attitude of indifference toward the customer by an employee

It is estimated that the average person who has a problem with a business tells 9 or 10 people about it. If one unsatisfied person tells 10 other people, and each of those people tells 5 others, then more than 60 people have heard about the problem and have a negative impression of the business. Additional bad news is that the majority of unhappy customers never complain directly to the business. The good news is that most customers who complain will continue to do business with a company if their complaint is resolved. And, happy customers who have had their complaints resolved will tell between 3 and 5 people about their positive experience.

It is important to appreciate complaining customers because they provide the opportunity to address problems and retain members. It costs five to six times more to attract new customers than to keep old ones. According to Gerson (1993), customer service is governed by the rule of 10s. If it costs $10,000 to get a new customer, it takes only 10 seconds to lose one and 10 years to get over it or for the problem to be resolved. Companies that focus on exceptional customer service will experience the most success.

THE BOTTOM LINE

Managers need to appreciate complaining customers. It is important to learn about customers' concerns and address those problems as quickly as possible.

Identifying Your Customer

Organizations have internal and external customers. **Internal customers** are all the people working in the same organization. The front-desk staff, personal trainers, group fitness leaders, program directors, maintenance workers, managers or team leaders, and any other people working for the organization are internal customers. By serving each other, employees of an organization create a positive atmosphere.

In a fitness center, the front-desk staff are the welcome committee, setting the tone for customers as they begin their experience. The front-desk staff may also be responsible for member sales and retention, customer concerns, problems or questions, and updating customers with information regarding current and future programs. These staff members provide a service to all fitness center employees by creating a positive feeling at the first point of contact and through new-member sales and member retention.

Group fitness instructors provide a service to other employees by conducting safe, effective, creative, and fun exercise classes. These classes provide a cardiorespiratory workout that creates less congestion on the cardio equipment during peak hours. Group fitness classes may include yoga, Pilates, kickboxing, step aerobics, and circuit training. The workout options available through group fitness classes give customers variety to keep them interested in getting and staying fit.

These are just a few examples of how the network within a fitness center can provide internal customer service that will affect the service provided to external customers. Providing strong internal customer service creates a positive atmosphere of teamwork and collaboration.

External customers are those people who purchase the services of a fitness professional or a fitness center. A satisfied customer will be a loyal member. A satisfied customer will also provide word-of-mouth marketing for the organization. An investment in customer service thus is a wise investment in short- and long-term marketing. Customer satisfaction is like an election that is held every day. Customers vote with their feet, and if they are dissatisfied, they will walk to the competitor. If they are satisfied, on the other hand, they will continue to walk through your door.

THE BOTTOM LINE

A customer is any person who requires or requests your services. An internal customer works for the organization, whereas an external customer purchases the services of the organization.

Understanding What the Customer Wants

In the fitness industry a customer may be called a *client, guest, patron,* or *member*. Whatever term used by the organization, it is essential to understand and respond to the wants and needs of the customer. The fitness industry is competitive and many options are available. If your organization does not meet or exceed customer expectations, the customer may do business with a competitor, purchase home exercise equipment, or not exercise at all.

Differences in perception between what a business thinks customers want and what customers actually want create poor service. It is necessary to keep in touch with customers through satisfaction surveys, advisory boards, focus groups, and wandering around and talking to customers to see what they are thinking about the services provided by your business.

The wants and needs of customers have great similarity, no matter what the business or service provided.

• *Customers want to feel welcome.* A warm greeting gives the customer an immediate sense of appreciation. Greeting customers with a friendly hello and a smile while making eye contact is the foundation of a greeting; addressing the customer by name is that little extra that can make a big difference. Customers need to be the first priority.

Visiting with a coworker, tending to paperwork, or completing tasks on the computer can send an unwelcome message if time is not taken for a brief and sincere welcome.

• *Customers expect a clean environment.* Equipment must be cleaned regularly by clients using the equipment and by staff working the floor. The base of treadmills, elliptical machines, rowers, recumbent bikes, steppers, resistance training units, hydraulic machines, and free-weight equipment can all accumulate dust, dirt, hair, and fuzz from carpets. Vacuuming and wiping down the equipment regularly keep the environment clean and welcoming for customers and increase the life of the equipment. An hourly bathroom check by employees is also a must. Placing a document on the inside of the bathroom door for employees to initial each hour as they conduct a bathroom check and quick cleanup assures customers of the commitment to a clean environment. A clean environment and a friendly atmosphere help to satisfy customers' need for comfort.

• *Customers want efficient service.* Most people have busy schedules and do not like to wait. Well-maintained equipment will help to create an environment of efficiency, and a quick and easy check-in system will keep membership records up to date and allow customers to access the facility without a wait. The facility should open on time and group fitness classes or personal training sessions should start and end on time. Peak hours should provide a system that allows all clients to have access to cardio equipment for at least 20 to 30 minutes. The system should be simple and monitored by staff so a customer doesn't have to ask another person to get off a machine. Guidelines should be in place to prevent the customer from doing multiple sets in a manner that may monopolize a piece of equipment during peak times. Of course, having an adequate selection of equipment during peak times is the ultimate in customer service, and budgeting to meet that goal is the best way to provide efficient exercise options during the busiest hours.

• *Customers appreciate solutions to problems.* Customers have a need to be understood. When they come to you with problems they have experienced in dealing with your company, it's your job to find a solution. For example, let's say a customer has purchased a 1-year membership and will have to be out of town for 6 weeks to 3 months. It is your job to determine an equitable solution through interaction with the customer. You may need to work with management to resolve the issue, but it is important not to pass the customer off without helping that person make the connection with the appropriate staff member. Customers like to be listened to when they have problems, concerns, or questions.

• *Customers expect a variety of programs that will help them reach their fitness goals.* When providing customer service at a fitness facility, it is important to consider why a customer is a member. A customer may want to lose weight, increase lean muscle mass, decrease body fat, reduce blood pressure, lower cholesterol, improve strength, increase flexibility, improve overall health, meet people, or a combination of these. Information gathered from a new member should identify goals, wants, and needs in an attempt to help that member succeed.

Weight loss is a billion-dollar industry, and people who want to succeed with a weight-management program on a long-term basis need to be involved in a regular exercise program. Sensitivity to a variety of body sizes and physical skills is important in a diverse market. Most people who become professionals in the health and fitness industry have typically been active in sport and fitness activities. People often pursue careers as personal trainers, group fitness leaders, or fitness facility managers because of personal passion for exercise and the health-related benefits associated with regular physical activity. However, this is not true for the majority of the population; for example, 60% of Americans are sedentary. In order for fitness facilities to succeed, it is essential to provide a customer service–driven environment with fitness programs that will attract a wide variety of people. A customer-focused, unintimidating environment will be more attractive to clients wanting to lose weight or change the way they look.

• *Customers expect knowledgeable, helpful staff.* It is important to make members feel comfortable when they walk in the door, and it is essential that they feel at ease as they enter a group fitness class, weight training area, or any other place in the facility. When an employee observes signs of confusion or frustration from a member, the employee should approach that member and offer assistance. Not many people are comfortable asking for help even if fitness staff members are readily available. Taking the initiative to help members who look confused can help them feel comfortable.

THE BOTTOM LINE

Understanding the specific wants, needs, expectations, and goals of a client provides an opportunity to meet and exceed them.

A staff that is well trained to meet the needs of a variety of customers is essential to the success of the organization. Every moment is a moment of truth in the fitness industry. Each encounter a member has with a staff member is important. When staff members meet the needs and wants of a customer, that person will become a loyal member.

Training Staff for Exceptional Customer Service

One of the common reasons for poor service is poor employee training. Providing excellent customer service does not cost the company much more than providing poor service. The company is already paying staff to work, and it is also spending money to train staff. Hiring positive employees and providing training specific to a customer-focused mission are key in preventing poor customer service. To prepare your employees to deliver exceptional customer service, it is important to train them to understand what exceptional customer service looks like, sounds like, and feels like, as well as how it will affect them and the company. Staff members who are well trained and deliver exceptional customer service will be happy and more likely to stay with the company. The cost of replacing an employee is much higher than the cost of training a new employee with a positive attitude.

There are a variety of training methods to prepare staff to provide exceptional customer service. The first step is to provide a visible and clear mission statement regarding the customer service philosophy of the company. Orientation of new staff should include comprehensive training of services provided by the organization that is linked to what customer service looks like in these areas. Continuing education can be provided with staff in-service sessions (conducted by a staff member or other professional), requirements to read specific material regarding customer service, attendance at training seminars, and requirements to listen to audio books or recorded seminars on customer service. However, modeling by leaders providing exceptional customer service is the best ongoing training. (For an overview of training techniques, see chapter 4.)

What to Teach

Customers will come away from every encounter with an employee feeling neutral, happy, or unhappy. To a customer, each and every employee

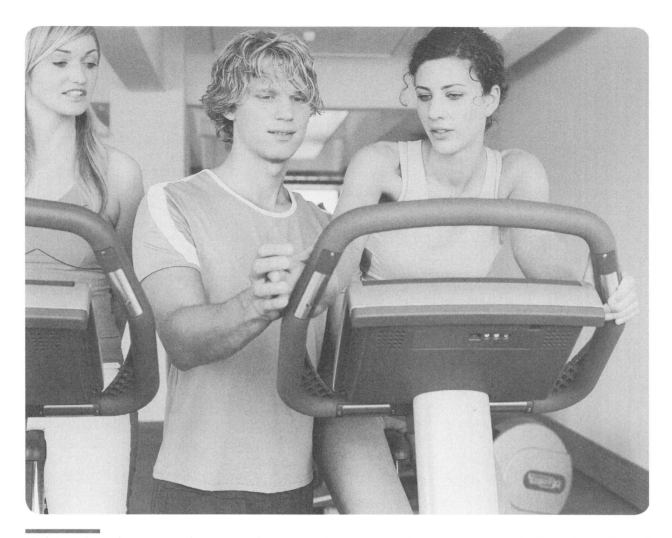

Understanding what your members want is key to providing exceptional customer service. Members of your club will certainly expect that the staff is knowledgeable and is willing to help them get the most from their membership.
© Getty Images/Joos Mind

is the company. A careless word or an indifferent attitude can ruin a customer relationship forever. On the other hand, if an employee is helpful, enthusiastic, and concerned, the customer will be impressed with the employee and the organization. All staff members have the power to make the organization successful or not based on how they treat people; thus, it is important for each and every staff member to be concerned with excellence in customer service. A fitness business will be only as good as the performance of every team member.

It is necessary to train staff on every aspect of the company that a customer may expect them to know. The staff must understand membership options, hours of service and services provided, club guidelines for safety and efficiency, emergency procedures, how to use equipment correctly, impor-

tance of exceptional customer service, and communication skills necessary to deliver that service.

Each staff member must have a thorough understanding of personal job responsibilities. These should be outlined in the job description, including position title, function of the position, department, personal and professional requirements of the position, responsibilities, and reporting relationships. Each job description needs to keep customer service as a focus. It is difficult to carry out a job without a good understanding of its responsibilities. (See chapter 3 for more on job descriptions.)

A **mission statement** with customer-focused beliefs and values sets the tone for employees. The fitness professional must know the focus of the organization, which can be identified with a well-written mission statement. If individual staff members do not understand the focus and purpose of the business, they will not have a clear understanding of why they are there and thus performance will suffer.

As mentioned, it is helpful to know what each department or employee is accountable for via job descriptions. A training checklist is also helpful to break down all job-related tasks and ensure that new employees understand what they need to do. This checklist may be as specific as smiling, using member names, and making eye contact as a member approaches the front desk.

Employee involvement in establishing customer service goals will increase commitment to achieving these goals. Customer service standards should be SMART—specific, measurable, attainable, realistic, and tracked regularly.

Accountability

Checklists for training and performance assessment ensure accountability. Accountability for customer service and other job-related tasks is essential to maximize employee performance and professional growth. Employees need specific and immediate feedback and should be rewarded when goals are met. Be consistent in catching employees doing things right and praise them immediately.

THE BOTTOM LINE

A training checklist with specific expectations will help focus service delivery.

Staff rewards can be simple and inexpensive. Positive and immediate feedback is often the best reward. Brainstorming with staff regarding desired rewards gives employees ownership in the plan. Rewards may include personal thank-you notes; a photo posted in the facility, newsletter, or local paper; a paid day off; movie coupons; a massage; lunch with the boss at a favorite restaurant; attendance at a local, regional, or national workshop; a free car wash; or a gift certificate to a local business. The best reward is often recognition and positive reinforcement for a job well done. (See chapter 5 for more on these kinds of incentives and rewards.)

When an employee continually provides inadequate customer service, it is necessary to document specific situations and provide opportunities for change. Giving feedback through conferencing can help get the employee on the right track to providing exceptional customer service. Generally, there are three types of **instructional conferences:**

- *Instructional conference that is used to accelerate growth and accentuate the positive.* The purpose of this conference is to identify and discuss the employee's customer service skills. This conference increases the probability of those behaviors continuing and improving and works best when the customer service skills are effective, the customer service representative is relatively new, and immediate feedback is possible.

- *Instructional conference that is used to address deficiencies and develop alternatives.* The purpose of this conference is to identify ineffective customer service skills and develop alternatives that will increase effectiveness and performance. Many times employees are unaware of their ineffective customer service skills and do not know how to correct the problem. The employee and manager brainstorm more effective ways to deal with weaknesses or the manager gives specific direction on how to improve. This conference is best used when the employee is relatively new or there have been observations or complaints of poor service.

- *Instructional conference that is used to ask why that employee is in the position.* The employee is creating unacceptable customer service and the situation is or may soon be out of control. The employee has made no attempt to correct the ineffective behaviors or skills. There must be an immediate action plan or else it is time to move toward job dismissal. This conference is to be used when the employee is not performing well and consistently provides inadequate customer service.

THE BOTTOM LINE

The most effective feedback is specific, immediate, and growth oriented, and it preserves the dignity of the person.

Communicating With Customers

Communication is a two-way sharing of information that results in an understanding between the receiver and the sender. Because each person filters everything that is heard and seen through a filter system of values, experiences, beliefs, and culture, perceptions of what a speaker says may be different from what the listener hears. Communication is 7% verbal, 38% intonation, and 55% body language. Most communication is sent through body language and other nonverbal forms of communication.

Be Aware of Nonverbal Communication

Nonverbal communication sends approximately 93% of the message. It is possible to communicate messages through body language and vocal inflection without even realizing communication is taking place. A person's facial expressions, eye contact, body posture, and gestures all send out messages. Vocal inflection can also alter the meaning of a message, and a sigh can suggest annoyance, frustration, or impatience.

It is helpful to be aware of facial expressions when communicating with a customer. A calm, concerned, and sincere facial expression can tell customers that an employee cares. Of all the things you wear, your expression is the most important. A smile sends a welcoming and friendly message. The only time a smile is not appropriate is when a customer is expressing anger—it may communicate a mocking attitude or indicate that the employee doesn't take the customer's message seriously. Facial expressions often affect inflection of the voice. A mirror placed by the phone with a reminder to smile can actually improve phone communication. The eyes communicate a great deal in conversation. Making eye contact indicates an interest in the customer and shows that the employee's attention is on that person. Rolling eyes can indicate disgust and should be avoided.

Employees should stand and sit straight and tall in a work setting. Slouching or putting feet up on an object or desk indicates an inattentive, disinterested, and overly relaxed attitude. It sends a "don't bother me" message. Maintain a nonthreatening, open body posture and make sure to stand far enough away so the customer's personal space is not invaded. Body movement can also affect perception of interest in a customer. Moving in a slow manner, especially when working with an upset customer or a customer who is waiting for service, can send a message of disinterest. Additionally, gestures can play a role in the interpretation of a message. Crossing the arms in front of the body is a more defensive stance and may suggest an unwillingness to listen. Resting the head in the hands indicates the employee is tired and unconcerned.

Chewing gum or eating when on the phone or in public in the fitness center should be avoided. Chewing gum can be distracting and irritating to a customer who is trying to communicate with an employee. A customer may be hesitant to approach an employee eating in public view because it is personal time to take care of a bodily need. Chewing food can also be noisy and give an unwanted view of chewing food.

Vocal inflection is 38% of communication. **Attitude** is projected through tone of voice, and people will respond more to how something is said than to what is said. A voice can sound welcoming, happy, confident, interested, or friendly, or it can sound angry, irritated, disinterested, bothered, or disgusted. It may be helpful to listen to your voice on a recording to see how you sound. Speak with a calm, interested, caring, and soothing voice when working with customers.

Personal habits of dress, grooming, and cleanliness also send out messages regarding professionalism. Hair, hands, fingernails, and teeth need to be clean. Clothing should be appropriate for the setting. Inappropriately showing skin and underwear is unprofessional and should be avoided. Body piercings are growing in popularity and are somewhat controversial. Tongue rings make it difficult to understand speech and can be distracting and noisy when played with during conversation. There should be policy regarding acceptable body piercing in the workplace.

THE BOTTOM LINE

It is not what you say, but what is heard. It is not what you mean, but what is understood. There is no one reality, only perception of what is said and heard.

Focus on Listening

The benefits of good listening are directly related to building the relationships that are necessary for success as a professional in the fitness business. **Listening** is the receiving part of communication. We receive information through the ears and eyes, attach meaning to information, and decide what we think or feel about that communication. Stephen Covey (1999) promotes seeking first to understand and then to be understood. It is common to wait for our turn to talk instead of listening for understanding; while another person is talking it is common to be formulating thoughts for a reply.

Listening for understanding is a valuable skill, and there are a variety of ways to improve listening skills. The first is to be aware of personal listening behaviors by identifying bad habits and good listening skills. Here are some suggestions for improving your listening skills:

- Stop talking.
- Check for understanding by restating; find out if what you heard was what was meant.
- Ask questions to clarify understanding of a message.
- Never make assumptions or jump to conclusions by attaching old meaning and experiences to a new situation.
- Focus on the speaker and be present. Avoid distractions.
- Watch nonverbal messages, and practice a body language of listening and interest with eye contact and an open posture.
- Listen with empathy rather than waiting for your turn to talk.
- Want to listen, and consistently think of the benefits of good listening habits.
- Make a listening action plan, identify bad listening habits, determine strategies for change, and set goals to improve listening skills.

Portray a Positive Attitude: The Power of One

As mentioned previously, each employee in an organization *is* the organization. Everything an employee does is a reflection of the organization and the person. One person can make a positive impact on the organization, and one person can make a negative impact. Unfortunately, it is the negative experience that will be most talked about and remembered. A positive attitude in customer service is essential for organizational success.

Attitude is a reflection of how you think about something or someone, and how you think about the customer is how you will treat the customer. If your attitude is positive, difficult situations are handled more effectively. To develop a positive attitude, it is important to realize that we all have control over our attitude. Attitude is a state of mind influenced by feelings, thoughts, and action tendencies; thus, it influences three things that you can control: what you think, what you say, and how you behave. We all choose our attitude about ourselves, other people, and work. An optimistic attitude is an essential attribute in providing exceptional customer service. The quality of an employee's work is a reflection of that person's attitude.

The hiring process is the beginning of employing people with positive attitudes. Fitness professionals and support staff need to genuinely believe in the positive benefits of fitness and have a desire to connect with people. Hiring people with an energetic, empathetic attitude will make it much easier for you to coach them and enhance professional growth. It is important to hire the right employees, be clear about expectations, train them based on expectations, and reward them accordingly. Job skills are easier to train than attitude—hire for attitude and train for skill.

Practice Emotional Intelligence Competencies

According to Goleman (1995, 1998), those with high emotional intelligence are the most successful in the world of work. A study conducted by Eckmann (2004) found that award-winning fitness professionals scored higher on the competencies of emotional intelligence than their non-award-winning peers. **Emotional intelligence** is the demonstration of self-awareness, self-management, social awareness, and relationship management at appropriate times. It is the ability to handle self and others effectively in a variety of situations. Research indicates that successful customer service representatives exhibit high self-control, conscientiousness, and empathy (Goleman 1998).

Self-awareness is the foundation of emotional intelligence. It includes accurate self-assessment, emotional self-awareness, and self-confidence. Accurate self-assessment is the ability to reflect on work performance and identify strengths and opportunities for improvement. Emotional self-awareness is the ability to identify feelings that may affect work performance. A person with emotional self-awareness understands the customer behaviors that may create frustration or anger. Self-confidence is confidence in personal and professional abilities. It gives employees the assurance that they have the skills and abilities to be effective in the workplace.

Understanding yourself is an important aspect of growing and learning to provide exceptional customer service. As mentioned, every person filters information through experiences, beliefs, values, gender, and relationships, and self-awareness helps you understand the factors that influence personal perception. For example, it is important to be aware that a customer's anger is not personal. Such customers may be angry about something happening in their personal life, a recent experience, or something about the organization you work for—it is not about you. This self-awareness can help to keep things in perspective.

Self-management is the ability to manage your feelings and act constructively in a stressful, fast-paced, highly competitive work environment. Strong self-management skills include awareness of your personal viewpoints and biases and your ability to respond to a variety of situations. Goleman (1995, 1998) includes achievement orientation, adaptability, emotional self-control, initiative, optimism, and transparency in the competencies that constitute self-management.

Achievement orientation is the drive to achieve excellence in achieving personal and professional goals. A person with a strong achievement orientation sets goals and works hard to achieve them. Adaptability is also an important self-management skill. It allows people to be flexible in the face of an ever-changing world. If there is any single competency needed in the fitness industry in this time of change, it is adaptability. Emotional self-control is the ability to understand your own emotions and manage them in the face of adversity. This skill is crucial in dealing with difficult customers and situations. Initiative is an essential skill of self-management. It is the ability to see and do what needs to be done to reach personal, professional, and organization goals. Optimism is the tendency to believe, expect, or hope that things will turn out well. An optimistic attitude facilitates persistence in pursuing goals despite obstacles or setbacks. Transparency is a character trait. The transparent person will keep promises, address ethical concerns, acknowledge mistakes, and act on values.

The competencies of **social awareness** include empathy, organizational awareness, and service orientation. Empathy is the ability to understand others and take an active interest in the concerns of others. The empathetic person can pick up on cues such as changes in tone of voice or facial expressions and determine how to respond according to varying moods or personality styles. Empathy is important in dealing with a diverse clientele. Service orientation is the drive to provide service to an individual, organization, or community and to make the world a better place. It is the ability to understand a customer's needs and concerns by listening and seeking understanding of the client's perspective. **Organizational awareness** is the ability to read the currents of emotions and political realities in groups and organizations. The person with organizational awareness understands the vision and mission of the organization and strives to help achieve the mission.

Relationship management comprises the competencies of change catalyst, conflict management, developing others, influence, inspirational leadership, and teamwork and collaboration. Effective professionals in the fitness industry are change catalysts. A change catalyst recognizes the need for change, removes barriers, and enlists others in the pursuit of new initiatives. It is essential to understand and facilitate change to assist others in reaching health and fitness goals. Developing others is the capacity to sense the developmental needs of others to help bolster their abilities. Fitness professionals with the ability to develop and influence others with inspirational leadership skills will provide the extra that makes a big difference. Teamwork and collaboration are also important competencies of relationship management, and the ability to work as a team demonstrates service to coworkers.

Dealing With Difficult Customers

Despite the best efforts, customer service will fail from time to time. It is best if the employee can respond on the spot to a dissatisfied customer, or as quickly as possible. Empowered employees can better serve the customer and resolve conflicts. Employees with an understanding of the importance of customer service and knowledge of how to effectively and efficiently resolve customer concerns will create an environment of customer satisfaction.

We have all heard the cliché, "The customer is always right." In actuality, the customer is not always right, but the customer is always the customer. Every customer complaint is an opportunity to create a positive relationship. The goal is to reduce the number and frequency of complaints, but complaints are truly an opportunity to improve the service of the club and build a positive relationship by turning an unhappy customer into a happy and loyal customer.

One of the most important strategies for dealing with an angry or difficult customer is to listen with empathy. Listening for understanding will often diffuse a difficult situation. Some people simply want to be heard and understood. In order to effectively listen, the employee must keep in mind that it is not a personal attack, although it may seem as if the customer is taking problems out on the employee. Listening is the skill that can have the most impact when dealing with an angry customer. You can't fix the problem until you know what it is, and if you are waiting for your turn to talk instead of seeking to understand the customer, you may miss the real problem.

As discussed previously, effective listeners are interested, patient, caring, responsive, not distracted, and not interrupting rather than impatient, uncaring, unresponsive, distracted, and interrupting. Effective listening requires you to let go of preconceived notions about the person and the situation and seek to understand the angry customer. People speak at approximately 125 to 175 words per minute (Slowik 2000); and we listen about four times faster, so a listener can easily think ahead and lose the underlying message being sent by the angry customer.

Listening to disgruntled customers can take you a long way. Working with them to achieve a win–win outcome is in the best interest of the customer, you, and the company. There will be times when angry customers are right about their situation. This is an appropriate time to go beyond listening for understanding and helping the customer to solve the problem; this is a time to go that extra mile with a complimentary service or an extension on membership. It is also important to follow up with a phone call or note to thank that customer for taking the time and energy to provide you with the opportunity to fix what went wrong.

When you are working with an angry or concerned customer, make sure that you do what you say you are going to do. If you are going to check on a policy or the possibility of another membership option, check it out and get back to the customer sooner rather than later. Prompt service is a key to customer satisfaction. It is also important to be flexible. Policies are necessary, but they can become outdated. Make sure to question the policies that often create customer dissatisfaction and anger. A policy that at one time had a purpose may no longer be necessary—don't lose people over a bad policy! Ask why the policy exists, if it still serves a purpose, and if it can be modified or thrown out to better serve the customers.

The job of the manager is to talk the talk and walk the walk of exceptional customer service. Employees often mirror the behavior of the organization leaders. A good leader is out there meeting, greeting, observing, and listening to customers. A good leader provides training for employees to prepare them to deal with difficult situations and people, and good leaders empower employees to make decisions in response to customer needs. A leader focused on customer service will consistently review policy and procedure to keep the organization focused on the changing needs of the customers and changes in the fitness industry.

Common reasons for poor service include uncaring employees, poor employee training, poor handling and resolution of complaints, employees who are not empowered to meet customer needs, and differences in what the organization thinks the customers want and what the customers actually want. Managers must stay focused on these issues to help to prevent difficult situations and angry customers.

There will be times when the angry customer is wrong and no matter what you do or say, that person is not happy. The angry, irrational customer can create a negative environment, making

Power Talking

No one likes to hear the word *no*. People don't want to hear what you cannot do for them. *Yes*, on the other hand is a powerful word that can turn a negative customer into a positive customer. A response that begins with a *yes* creates a positive perception. *Yes* sends a message that the service representative is working to accommodate the needs of the customer. Power talking is getting to *yes*—it is focusing on what can be done, as you can see in the following sample phrases.

Power talking is a way to use positive words to tell the customer what you can do. It involves avoiding blame and striving to understand the listener.

Instead of these phrases	Use these phrases
Your problem	This situation
You have to	I'd appreciate it if you'd
Don't forget	Please remember
I'll have to	I'll be glad to
I can't	I can
But	And
Spend	Invest
I disagree	I understand
You'll have to ask	I can help you by

employees and other customers uncomfortable and unhappy. Everyone seems to know this person and has the same feeling about the negative attitude that permeates the climate of the club when this person is present. It is up to the leaders in management positions to address the ongoing conflict and suggest that the customer may be happier elsewhere. The key is to recognize that the employees and organization have done everything possible to meet the customer's needs and it has become a lose–lose situation. It is best to cut ties with that customer or else lose other customers.

Monitoring the Effects of Customer Service

Everyone in an organization is responsible for delivering and measuring customer satisfaction. There are a variety of ways a business in the fitness industry can know whether its customer service is working. For starters, each new member should be asked to fill out a quick form to determine how that person learned about your business. (See chapter 8 for additional discussion of guest cards.) There may be a checklist that identifies how that person heard about the club, including the following options:

- Friend, coworker, or family member
- Radio advertisement
- Newspaper advertisement
- Television advertisement
- Local event
- Billboard
- Other _____

When customer service is working, member referrals will increase. Word of mouth can be a positive marketing tool when customer service is exceptional. Current club members will use the club more often and for longer periods of time if they feel welcome and comfortable in the environment. Former members are more likely to return if they have established relationships with club staff through positive customer service experiences. Club members and staff will be smiling and laughing if the environment is conducive to having a good time and people are happy. Members will take pride in their club. You will see members wearing club T-shirts and hats or carrying water bottles with the club logo.

When customer service is working, there will be more positive comments and fewer complaints in the suggestion box. Focus groups will come up with creative new ideas rather than dwelling on what is wrong at the club. Customer service surveys will focus on the positive experiences more than the negative ones.

Staff members are more involved in a customer service–driven organization. They take pride in the club and create a team atmosphere when customer service is working, and there are fewer problems with absenteeism and less staff turnover. Here are some ways to measure the effectiveness of customer service:

- *Focus groups.* Conducting focus groups of about 10 people who provide the club with general performance feedback or share feedback related to specific issues is a great way to improve customer service and increase retention. Focus groups can offer valuable ideas for your facility and build strong relationships with club members as you include them in the improvement process. Listening to club members in a focus group sends the message that customer opinions are important. Make the focus group experience valuable by following these guidelines:

1. Write clear goals and objectives for the meeting. Know what you want to accomplish and what open-ended questions you need to ask.

2. Select 8 to 10 people to participate in the group. It is wise to brainstorm with staff to identify between 10 and 20 people. The group should include clients who are regulars and those who come less regularly, people of different ages, men and women, and people with different ethnic backgrounds. A diverse group will provide a wider perspective.

3. It is wise to offer simple incentives to those who participate. For example, members of the focus group may receive healthy food and beverages during the group meeting and a $5 membership discount or gift certificate from the pro shop.

4. Focus groups are more likely to be honest and share thoughts and ideas if a facilitator conducts the group. The facilitator will keep the conversation focused and flowing in a nonintimidating manner.

5. Thank the focus group at the end of the meeting and with a follow-up note informing them of the action taken in response to the meeting. Meeting notes can be posted on the club bulletin board or in the newsletter.

• *Customer satisfaction surveys and inventories.* These can provide an opportunity to know what customers are thinking. They can be specific or general depending on what you want to know from the customers. It is important to follow up with those completing the surveys and inventories to show that the input they have taken the time to give you has been heard. An action plan to implement legitimate suggestions and address common concerns can help build trusting relationships with customers.

• *Advisory boards.* Advisory boards made up of club members can offer effective feedback on a regular basis to allow club owners, team leaders, and staff members to see the club from a member's perspective. An advisory board may comprise between 10 and 20 people with diverse backgrounds and a wide age range. The advisory board term may be from 1 to 5 years, and meetings may be held quarterly or monthly. Board members should receive an agenda before the meeting so they can provide input on topics generated by management and staff and consider other topics of concern or ideas for improvement. Board members should receive recognition in the club, verbal and written thanks, and a small gift for their efforts.

• *Management by wandering around.* This is a common leadership practice of successful businesses. Managers and owners must do more than talk the talk of customer service. Walking the walk of exceptional customer service by setting an example through visibility throughout the facility should happen daily. Managers, owners, and team leaders should walk around the club to provide performance feedback to staff and build relationships with members. Management by wandering around is one of the best ways to train staff, provide immediate feedback on staff performance, and consistently monitor customer service. A leader's mood and modeling can send a powerful message to employees.

• *Suggestion box.* A suggestion box is a good way to measure customer service efforts and find ways to improve service. The front desk is a good place for a suggestion box. The box should be emptied daily and given to the person in charge of following up on suggestions with members and staff. It is important to address concerns in a timely manner.

Measuring customer service quality and customer satisfaction helps to improve service and increase satisfaction. Everyone working in an organization is responsible for delivering and measuring customer satisfaction. Anything and everything that affects the customer should be measured. Performance standards and criteria that are quantifiable and that can evaluate performance via hard data are essential in order to effectively measure improvement and apply the process of continual improvement.

KEY TERMS

attitude

communication

customer

customer satisfaction

emotional intelligence

exceptional customer service

external customers

instructional conferences

internal customers

listening

mission statement

nonverbal communication

organizational awareness

relationship management

self-awareness

self-management

service

social awareness

REFERENCES AND RECOMMENDED READINGS

Blacharski, D. 2006. *Superior customer service: How to keep your customers racing back to your business.* Ocala, FL: Atlantic.

Carlaw, P., and K.V. Deming. 1999. *The big book of customer service training games.* New York: McGraw-Hill.

Cherniss, C., and D. Goleman, eds. 2001. *The emotionally intelligent workplace.* San Francisco: Jossey-Bass.

Covey, S. 1999. *The seven habits of highly effective people.* New York: Simon & Schuster.

Eckmann, T. 2004. *The emotional intelligence of award winning fitness professionals.* Doctoral Dissertation. University of North Dakota.

Evenson, R. 2005. *Customer service training 101*. New York: Anacom Books.

Gee, V., and J. Gee. 1999. *Super service: Seven keys to deliver great customer service*. New York: McGraw-Hill.

Gerson, R. 1993. *Measuring customer satisfaction*. Menlo Park, CA: Crisp.

Goleman, D. 1995. *Emotional intelligence*. New York: Bantam Books.

———. 1998. *Working with emotional intelligence*. New York: Bantam Books.

Kamin, M. 2006. *Customer service training*. Burlington, MA: Pergamon Flexible Learning.

LeBoeuf, M. 2000. *How to win customers and keep them for life*. Berkeley, CA: Berkeley Trade.

Morgan, R. 1989. *Calming upset customers*. Los Altos, CA: Crisp.

Nulman, P. 2000. *Just say yes! Extreme customer service: How to give it! How to get it!* Franklin Lakes, NJ: Career Press.

Slowik, D. 2000. *Upset citizens and customers: How to deal with the angry, difficult, and demanding public*. Evergreen, CO: Evergreen Press.

ten

Retaining Members Through Program Management

Sandy Coffman

After studying this chapter, the reader will be able to

- turn every program into a retention program,
- apply the 10 keys that will turn new members into retained members,
- develop a retention plan using the logical progression of programming,
- use one program to promote another,
- use a checklist with the five steps to successful programs, and
- follow a complete programming agenda.

Tales From the Trenches

A multipurpose health club was experiencing a decline in member sales as well as an increased attrition rate. They did a major renovation that was costly and consequently had a substantial increase in dues. The renovation was done to bring in more members and to retain new and existing members.

The initial response to the renovation, as expected, was positive. But the general manager and the membership and marketing director of the club soon found that the growth stopped. They realized that they needed an upgraded service program, a more productive and sophisticated integration program for new members, a follow-up retention program, and a structured accountability program.

The original orientation program for new members consisted of a knowledgeable group of trainers who invited new members to meet for an hour to discuss their goals and to get a fitness evaluation or assessment. Members were then shown how to use six pieces of equipment and were provided with a fitness card that could be used to track their workouts. After 6 weeks, members were to contact the trainer to get an updated workout card.

The club called in a program consultant to fix the problem, who took the opportunity to educate the staff on how to professionally greet new and prospective members, how to promote sign-ups, how to track the results, and how to get the participants into the follow-up 6-week program called WOW (Work Out on Weights). This was significant in that the club had to be realistic about who they hired in the first place, as well as what and how they trained employees in communication skills. Needless to say, the first step was to get the right staff in place.

Next, they set up a huge orientation board listing the days and times that equipment orientations would be made available. Members could choose orientations on either the cardio equipment or the strength training equipment. There were five differences between the original orientation program and the new and improved program.

- The new orientation encouraged group participation instead of individual workouts with the trainer so that 4 to 12 participants could sign up for one time slot.

- Because two types of programs were offered, the new member would sign up for the first choice but then be encouraged to sign up for the second orientation.

- The instructors were trained in role-playing sessions on how to professionally run group activities that provided fun, camaraderie, and sociability along with education.

- It was imperative that the sales department join in. They needed to be in on all the training and retention sessions. All membership employees were to sign up every new member and prospective member to one of the orientations. This was done effectively during the tour. Even if prospective members didn't join on the spot, they were invited to attend a group orientation program and therefore become a better prospect for membership.

- The trainers had goals to meet. Their first goal was to provide a fun, social, educational experience. Their second goal was to get the participants to sign up for the second orientation. Their third goal was to get the new members to sign up for program such as WOW that would serve as a follow-up program in a group setting twice a week for 6 weeks.

Within a 2-year period, the average attrition rate dropped 12.5% lower than before the program started. The average number of sales at the club was approximately 100 per month. Within that time, the number of new members participating in the 6-week WOW program grew from 280 to 400.

A retention program like this one will only be successful if you understand and appreciate the nuances of the new member. Be realistic. Be empathetic. Be caring and compassionate. Don't take your new members for granted and assume that people automatically take on the responsibility of exercising regularly just because they joined your club. Educate yourself on your members first. Then you will have the opportunity to educate your members.

Although people know they should exercise, want to exercise, and even join a club to exercise, they will not continue to exercise if they aren't enjoying the experience. The majority of people, if left alone to exercise without encouragement or recognition, eventually become inactive and quit the club. The excuses we've heard for years are, "I'm not using the club enough," or "I don't have time." Members are not exactly lying with these excuses, but the reality is that they are not using the club and can't find the time to exercise because the experience they have at the club is not of value to them. This is perhaps a perceived unmet value, but perception is reality, and we have to deal with these perceptions. Most members who are left to fend for themselves and work out alone with little or no direction do not realize a club experience. The value of a club membership is in sociability, camaraderie, friendships, relationships, leadership, and group experiences—all things that programs provide.

Retention occurs when you have a variety of programs that offer different experiences and challenges that will keep members active and excited month after month, year after year. Members will become bored with the same routine. In essence, exercise is our product, and we package our product in various packages called *programs*. We must sell many different programs over the course of a year to keep members committed and returning to the club regularly. It may take up to six or eight different programs in a year to get a member committed to a club and a lifestyle of health and fitness.

The goal of programming is retention, so the objective of every program is to get members to use the club, enjoy the club, and therefore come closer to becoming a retained member. The words *programming* and *retention* go hand in hand, and although they are two of the most important words in the business, they are also two of the most underachieved words. If we put as much time, effort, and energy in programming plans for retention as we do in sales and marketing campaigns, we would significantly increase the bottom line. Studies show that it can cost up to six times more to get a new member than to keep an existing one, and if clubs can decrease their attrition rates by 5%, they may be able to double their profits!

The more attention you pay to members, the more they will use the club. When members make friends in the club and work out with others like themselves, they have a much more enjoyable experience than when exercising alone. If you provide programs that bring people together in a fun, social environment, the number of refer-rals increases, retention increases, and attrition decreases. Programs must be developed with systems that guarantee these experiences, thus resulting in retention and growth.

Establishing the Purpose of Programming

Every program must be able to benefit the member. The member should enjoy the experience, gain a sense of belonging, realize some personal achievement, and acquire confidence in taking on new challenges. To make sure this happens, a staff member should be assigned to track participation, give recognition for performance, and promote the next program. You must keep track of who is coming to your club, when they are using the club, and if they stop using the club (so that you can invite them back). This will keep them from becoming inactive and eventually dropping out of the club because they aren't using it. Your responsibility in running a professional program is to help members meet other members who have common interests, schedules, and abilities so that they develop a sense of belonging and commitment with other people like themselves while experiencing a sense of achievement and purpose.

The success of professional programming for retention is dependent on training the right staff with the proper procedures, teaching the staff to use specific tools to accomplish goals for every program, and holding the staff accountable for completing every requirement to reach those goals. Why are *programming* and *retention* two of the most underachieved words in our business? Perhaps it's because staff members have not been given the tools, training, or systems to guarantee successful programs. The real work begins after the member buys the membership.

Before we begin, you should understand that it takes a full year of programming before a member can be considered to be retained. During that year of programming all of the following must occur:

- The member should be using the club or facility at least one or two times per week.
- The member should be participating in a scheduled program every week.
- The member should be participating in a group program with people of similar interests, skill levels, schedules, personalities, ages, and gender. In other words, members

are more likely to become retained members if they form relationships along the way.

- The member should be using the club or facility on the same day, at the same hour, with the same people, and with an instructor every week.

- The member should feel loyalty to one or more of your staff members. An instructor, trainer, supervisor, or receptionist who welcomes a member as a returning friend creates loyalty, trust, and a comfortable familiarity, all of which contribute to retention.

- The member should experience more than one program within the year. After a full year of enjoying the club and its programs on a regular basis, such members will have put your facility into their daily or weekly schedule. Exercise and your club will be part of their lifestyle, and they will become retained members of exercise as well as of your club.

How the new member is turned into a retained member depends on the programs offered by the club. Populations can be categorized by gender, age, interests, skill levels, schedules, personalities, and lifestyles. Among these subdivisions, all members must be placed in four main groups for programming:

1. New members
2. Active members
3. Inactive members
4. Potential members

The purpose of every program, then, must be to integrate new members, diversify active members, offer a new beginning to inactive members, and create the initial interest in potential members.

Retaining Your Members: Ten Keys

After establishing the purpose of a program, use these 10 keys for implementing programs that will turn new members into retained members.

1. *Communication with new members.* It's necessary to personally contact every new member who joins your club. At the very least, new members should be contacted within the first week of membership. It has been proven time and time again that most new members quit a club before they ever really start using the club on a regular basis. Even with the best intentions, it is difficult for a new member, especially an inexperienced one, to enter a club alone and feel perfectly comfortable walking into a group exercise class or getting on a piece of equipment. A personal invitation to a specific event at a specific time is the most effective form of communication you can use. You can send a reminder postcard or an e-mail, but a sincere phone call is best. Members who are intimidated or inexperienced will probably not come in without it.

2. *Follow-up.* Just because you called and invited the member to a program or event, don't think your work is done. Professional communication includes the responsibility of following up on your invitation or promise. You should call again, perhaps up to three times, especially if there is an indication that the person is not sure about participating. Even after the invitation is accepted, a confirmation call 12 to 24 hours in advance of the program is necessary to ensure participation and avoid a no-show. The follow-up phone calls show that you are taking responsibility for inviting the new member to the program.

3. *Recognition of participants.* It's imperative to give personal recognition to every new member who participates in a program or activity. People need to feel important. Recognition can be given for achievements, such as an award, ribbon, or trophy for excellent performance, but it can also be given for many other reasons that are far more important to the new member. Giving a compliment, taking a picture, or extending a sincere handshake can be just as effective. The most important thing to remember about recognition is that it must be given by the leader in front of the member's peers. Programming essentially is tracking—by keeping track of a member's attendance, you have an opportunity to give recognition for participation. You can always find a way to make people feel important.

4. *Sociability.* When people join a club, they want to be with others like themselves. If you get people in a group situation or program, they are more likely to enjoy themselves, meet others like themselves, and form friendships. Most members join clubs for fitness, but they stay for the fun. Sociability, camaraderie, and friendships are all key ingredients to a club experience. Group programs provide sociability, which is a major factor in retention.

5. *Commitment to a schedule.* Certainly new members must be committed to the program, to

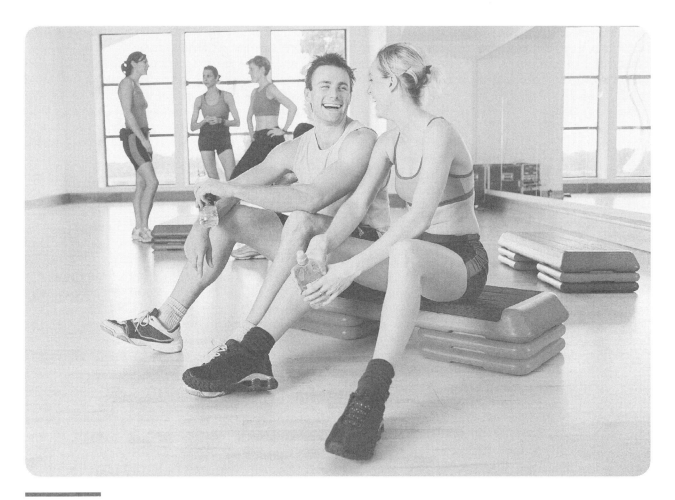

An important key to retaining memberships is to implement group programs that foster the formation of friendships.
© BananaStock

exercise, and to a new lifestyle, but there are other commitments that must be established before that happens. Some say a member's commitment is to the activity itself, the leader, or the other members of the group. These are all good commitments and if they occur, new members are sure to feel the sense of belonging that will keep them coming back. The commitment that will be the key to retention, however, is a commitment to a specific schedule or time frame. Retention occurs when the members put your club into their lifestyle, coming to the club on the same day at the same time every week. There are three main time frames for programming:

- Peak hours (weekdays from 5:00 p.m. to 7:00 p.m.)
- Off-peak hours (daytime hours, weekdays)
- Weekends

6. *Diversification of activities.* A huge factor in retention is providing diverse activities. People get bored doing the same routine over and over, so new challenges, goals, and experiences will keep them interested or renew their interest in exercising. Cross-training is another reason why diversified programming is so important. Cross-training gives better fitness results, so diversified programming is mentally, emotionally, and physically beneficial as well. Diversification can come in the form of a higher level of achievement in the same program, such as moving through beginning, intermediate, or advanced levels of performance, as well as in different types of programs. Diversified programming is especially important for existing members who are already active. It will keep them coming back, and that's the goal of programming.

7. *Progression of programs.* Progressing through a series of programs is the objective of the wheel of logical progression (explained in fuller detail later in this chapter). It ensures retention through a year of diversified programming. New members begin their membership with an introductory program

and progress to instructional opportunities, which prepares them for regular involvement in programs such as sport leagues, fitness clinics, circuit sessions, or group exercise classes. Participation in progressive programming is essential to keeping members active, interested, goal driven, and successful in their efforts. The wheel of logical progression provides an ongoing check on every phase of programming for every member. Always use one program to promote another, and the progression will continue. The objective is for all members to become integrated in the club through introductory programs, become familiar and comfortable with activities, and finally to commit to a schedule that puts your club in their weekly routine.

8. *Promotion of programs.* Members are not considered to be retained until they are using the club every week for a full year. Professional promotion starts with a calendar of events that is posted at the beginning of the year and offers a variety of activities and programs that remain consistent throughout the year. The promotion of these and other programs must include posters, bulletin boards, and flyers promoting the onset of the programs no less than 3 weeks in advance. In addition to the readable promotions, telephone campaigns inviting members to a specific event at a specific time are productive if done no less than 3 weeks in advance and followed up with confirmation calls 12 to 24 hours before the program. Most programs need to be promoted verbally throughout the club, too. For example, the front desk has the opportunity of promoting a program to every person who walks in the door, group exercise instructors can promote programs in their classes, and fitness trainers should be promoting programs to their clients for cross-training purposes. All promotions must be scheduled and monitored as much as the programs themselves, and a full staff effort must be organized to make sure all promotions are put in place on a timely schedule.

9. *Reliability of the schedule.* Reliability is a crucial issue that is most often misunderstood or ignored altogether. Reliability means that you set a precedent within the programming schedule that is not only reasonable to get started with, but, more importantly, easy to progress with. For example, a programming schedule that offers a beginning program on a Tuesday and an intermediate level of the same program on a Thursday should maintain that schedule for at least 6 months and preferably a year or more. Members need to plan ahead, and your club must remain consistent in its core program offerings to allow people to adjust their schedules to make room for your club and their program of choice. If you constantly change the same program to a different time and day, you eliminate the members who spend weeks preparing their schedules to make room for a class at 9:00 a.m. on Tuesdays only to find that it has been changed to Wednesdays. Keep a number of core programs on a consistent calendar of events to set a reliable precedent for members.

10. *Accountability for growth and retention.* Every program must have a leader who is held accountable for all 10 keys of retention. The accountability structure of programming, if managed efficiently, is worthy of a program director's position. If the specific role of program director is not feasible, there must be a leader assigned to each program who is capable, responsible, and held accountable for taking the program through all 10 keys of program development. At the end of the day, the success or failure of a program will be linked to how well the 10 keys were implemented. A program cannot run successfully without accountability for its presentation, growth, and retention. Professional programming is the heart of membership growth and retention. Never run a program unless you are going to run it 100%.

THE BOTTOM LINE

Retention is not only a goal—it's a vision.

Programming by Logical Progression

Simply put, a **program for retention** is a step-by-step plan to take every member in your club from orientation to involvement to commitment. Instead of concentrating sales efforts on replacing people who leave the club or quit using the club every month, you should concentrate on promoting various programs to members to keep them interested, excited, and active. Retention means repeat business, and in the fitness industry that means repeat sales of programs. This sale may or may not mean that an extra fee is necessary for a program, but selling the program means getting a commitment from the member. The sale of programs must be ongoing—as mentioned, the real sale begins after the sale of the membership.

The goal of every service organization is retention, whether it be retention of a new member, a regular participant, or an inactive member wanting to get involved again. In this industry, however, it's not only a goal, but a vision as well. The vision of health clubs is to provide opportunity, education, and leadership in a clublike atmosphere that ensures an ongoing program of activity resulting in fitness, exercise, and health. The operative word is *ongoing*. Unfortunately, working out regularly for 3 months will not provide the lifetime of fitness members need, yet that's the scenario commonly experienced by the majority of people who join with the idea of a lifetime commitment to exercise. Let's take a look at how we set up the programming business to achieve the goal of retention. Programming sets up a club experience for the member, an experience that is enjoyable and sociable as well as health inspired and physically beneficial.

The **wheel of logical progression** is based on the theory of applied creativity used in the business world. It means that a logical progression of activities or programs needs to be followed to ensure that people will keep coming back for more. The theory is best illustrated by a wheel with six spokes (see figure 10.1). All the spokes must be in place for this wheel of retention to turn.

The logical progression of programming includes the following:

- *Three stages of retention.* When people join a club or any exercise program, they go through three major stages of development within the first year.
  1. Integration stage
  2. Acceptance stage
  3. Commitment stage

- *Six programming phases.* These programming phases within the three major stages include programming opportunities that lead to retention. The integration stage includes the introduction and instruction phases; the acceptance stage includes the involvement and achievement phases; and the commitment stage includes the improvement and fun phases.

This system is adaptable to any facility, recreational activity, fitness program, or ability level of participants. For example, people who are new to exercise or sport can begin their participation on the wheel of progression and continue on. In addition, a person who is experienced, active, and fit will find that the wheel offers the exact experience necessary for beginning a new activity or sport and will allow the progression to occur at a higher degree of ability, experience, or skill. The steps to retention remain the same.

1. **Introduction**
   - Develop a new interest
   - Have fun
   - Experience success
2. **Instruction**
   - Learn more
   - Get better
3. **Involvement**
   - Leagues
   - Sessions
4. **Achievement**
   - Recognition
   - Award presentations
5. **Improvement**
   - Competition
   - Education
   - Diversification
   - Advancement in skills
6. **Fun**
   - Social events
   - Special events

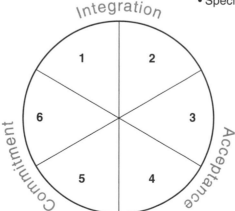

Figure 10.1 The wheel of logical progression.
© Sandy Coffman

The next section provides an outline of the three-stage, six-phase programming system that each member should complete during the first year of membership or participation. Chances are that you are already doing some of these programming activities. The key is to identify any gaps in your programming system that can cause members to drop out. You will see where you can fill those gaps with the appropriate programs.

This gap concept is important. One of the major mistakes made in the industry is skipping programming phases. Skipping phases will result in lack of achievement, poor performance, or just plain frustration. It's important, for instance, to begin at step 1, not step 4, or not to skip step 4 and go from step 3 to step 5. The majority of people who drop out of a program or club quit before they ever get started because they don't join a program that automatically leads to another level or program, and then another, and then another. Every program should be designed to promote and inspire participation in a follow-up program. This is more likely to occur, of course, if the programs are enjoyable, achievable, and successful.

No doubt, you are beginning to see how the sale begins after the sale. Our definition of *retention* indicates that each programming phase must be promoted and sold to members after they have bought the membership. Note the importance of the program director, instructor, trainer, or leader in this stage. The program director must be held accountable for selling the idea of progressing from one level to the next and for keeping the members involved in a program or series of programs throughout the year.

First Stage: Integration

The **integration stage** is often called *orientation*, and it gives members a beginning experience, but it must also be designed to encourage further participation and thus improve retention. Most clubs have some sort of system to introduce members to a new activity or program but then expect members to be comfortable being on their own and to call on the leaders when improvement is needed.

Realizing that the majority of members quit using a club within the first 90 days, most clubs make an effort to set up a system through computers or workout programs to track member participation for the first 3 months of membership. But setting up individual workout programs for members does not particularly create a club atmosphere, and it doesn't provide enough guidance and encouragement from the leaders or others to continue. New members receive their initial orientation, have a goal-setting session, and then are left to fend for themselves. The problem is that these members won't use the facilities frequently, and eventually they'll drop their membership. To prevent this, you need to give members a variety of reasons to keep coming to the club. The integration stage begins that process.

The two phases in the integration stage are introduction and instruction.

Introduction Phase

The **introduction phase** of the integration stage is the most important phase and usually the most poorly implemented. The biggest mistake made in the introduction program is that an instructor typically gives too much information. Think of the words that are important here—*integration, orientation, introduction, new beginning*. They all refer to getting new information and learning or trying something for the first time. Do not try to teach too much too soon.

The introduction phase has three objectives. The participant must

1. develop a new interest and learn something new,
2. have fun and be encouraged and complimented by the leader, and
3. experience some degree of success.

The introduction phase might consist of a one-on-one orientation, an introductory class, a new-member party, a beginners' clinic, or some combination thereof. The best advice is to keep it simple. This is not the time to show off, try to impress members with an enormous amount of knowledge, or rattle on with unfamiliar terminology. The participant already has your attention and appreciates your knowledge. The goal of the introduction phase is to create an environment that makes the participant eager to come back and learn more.

Once again, the goal of programming is retention, so members must feel confident, educated, and accomplished. An introduction program must leave the participants feeling at least somewhat successful. Don't confuse them and don't overwhelm them, but do compliment them and find a reason to applaud their efforts.

Instruction Phase

In the **instruction phase,** the two objectives for the participant are to learn more and to get better. The instruction phase introduces members to goal setting and gets them to start using the club on a regular basis. During this phase you want to establish a specific workout schedule and begin the members' education, including terminology, safety, correct form, and general dos and don'ts.

At this point, we have to consider the instructor's teaching expertise. The all-important introductory and instruction phases will fail if the instructor does not establish rapport with beginners. Instructors must have empathy for beginners and a sincere understanding of their frustrations and fears. The biggest fear, of course, is failure, and this is not the time to let them fail or even have the perception of failure.

For example, take an introductory racquetball clinic. If the instructor happens to be the local or state champion, that's fine, but being the best player has little to do with being the best teacher. The best player often doesn't have the empathy or the desire to teach and promote the sport in any other aspect than its technical skills, and this is not what will get the average person out on the court.

More Than a Clinic The instruction phase should be more than a one-time clinic. You want new members to commit to a series of lessons so they will keep coming back to learn more. A series of lessons over 4 to 8 weeks is ideal. Less than 4 weeks doesn't give enough momentum to the series and more than 8 weeks becomes redundant and boring. You will find that the dropout rate increases dramatically after 8 weeks.

Sense of Belonging Another great reason for the series of lessons is that in 6 to 8 weeks the participants feel a sense of belonging that encourages commitment. For instance, if the program is in a group setting, some of the participants will develop friendships, which are a key to retention.

Second Stage: Acceptance

The **acceptance stage** of the year of retention is the second of the three stages. They have gone through the introduction phase, become familiar with the activity, met other people like themselves, gained respect for the instructor, gained a little self-confidence, and learned more and gotten better.

If you have been tracking their attendance and encouraging their performance, they have developed a sense of belonging and are eager to continue their efforts. The acceptance stage is when the member gets involved in an ongoing program and subsequently can be part of a recognition event or even participate in a competition and win an award for personal achievement.

Involvement Phase

Now it's time for the member to enter the **involvement phase** and start using the club on a regular basis. At this point, retention is really starting to occur. In an involvement program, members make a commitment to a specific program on a specific day of the week and a specific hour of the day for a certain number of weeks. Involvement programs include any type of league or series of classes, meetings, or clinics.

A league program is a good example of an instruction program. Once you learn something new and start getting better at it, you will want to continue with the activity. For instance, introductory clinics or lessons in racquetball, tennis, or volleyball will encourage players to join a league whereby they will meet with other players every week and compete for a prize at the end of 6, 8, or 10 weeks of activity. Leagues are fun, social, and competitive, and they get members to put your club or program into their schedule of events.

For example, a racquetball or tennis league will meet at the same time on the same day every week with the same people playing each other. The players look forward to seeing familiar faces, competing with them, and talking about the game afterward. This sort of experience is eagerly anticipated and members will make it a priority. It's easy to see why the involvement program is critical to achieving retention: It truly offers a sense of belonging.

Another form of involvement programming is offering sessions or a series of classes such as group exercise or circuit training sessions. Again, the group program will consist of a variety of classes and exercises. Each class will have its own time slot every week with the same instructor. The majority of participants in that class choose to come to the same class every week, setting that time aside in their schedule as a priority.

The quality of the program and the quality of the instructor will, of course, be the deciding factors in whether the participants continue on a regular basis. The basic premise here is the significance of the regularly scheduled activity as an involvement program in the acceptance phase of the wheel of logical progression.

The points to consider in the involvement program are as follows:

- The program is offered on the same day and at the same time every week.
- The program will have the same instructor or supervisor directing the activity during each session.

- The majority of participants will be the same people, who thus have an opportunity to create friendships.
- New participants will be encouraged to return.

Achievement Phase

The introductory program has created an initial interest and members have had fun participating. The instruction program was successful if the participants were eager to learn, if they had fun, and if they truly felt that they got better at what they were doing. The logical progression of programming is under way and everyone gets involved in leagues, sessions, or clinics on a regular weekly schedule. Now it's time for the **achievement phase,** to give recognition for performance or achievement. The objectives of the achievement phase include recognition for participation or competition and award presentations by the leader in front of peers.

The achievement program is the pivotal program within the wheel of logical progression. The participants at this point are feeling good about themselves and their new experience, but they need encouragement and recognition from the program directors or instructors. The objective of this phase is to encourage a desire for more activity by taking time to recognize the accomplishment that members have made in the involvement phase. As a result, you raise the self-esteem and comfort level of members.

Recognition for Personal Achievement   This important phase is often eliminated because clubs have a tendency to rest on their laurels and assume that if the members get involved they will remain involved, and because awards and recognition events take time and money and clubs feel they can't afford either one. Not only is it wrong to think that you can't afford to give out awards, you can't afford not to give out awards. Everyone wants recognition for something and nothing makes a person feel more important than getting recognition for personal achievement.

The best achievement programs will be in the form of award ceremonies or at the very least, visible and memorable presentations. Personal achievement needs to be recognized by the leader and demonstrated in front of peers in order to have the greatest impact. The good news is that the awards need not be expensive. Ribbons, small trophies, or T-shirts are as appreciated as more costly items. Recognition for achievement can be as simple as giving out ribbons,

posting names on recognition boards, featuring members' names or pictures in your newsletter, or even giving an enthusiastic handshake and asking for applause from the other participants.

Performance Measurement   Awards need not be given strictly for the biggest, best, fastest, or fittest winners. Indeed, giving recognition on a competitive basis may actually leave out the participants who want and need the experience most. For example, presenting an award based on attendance rather than performance will provide a wonderful experience to someone who may not ever get a chance to receive an award for achievement based on performance alone. The bottom line is to be creative and find ways to recognize everyone for something. This is the ultimate goal of the achievement phase.

Third Stage: Commitment

We know now that retention will occur only when the member becomes committed to the program, the lifestyle, and the club. We've learned, too, that it takes a series of programs and activities to achieve that commitment. Without setting up the cycle of programming described here, many clubs scramble to sell enough memberships every month to replace the people who leave. While that is happening, members who joined a few months earlier stop using the club on a regular basis, which is one step before quitting.

The object of the **commitment stage** is to enhance the member's commitment to the club by creating a deeper level of socialization and bonding between members and staff. During this stage, members get involved in a clubwide event, such as a holiday party or other social function, competition, tournament, seminar, or health education.

Improvement Phase

It's important to elevate your members to a higher level of accomplishment and achievement as they progress in their exercise routines or sport activity; thus, you must create in members the desire to improve. That desire will be evident if all of the objectives were met in the introduction program, instruction program, involvement program, and achievement program. You'll want to help establish new goals and diversify activities. The beauty of getting to the **improvement phase** is that it provides you with another opportunity to recognize achievements and continues to build a sense of belonging that will lead to retention.

When people are comfortable and confident in their ability levels, even if it is at a beginning level, they are ready to learn more and accept new challenges. Improvement programs add new dimensions to previous programs. As participants gain confidence, they also get a heightened competitive edge. Even those who declared themselves to be noncompetitive will enter the improvement phase of programming comparing themselves with others in the program. The quest for improvement is exciting and will solidify members' activity even further.

It's essential to be aware of the psychology behind the improvement phase. The members have experienced a good deal of success by this time. If they had not gone through the first four phases of programs, the club may have left them feeling unfit, unknowledgeable, and uninspired. It's exciting to see a member willing to take on a new challenge with confidence and a positive attitude. At this point you know you've done your job. You've traveled yet another mile down the road to retention.

Improvement programs include competitions, education, seminars, and clinics; diversification (new programs or activities); and more advanced play or exercise programs.

Fun Phase

The last phase of the wheel of logical progression is the **fun phase,** or the social events. At the end of the day, it's all about enjoying what you are doing and having fun. Making fitness fun has been a mantra for the health and fitness industry for nearly 10 years, and it is one of the most difficult parts of the business to accomplish.

If you run an all-club event such as a holiday party or a member appreciation party, the scenario is almost always the same—about 90% of the attendees are already active members who have been using the club regularly for more than a year and who have already made friends with other members or even with some of the staff. An all-club event, party, or program should be attended by new members who need to feel wanted, accepted, and comfortable before they become inactive or quit altogether. The existing, active member will come with ease and enthusiasm. The new member needs to invited and encouraged.

Participation of New Members   Even though a club party or special event is designed to be social, friendly, and fun, the newest members will not participate if they have not felt needed, wanted, or appreciated. They will not participate if they have

not been introduced to others like themselves, participated in a regularly scheduled activity, gotten rewarded for their achievements, and acquired confidence and familiarity along the way. You can't simply announce that you are having a party or a special event and expect new people to participate without having had a friendly, fun experience in the club.

On the other hand, if the members who have joined the club within the last 3 or 6 months experienced an introductory clinic with other new members and have been participating in a regularly scheduled program every week, they will likely feel comfortable enough to attend an all-club event. If they do, you know that your programming efforts are working with the members who would normally be the most likely to quit and certainly the most likely to not attend an all-club function. You

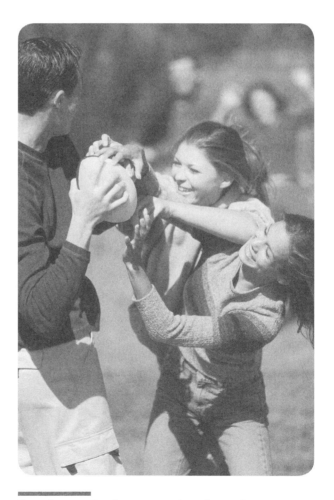

Social events that focus on making fitness fun are a part of the commitment stage during which members become committed to the program, the lifestyle, and the club.
© PhotoDisc

have nurtured their experiences with a systematic calendar of programs that included physical activity, recognition, education, productivity, and camaraderie, all of which has led to retention and a sense of belonging. Your members will be committed to your club and their new lifestyle.

Clubs Within Clubs   The programs leading up to an all-club event or party must be part of the wheel of logical progression. The experiences in the programs must be positive and fun. The leaders must be enthusiastic, professional promoters. Each program then will be a club within the club, and as they progress through the programs, members will experience all three stages of retention: integration, acceptance, and commitment.

Your members will also experience all six phases of programming: introduction, instruction, involvement, achievement, improvement, and fun.

THE BOTTOM LINE

Always use one program to promote another in order to increase retention.

Developing a Successful Program

There is no reason for any program to fail!

That is a bold statement to make, but it is true. Some programs may be better than others, of course, but no program need be cancelled. Almost every unsuccessful program did not fail due to the program itself. Most programs have potential; it's all a matter of how they are presented to the member. After a program is dubbed a failure, you may hear excuses like, "The members didn't like it," "The members didn't want it," "No one showed up," or "No one signed up." However, invariably the failure is directly due to a lack of effort and poor follow-up on the part of the programming staff. Any club that thinks a program needs only to be presented with a sign-up sheet or an announcement in a newsletter will become very good at finding excuses to explain program failure.

The most important information on retention offered here is in the systems, agendas, checklists, parameters, promotions, marketing techniques, communication skills, agendas, evaluations, and follow-up procedures that must be followed for every program. The systems work, so if you work the systems, there is no reason why any program should fail.

As discussed, the battle to turn a new member into a dedicated club user begins after the sale is made, and the main weapon in that battle is programming. The problem is that too many club managers rely on an orientation program alone to achieve the goal of increased retention. After the initial 6-week period is over, they expect members to find their own friends, establish their own schedules, and seek out additional help as needed. An orientation program, usually introducing four to six pieces of equipment, is relied upon to help members initiate a lifetime of exercise independence, but most members who quit by the end of the first year actually quit using the club within the first 3 months.

For example, many club managers and program directors still don't understand how to put together a successful program. For many of them, the programming scenario sounds something like this: (1) Get an idea, (2) put out a sign-up sheet, (3) announce the program in the club newsletter, (4) talk it up, and (5) sit back and hope it flies. Even programs that are great ideas will fail with that system. The correct steps to achieving a program that will attract a high level of participation and have a positive effect on your club's retention rate are as follows: (1) Define a purpose, (2) set a goal, (3) develop a marketing plan to reach the goal, (4) measure the results, and (5) implement a follow-up program.

Define a Purpose

An example of the purpose of a program may be to get new members committed to an 8-week cardio circuit program. They will meet other new members like themselves and gain stamina, endurance, and satisfaction by completing the program. A staff member will be assigned to track participation, give recognition for performance, and promote the next program. Members will have enjoyed their involvement and gained a sense of belonging, a degree of personal achievement, and a comfort level to take on a new challenge.

Set a Goal

A program is a club project that directly affects the bottom line, and a good business doesn't undertake a project without having a clear goal in mind. All too often you get a good idea for a program, put out a sign-up sheet, and wait to see how many people, if any, will sign up. The success of a program is first measured by the number of participants.

What is a realistic number to expect if the purpose of the program is clearly beneficial to the club and to a specific group of members? Let's continue with the new-member cardio circuit program as an example. If a club is selling an average of 50 new memberships per month, it is reasonable to think that 20% to 30% would be good candidates for a cardio circuit program. Conservatively, 20% or 10 new members in the last month would enjoy the program and benefit from it. If you consider that members are considered new for the first 3 months of membership, new members from the previous 2 months would be good candidates for this program as well. That would give another 20 potential participants, or 30 total, for the cardio circuit program. You should always set an attainable goal, one that is easily reached and possible to surpass. The set goal, however, must be reached. In this example we will set our total goal at 20 participants.

Develop a Marketing Plan

Up until now, the sign-up sheet was the major marketing tool for programs. There are two things to remember about sign-up sheets: They are absolutely necessary, and absolutely worthless! A sign-up sheet is necessary because it is a good promotional tool; it will create an initial interest in a program. However, it is unlikely to attract the type of member that the program is designed for, and it is unlikely to result in the goal number of members needed to make the program a success.

The program marketing plan must resemble that of the sales plan for marketing to new prospects. All the programmers, trainers, and instructors for the program must be able to verbalize the positives of the program, including its features, benefits, and purpose. Second, they must be able to overcome objections, such as, "I'm too busy," "The program costs too much," and "I don't want to make a commitment right now." Third, a good salesperson must ask for the sale three to five times. Asking may consist of a postcard, an e-mail, and, most importantly, up to three phone calls delivering a personal invitation to the member. How often do your programmers ask a member to participate in any given program? The sales team is trained to ask a potential member for the sale at least three to five times before closing the sale. Your programmers must do the same thing when asking a member to participate in a program.

Measure the Results

If you follow a system of programming by defining a purpose, setting a goal, and developing a marketing plan, you will be able to measure the results.

In our example, we have now established that the program is good for members, and we have designed it for a specific type of member, in this case the new member. We've set our goal and followed our marketing plan. Now we must measure whether the result is good for the bottom line.

- 50 new members join per month.
- 10 new members (20%) get involved in a new-member program (cardio circuit) per month.
- Each member pays $40 in monthly dues, or $480 per year.
- The program delivers enjoyment, friends, staff recognition, and a follow-up program.
- Each year, 120 new members who would have potentially dropped out or quit are now retained, active participants delivering $57,600 in annual revenues alone (10 new members per month = 120 members per year; 120 members × $480 yearly dues = $57,600).

Isn't that the result we are all looking for? It starts with the first program and continues only if all the participants complete the program. Again, that will be the result of constant communication, promotion, and recognition by the programming staff. The program is only as good as the way it is managed.

By the way, active, happy new members in their first year of membership are most likely to bring in 60% to 80% of your new business by word of mouth. A professionally trained programming staff with a well-planned program calendar should be able to run six to eight different programs, six to eight times per year. Well-managed programs keep hundreds of members enjoying themselves and using your club regularly.

Develop Follow-Up Programs

Retention doesn't occur automatically after the first 6- to 8-week program. If you want your new members to become active club users, then timely, well-designed follow-up programs are crucial. The programming calendar must include activities for everyone—men, women, juniors, seniors, first-time exercisers, and competitive athletes. Professional programming involves leagues, lessons, clinics, contests, classes, seminars, and tournaments, all carefully targeted to different groups of members sharing similar interests that will bond them together in a congenial atmosphere. You must sell each of these

Programming Agenda

The programming agenda presented here is an outline of the steps and considerations necessary for developing programming that turns new members into retained members. Use it as a checklist to ensure a successful program. It will help you remember that you should never run a program if you don't run it 100%!

1. The program leader is responsible for the event and its result.
2. Every program should do the following:
   - Have a purpose—Define how the program will benefit the club and the member.
   - Have a goal—Know the number of participants needed for success.
   - Have a plan—Create a written agenda including marketing and promotional procedures, staff assignments, and deadlines to reach the goal.
   - Follow up—Always have a follow-up program ready to promote.
3. Consider all four groups of members for programs:
   - New members
   - Active members
   - Inactive members
   - Potential members
4. When introducing a program, it is a good idea to offer it in all three time frames in order to reach the majority of members.
   - Peak hours
   - Off-peak hours
   - Weekends
5. Be able to place each program in a spoke on the wheel of logical progression.
   - Integration stage—introduction phase and instruction phase
   - Acceptance stage—involvement phase and achievement phase
   - Commitment stage—improvement phase and fun phase
6. Have introductory programs to create interest and to integrate new members.
   - Promote camaraderie.
   - Qualify skill levels.
   - Categorize personalities.
   - Recognize individual achievements.
   - Promote involvement in follow-up programs.
7. Review the 10 keys to successful programming and have a written example of each key before running the program.
8. Always use one program to promote another. Have the sign-up sheet ready, as well as flyers, available schedules, rules, costs, and so on for follow-up programs.
9. Every program must have a sign-in procedure (name and phone number) for follow-up and program analysis.
10. If a program is worth doing once, it is worth doing again. Have a consistent schedule in a calendar of events to present to members.

programs as a new challenge or a new beginning, and always use one program to promote another in order to keep the retention ball rolling.

Recognizing the Importance of Program Directors

You should have special events to lure back inactive and former members, recognition programs to keep new members active, competitive programs to keep dedicated exercisers interested, social programs to get members involved, and educational programs for those who are misinformed or confused about health and fitness concerns. All this should be done in an environment that's fun and comfortable, and it should be orchestrated by a leader with good communication skills. Increasingly, the most successful clubs are those that have professional programming—programming with a purpose, goal, marketing plan, result, and system for continued success and growth.

The goal of programming is retention, and the program director is ultimately held accountable for retention. Is a program director worthwhile in your business? Many clubs debate this issue, but a look at the numbers should convince you that a program director will increase retention and decrease attrition.

Let's look at a potential situation. What do we know?

1. Retention is vital to your bottom line. Industry statistics say that it costs four to six times more to get a new member than it does to keep one.
2. The goal of programming is retention. Programs keep members active and happy.
3. Word of mouth (referrals) accounts for 60% to 80% of your new business. People who are enjoying your programs and using your club on a regular basis will refer new members.

The bottom line is clear. Can you afford not to have a program director?

Here is a typical club scenario as an example.

- Total number of members is 2,000.
- Monthly membership rate is $40.00 per month, or $480 per year.
- The difference between getting 10 new members per month, or 120 per year, involved in a program instead of allowing them to fend for themselves and likely drop out is $48,000 per year in membership fees alone (120 new members $\times$ $480 yearly dues). A program director's salary is certainly justified when these numbers are achieved.

Business is measured in terms of results, not just activities. Every business needs leaders to be accountable and to keep others accountable. The role of the program director does just that.

KEY TERMS

acceptance stage

achievement phase

commitment stage

fun phase

improvement phase

instruction phase

integration stage

introduction phase

involvement phase

program for retention

wheel of logical progression

REFERENCES AND RECOMMENDED READINGS

Coffman, S. 2007. *Successful programs for fitness and health clubs: 101 profitable ideas.* Champaign, IL: Human Kinetics.

LeBoeuf, M. 1987. *How to win customers and keep them for life.* New York: Putnam.

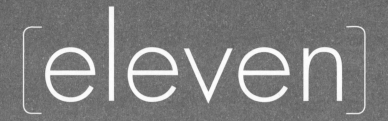

Generating Revenue Through Profit Centers

Cheryl Jones

LEARNING OBJECTIVES

After studying this chapter, the reader will be able to

- identify different types of profit centers,
- understand operational expenses involved in profit centers,
- determine profit centers with the highest net operating income,
- identify common pitfalls in the development of profitable programs, and
- appreciate the importance of hiring staff with specific competencies and technical skills.

Tales From the Trenches

A young health club owner was concerned that his club was not meeting its monthly membership sales targets and therefore not attaining the profitability expected. He had been reading industry publications and noticed that many articles described revenue sources other than membership that contributed to the bottom line of clubs. He called a meeting with his management team to brainstorm some revenue-generating initiatives. After a few hours, the team had come up with several fee-related services they could offer to generate additional revenues.

The managers were so excited about these new initiatives that they soon added classes on cooking, health and wellness, feng shui, tai chi, social dancing, and much more. They decided to pay top wages in order to attract the finest instructors in the area. The club produced a 16-page brochure with beautiful color photos advertising the exciting new programs and mailed them to all 2,000 members. The cost to produce, print, and mail the brochure was fairly expensive, but everyone knew that you had to spend money to make money.

After a few months, the business owner queried his staff about the amount of interest these programs had generated and their response was a resounding "Lots!" The club offered the classes at all different times of the day in order to accommodate every interested member's schedule, resulting in an average class size of three participants. It was a struggle to staff all these programs and classes, but the participants really liked their time slots.

Membership sales continued to drop and customer service complaints started to increase. The owner noticed that his management staff was being pulled away from their main membership sales and customer service responsibilities, so he hired an independent contractor to manage the programming. This new manager had made a name for herself in the community for programming and she brought a following with her to the club. She had been known to be somewhat difficult to work with, but her following would be well worth the conflict she tended to create. Since the owner believed his managers should have the freedom to develop their programs with little interference, he allowed his new program manager to run the show. After all, she knew how to run the programming business better than he did.

The business owner was busy with ventures outside of the club, so when he finally took the time to look at the finances of the club, he noticed that his revenue was higher than last year, but his profitability was considerably less. When he took the time to analyze his profit and loss statement, he was shocked that his payroll and direct expenses were at an all-time high and the new revenue did not make up for the increase in expenses. After further investigation, he noted that in aggregate, many people were involved in his programs, but the original pricing for the programs had been lowered and more classes were added to the schedule. Instructor pay rates were way above the market and the program manager was teaching a lot more classes than managing since she wanted to make more than her basic salary. Additional staff members were hired to work the front desk and take program registrations, and housekeeping hours had been increased due to the additional club usage. The member cancellation rate had increased and the major complaint was that management didn't care about their members anymore; they just wanted to take time and space away from them to accommodate more programming.

In summary, the club's expenses were too high to support the incremental revenue they drove. Net profit was down and their core business—membership—was negatively affected due to poor customer service.

Profit centers offer opportunities to increase the profitability of an organization. Ancillary revenue-generating programs can enhance a brand, improve member retention, increase revenue per member, and add profit to the bottom line. In this chapter, we review the operation of four profit centers that are common in many fitness settings, including personal training, group programs, spa services, youth programs, and child care. You will begin to understand how a new profit center may add value to your memberships and improve membership net gain. Certain gauges will be provided to assist in determining what types of profit centers add significant money to the bottom line. Once a profit center is identified, initial investment costs, ongoing payroll and expenses, and appropriate operational support will be reviewed. (See chapter 17 for additional information on evaluating profit centers.)

Managing a health club in any setting has become a highly complex and demanding task. No longer can club operators simply expect initiation fees and dues revenue to guarantee success and provide ample profit for the long run. When prices are dropping in the market and the competition is opening facilities with shiny, new self-service equipment in contemporary spaces, the club with the lowest cost and leanest operating structure has a far greater advantage. Yet constantly competing on price leaves your business vulnerable year after year. The threat of becoming a commodity in an overbuilt market will leave the clubs with limited services and marginal programming in the dust.

Profit centers are necessary to drive profitability by creating additional revenue and adding value to attract memberships. As stated in *IHRSA's Guide to Membership Retention* (McCarthy 2006), "The more they pay, the longer they stay. Members who spend more money at the club (in nondues revenue) have higher retention rates than members who spend less. As a result, there is a correlation between clubs that have a high percentage of nondues revenue and clubs that have higher retention rates. In general, clubs that have nondues revenue that is 25% or more of total revenue will have higher retention rates than clubs in which nondues revenue is less than 25%." Hence, it may be that the quest for improved member retention drives the decision to add profit centers. Within each facility lies the opportunity and financial necessity to create additional programming and services to generate profit. These profit centers will not guarantee financial success, but if run properly they can have a positive result on the bottom line as well as differentiate your club from the competition.

Development and Organization of Profit Centers

Profit centers are programs or services offered within club operations that provide additional revenue and profit to the bottom line. Financially, these profit centers can run as separate entities within the global profit and loss statement of the facility. Operationally, most profit centers are run as separate departments within the scope of the organization. That said, intraclub awareness among management, club departments, and field staff (e.g., front-desk staff, membership consultants, fitness staff) is critical to success. No doubt the ability of the facility manager to plan, organize, and communicate the purpose of the new business within the global organizational mission will contribute to the financial success of the operation. IHRSA's *Profiles of Success* (2006) indicates that the median percentage of profit centers in multipurpose clubs contributes to 32.9% of total revenue. In clubs

with 60,000 square feet (5,574 square meters) or more, the median percentage is 41.1%, and in clubs between 20,000 and 34,999 square feet (1,858 and 3,252 square meters), the median is 23.6%. Clubs reported a steady increase in nondues revenue from 30.9% in 2001 to 34.8% in 2005.

Developing and operating successful profit centers is a demanding responsibility of the facility manager. The types of profit centers and their daily operation can vary greatly not only from each other but also from the general operation of the facility.

The steps to initiating a profit center are in many ways similar to the steps to planning and developing a fitness center. First, determine the purpose of the profit center. Will it exist to generate a predetermined flow-through profit, or will it exist as a value-added service that breaks even in profitability yet enhances the value of the membership, thereby improving sales and retention? Make sure the profit center is a good fit for your club and its membership. If it is too specialized, the operations might be too complex and the resources too scarce. If it is a free commodity in the typical health club, members will feel as if their club is taking advantage of them and charging them for every little service and amenity. Can you establish awareness so that your program or service has TOMA among your consumers (see chapter 7)?

Once you have decided on the right profit center, determine specific, measurable goals and objectives for the operation. After researching areas such as competition, market demand, consumer interest, income, and price considerations, develop a marketing plan with an identified target market, typically the existing membership and local community. Often an informal member survey can provide a great deal of information for this aspect of the business plan. Ask yourself these questions: Will members see the value outside of their membership? Do you have a family-oriented membership base, or is it primarily composed of students with limited funds? Will you offer these programs and services to nonmembers, and if so, will they travel to obtain them? How far will they travel?

THE BOTTOM LINE

Developing a detailed business plan that defines the purpose of the profit center and includes a market analysis, goals and objectives statement, marketing plan, management plan, and financial pro forma is vital for a successful venture.

A management plan that considers issues such as staffing, space allocation and design, equipment needs, vendor management, operating procedures, and sales procedures is the next logical step. Finally, develop a **financial pro forma** evaluating the capital investment needs, operating expenses, tax and insurance considerations, accounting procedures, documentation, and potential profitability. Establish desired return on investment and profit margins. Many a well-intentioned club operator has implemented multiple ancillary programs with complex operational systems that generate minimal profit. The realistic evaluation of your business is required to determine major areas for profit and provides a road map for developing a successful profit center. Are you a small club with limited space and equipment? Do you have a multipurpose facility with a swimming pool and tennis, squash, or basketball courts? Can your group exercise studios provide an area to generate revenue during off-peak hours? What other spaces in the club can be utilized or expanded? What type of staff training is needed? Do you have access to those staff resources or do you need to outsource or train within?

Before starting a profit center, the club operator should select a member of the existing staff or hire a qualified person to oversee the development and operation of the endeavor. Identifying a person with a background and interest in the venture relieves much of the start-up burden from the already busy club manager. The person selected should have direct access to the club manager and the business plan for continued advice and direction. Link the compensation to the successful launch and operation of the profit center along with a bonus structure that drives achievement beyond 100% of the goal. This profit-center manager should also be responsible for making the existence of this new service or product evident to the membership and for clearly articulating the differentiation between fee and free programming to membership consultants and field staff. Use the marketing and advertising strategies identified in the marketing plan to assist in this effort.

THE BOTTOM LINE

Selecting a qualified and motivated profit-center manager with great communication and sales skills will enhance the potential for success.

Four Common Profit Centers

There are various profit centers that you may want to implement depending on facility space available, club location, and demographics. Personal training, group training, physical therapy and rehabilitation, sport performance training, youth and adult programming, spa services, tanning, food and beverage, and pro shops are several choices. Evaluating the operating model, expenses, and revenues of each will determine which profit center has the highest financial return and adds the most value to the membership.

Personal Training

Twenty-five years ago, most people were not aware of personal training, but today it is a household term. In 2005, 6.1 million Americans paid for the services of a personal trainer, a 53% increase from 1999. For commercial clubs, the incidence of personal training is 13% (International Health, Racquet, and Sportsclub Association [IHRSA] 2004).

THE BOTTOM LINE

A strong personal training business correlates to improved member retention since people who participate in personal training remain members longer.

Personal training can be defined as a one-on-one workout program with a certified fitness professional. According to the International Health, Racquet, and Sportsclub Association (IHRSA), more than 50% of health clubs listed personal training in their top five profit centers. Entire books have been written on the theory and practice of personal training, but in this section we will simply touch on the key elements that any club owner or operator needs to be familiar with in order to manage a successful personal training business.

Location

In most facilities, personal training occurs on the main fitness floor among other members, but some clubs have dedicated areas for personal training clients only. These areas are constructed separately or roped off from the main membership traffic in order to create a sense of exclusivity and perceived value to the individualized attention and training. Specialized equipment, free weights, cardio equipment, and props can be provided for the sole use of clients.

Customers

All members are potential customers, whether they are new members or existing members. People who are pressed for time, want to learn new techniques and proper use of equipment, and are in need of motivation are all prime candidates for personal training, and 1.5 million of the 3.6 million members who belong to a health club and use personal training are first-time members of the club (IHRSA 2004). Personal training is a great vehicle for the new member to get oriented to the club and started on a fitness program the right way, right away.

Weight loss and toning are among the top goals of personal training clients, but taking the time to ask the right questions in a needs analysis with new clients is the only way to determine their goals. Until you understand what the member wants, you cannot provide a solution to get there. It is important that your sales and fitness team does not make assumptions and prequalify a member's interest in personal training without first doing an analysis of the member's needs. A fit member could be bored with her current routine and need some new training tools to reenergize her workout, or a student might find a way to afford getting in shape for a special event he will be attending. The club manager should focus on building a strong team of membership consultants and personal trainers, and an understanding of how these two roles can work together to achieve membership and personal training goals is key. Membership consultants who introduce prospective members to a personal trainer create a sense of comfort and exert a favorable influence on the decision to purchase a membership. This also creates an avenue for the personal trainer to establish a relationship with a new member that could lead to a new personal training client.

Point of Sale

There are many methods of introducing new members to the idea of personal training. Giving new members a taste of the product can go a long way toward their decision to purchase training. A free personal training session or fitness assessment with a trainer is an added benefit to membership and can give the trainer the opportunity to develop a rapport with the member. Trainers can be assigned **conversion goals** for converting free sessions or assessments to personal training packages sold. Bonuses for meeting these goals can be an added incentive.

A phone call congratulating new members on their commitment to get fit is another way a trainer can start building a relationship with the new member. Some companies **bundle** personal training into different membership options, offering one or more sessions in a tiered pricing format (e.g., basic, premier, elite). Other clubs assign personal training quotas as well as membership quotas to their sales consultants in order to promote personal training at the point of a membership sale. Whatever method you choose at the point of sale, linking sales consultants' compensation to the sale of personal training is necessary to drive them to include this product sale in an often-lengthy membership sales process. If this quota process is not monitored and enforced with some rigor and the commission is too small to make an impact, sales consultants will stop selling at the point of membership.

Existing Customers

Once you have established a base of personal training clients, methods must be in place to retain them. Satisfied customers return to buy more sessions. Inspecting the delivery of the personal training product is necessary to maintain the business. Phone calls by the manager to current clients and clients who have not renewed will help the manager assess the quality of the training experience. Not all club operators are trained in the exercise science behind personal training, but there are certain observations they can make to evaluate safety and customer service.

Every trainer should keep a written program card to chart the progress of clients toward their goals. This is not only a good safety practice, but a tool to inspect a well-thought-out, progressive program. Discuss this progressive plan with the trainer. What is the goal of the client and why were these exercises selected? Trainers should be able to articulate their methodology and rationale. Are there changes in weight, equipment, or types of exercises from week to week, or do they remain the same? Every good program should include a warm-up, core training, resistance training, cardiorespiratory conditioning, cool-down, and flexibility. Does the trainer look engaged with the client and does the client look motivated? These are simple areas of validation and inspection that are important to the maintenance of personal training clientele.

THE BOTTOM LINE

As with membership sales, there must be a constant focus on the front door, driving in new business and attracting new clients while also keeping a steady eye on the back door, retaining and serving existing clients.

Package and Program Types

A personal training business may have a menu of personal training packages and programs. Single 1-hour sessions and various-sized packages of 5, 10, and 20 are standard. Thirty-minute and 45-minute sessions are becoming increasingly popular due to the increasing time constraints of clients. If clients are looking for a lower-priced alternative, packages with a ratio of two clients to one trainer are an appealing option. Other affordable and time-efficient programs can include minisessions, with progress evaluations from the trainer at specific points during a prescribed program while the client independently follows the program. Solution-based programs that are tied to a specific desired result are on the rise. Weight loss, event preparation for reunions and weddings, and sport-specific performance programs for golf, tennis, running, and so on are popular choices.

Determining the needs of your customers will help identify what types of programs and packages you want to offer. Execution and accountability of predesigned programs are hard to monitor and trainers can tend to veer off their own course of delivery. If these predesigned programs are a component of your training business, then an ongoing training and inspection plan needs to be in place. Buy-in from the trainers is critical to the successful implementation of any personal training packages or predesigned programs. Time spent coaching and working with your trainers is invaluable to this process.

Cost of Sale, Profit Margins, and Metrics

After a competitive analysis of personal training, pricing can be determined. Standard overall profit margins range from 35% to 50%. Expenses include trainer payroll and taxes plus commissions and any advertising and promotion costs. Single-session pricing can vary based on the certifications and skill level of your trainers, but they are usually priced higher than multiple-session packages. A single hourly session based on demographics and cost of living can range from $50 to $90 a session. Specially priced introductory packages of 3 or 5 sessions can be created to entice members to try personal training.

Types of **industry metrics** used to monitor the growth of the business are percentage of personal training revenue to total membership revenue, penetration percentage of personal training clients to total membership, and percentage of personal training to member usage, as well as average amount spent on training per member. The number

of **active clients** (unique users who have trained in the past 6 months to 1 year), percentage of new clients, and percentage of repeat clients all warrant tracking and review.

Guidelines

After your personal training menu and pricing is complete, the guidelines and policies for purchase and use need to be constructed. Determine expiration dates for personal training programs; expiration dates can vary from 30 days after purchase to 1 year. A tracking report or system for identifying expired sessions should be developed. Establish a cancellation, refund, and makeup policy and adhere to these policies. Sometimes trainers can be their own worst enemies when building a solid training business. In a fledgling business where their schedule is not yet in demand, they may be uncomfortable charging their clients for missed sessions or may empathize with their clients' problems and consistently allow them to cancel with less than 24 hours' notice. The manager may have to enforce these policies until the trainers become more confident and self-assured.

Equipment

The investment in equipment is minimal when using existing equipment, free weights, stability balls, and tubing from your health club. All trainers have a favorite prop they like to use for core training and resistance training.

Operations

Several types of business models can be used when structuring a personal training business in a health club. The club owner needs to decide if offering free fitness services on the floor adds value to membership and a point of differentiation from the competition. With the rapid growth of one-on-one, stand-alone personal training facilities, many health clubs offer personal training as the only vehicle for members to orient themselves to the club and learn how to use the equipment. Employing an independent contractor or an on-staff personal training manager can be used in this type of structure.

Sometimes members perceive the personal training–only structure as a high-pressure sales model whereby they cannot get assistance on the fitness floor without paying for it. If the expectation is to provide a free fitness service (initial fitness assessment, program design, guidance on the fitness floor) and provide personal training for an additional fee, then several types of management support can be used. In some cases, a fitness manager is employed to staff the fitness floor and drive personal training revenues. In other instances, a fitness manager is assigned to provide floor service and a personal training manager is assigned to drive personal training sales. Roles, responsibilities, and priorities need to be defined as well as overhead expenses and commission structures. Are you in the service business or sales business? How do you operate successfully and economically? Will one manager be able to handle the service in a high-usage club and still coach and hold trainers accountable for meeting their training quotas? Will members understand the difference between personal trainers and floor staff? How will they know how to ask for assistance?

Staffing

After deciding upon your business model, you can establish staffing roles, responsibilities, job requirements, budgeted floor hours, pay rates, and commissions. Will trainers be required to work a certain number of floor service hours? Do they need to train a minimum amount of sessions and do they have a specific time frame in which to achieve this? Will you hire only full-time employees or have different standards for part-time employees? Floor rates can differ from personal training rates, commissions can be assigned for personal training sales, incentives can be used to increase the amount of sessions trained, and advanced certifications and continuing education can command higher pay rates. What's the right structure for your company to build this profit center and attract and retain staff? A strong short- and long-term strategy that is in line with your business goals will point you in the direction of success.

Now that your structure is in place, you can define the type and number of employees you need to drive the business. Unless your top sales consultants are selling all of your personal training programs, you need to find motivated, positive people with good communication and people skills and then train them on technical aspects of personal training. Within recent years, personal training has become a true sales business. Personal training certifications provide knowledge in exercise science, physiology, and program design but do not provide the practical skills to build a business. Practical skills include time management, customer service, and sales proficiencies. A trainer with great fitness knowledge does not necessarily equate to a productive trainer. The initial excitement and passion for fitness may wane when confronted with the realities of the club environment and struggles to attract clients. Trainers need to be trained in the sales process. Successful trainers always have goals, and these goals translate to new business and repeat business goals.

After overall budgets are finalized, all trainers need to sign up for their contribution to the overall sales and revenue goal. **Personal training sales** will be defined as the number of personal training sessions sold and **personal training revenue** will refer to the number of personal training sessions used.

Management should meet with trainers to discuss a realistic business plan that projects sales and revenue based on repeat purchases (existing clients) and new purchases (new clients). Tracking client training patterns (e.g., one time per week, two times per month) and the number of sessions left on a client's package makes it easy to determine when and what that client will purchase next. Subtract repeat business from the overall sales budget and the negative variance will determine how many dollars are needed in new client sales. The manager should know the sales abilities of the trainers and, after a time, create a conversion ratio (number of leads, contacts needed to create a sale) to help assign individual trainer quotas. Trainers should be able to articulate where and how they will attract new business. The next step will determine the number of sessions that will be trained based on existing client training patterns and average training usage of a new client. Trainers should always consider holidays and vacations in predicting current client usage.

Recruitment

It will always be a challenge to find qualified, outgoing personal trainers. Identifying a loyal member with a positive attitude and passion for introducing people to fitness is a great way to build the trainer to fit your model. Other areas of recruitment are Web sites, career fairs, certification lists, and colleges.

THE BOTTOM LINE

The right personality is the most important qualification for a successful personal trainer. Training the person to have the necessary technical skills (personal training certifications) is the next step.

Certifications

More than 80 organizations offer personal training and fitness certifications in the United States. Aligning the club with a narrow list of certifications or one certifying body can create consistency in training methods on the fitness floor. This consistent methodology eliminates confusion in the eyes of the member as to the proper way to train. Some facilities create their own internal training programs in order to provide new trainers with basic knowledge and skills and assistance in successfully completing a nationally recognized certification. The investment of time and resources to develop an internal training program may be prohibitive for a single health club, however.

The average national certification costs $250 to $500 and requires current CPR and AED certification. In this litigious culture, it is advised that your trainers hold at least one national certification or college degree in a field related to exercise science. Specialty certifications in sport performance, flexibility, special populations, nutrition, and so on broaden a trainer's scope of practice and appeal to clients with specific needs. Some of the top national training certifications are as follows:

- American College of Sports Medicine (ACSM)
- National Academy of Sports Medicine (NASM)
- Cooper Institute
- National Strength and Conditioning Association (NSCA)
- Aerobics and Fitness Association of America (AFAA)
- American Council on Exercise (ACE)

Client Safety

IHRSA has recently established certain personal training principles to protect the health and safety of clients. Client safety should be the governing principle of personal training, and when it is not, the risk of harm increases. Personal training can never be effective in achieving improved physical fitness if it is not first and foremost safe for the client, and 10 Commandments for Personal Training on page 209 are intended as guidelines for club owners to ensure that the safety of their members is paramount in their personal training program.

With all the investment in coaching and mentoring trainers, a company may still be at risk if it does not build a solid bench of trainers who are progressing in skills and sessions trained. People relocate, experience poor health, find new jobs, and start their own personal training business. Time, appreciation, and recognition build a loyal professional. The personal training business is entrepreneurial; successful trainers quickly identify their strengths

and ability to attract and retain clients and want to take home all of the profit. Since the equipment investment is minimal, they can design their own schedule and train out of their homes, in their clients' homes, or in rented space. Spending the time with a new hire to explain all the benefits of working in a club environment is time well spent. They have access to the entire member base; they may receive benefits; the heat, lighting, rent and equipment, advertising, and promotions are paid for; and they get to network and learn from their peers. Knowing your trainers is an important part of maintaining a loyal workforce.

THE BOTTOM LINE

A solid personal training business cannot be built on skills and performance of only a few trainers.

Advertising and Promotions

Creating awareness and attracting attention will benefit the personal training business. Market positioning to show members how personal training will satisfy their specific needs is a smart business initiative. New-member programs, discounts to new members and new clients, and client loyalty programs are good methods to foster awareness and appreciation among members. Posters, direct mail, referral programs, trainer biography boards, and business cards are other ways to promote your business.

Group Training Programs

The 2004 *IDEA Fitness Programs and Equipment Survey* stated that among the most noteworthy programming trends uncovered during the year was diversified partner training involving 3, 4, or 5 clients, with more than 65% of those polled engaging in partner or small-group activities to improve social interaction, reduce customer costs, and boost training efficiency. In IHRSA's 2004 *Global Report*, David Patchell-Evans, founder of GoodLife Fitness Clubs in Canada, states, "Clubs that are focused on the individuality of their members will be driven by personal training and group exercise. That is to say, focus on programs specific to the individual programs that take into account a member's individual requirements in terms of exercise, diet and lifestyle. These clubs are built around treating members as individuals, not as a 'number.' The other side of this coin is placing emphasis on sociability through offerings such as group exercise or clubs within a

10 Commandments for Personal Training

1. Personal trainers shall not diagnose disease or treat injuries, except for the preliminary treatment of an injury following basic first aid measures.

2. Personal trainers shall not recommend specific supplements, medicine, or curative practices to clients for specific illness, injury, or health conditions unless the personal trainer has additional appropriate credentials to make such a recommendation.

3. Personal trainers shall not train clients with a serious, diagnosed, chronic health condition unless they have been specifically trained and certified to provide training to people with such conditions or are following the procedures prescribed and supervised by a physician.

4. Personal trainers shall not begin training a client before they have received and reviewed a signed, comprehensive health history from the client.

5. Personal trainers shall ask clients before each training session if they are currently experiencing any specific pains or health problems or if they are taking any medications that might be affecting them.

6. Whenever a personal trainer becomes aware of an undiagnosed illness, injury, or a risk factor, the trainer should immediately advise the client to contact the appropriate medical or allied health practitioner.

7. Personal trainers shall not offer specific and individualized nutritional advice unless specifically trained and certified to do so.

8. If, in the course of personal training, a client experiences any unusual pain or discomfort, the trainer should immediately discontinue the training session and advise the client to see a physician or appropriate medical professional.

9. Personal trainers shall not engage in personal training unless they have had first aid training and certification to use CPR and AED (if an AED is available on site for use).

10. Personal trainers should be certified or be licensed in a related field such as physical therapy or athletic training.

Adapted, by permission, from IHRSA.

club. By the latter I mean specialty programs like running clubs or get-ready-for-golf clinics." These trends point to new opportunities for driving personal training revenues through structured group formats.

Many club members pay for programs that are offered outside their health club and may even pay another membership fee in order to access these specialty programs or studios like yoga, Pilates, boxing, and martial arts. Programs that require specialized equipment and specifically trained instructors help the consumer understand their value-added expense. Group training programs such as these can easily be delivered in an existing group exercise studio in a health club, but the impact of these programs on total profit will be commensurate with the amount of space available on the schedule. Available prime-time classes will be limited due to the number of free programs offered.

Aging fitness enthusiasts from professional golfers to suburban housewives have embraced Pilates, a form of resistance training that strengthens muscles and reduces tightness through precise, demanding exercises and movements performed on mats and elaborate equipment. Pilates has become one of the fastest-growing fitness activities in the country, especially among baby boomers worn out by years of running and tennis. Some 9.5 million people participated in Pilates in 2003, the latest year figures were available, up from 2.4 million in 2001 (Sporting Goods Manufacturers Association [SGMA] 2003).

According to a recent industry survey conducted by the IDEA Health and Fitness Association, 60% of responding program directors now offer yoga and 63% offer Pilates. The survey also showed that these programs are going to continue to grow in popularity. In 2004, there were 1.285 million health club members who participated in Pilates, a 203% increase since 2000 (the first year IHRSA started collecting data on Pilates). In a generation made up of 40 million female baby boomers who are obsessed with staying healthy and looking good and who control two-thirds of consumer spending, a profit center that appeals to their sensibilities should be

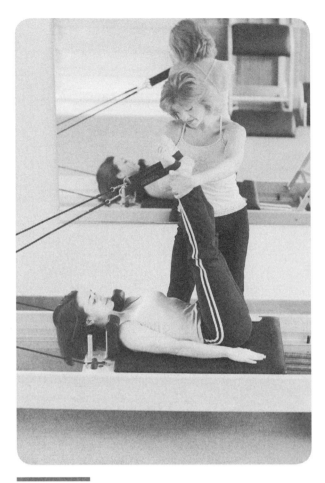

Pilates is one of the fastest-growing specialty programs in the fitness industry. The specialized equipment and training needed for the program are a perceived value to the consumer who understands the need for the additional fee usually required for participation.

© Copyright Rick Gomez 2004/Corbis

a significant revenue source. As written in a 2004 article from *Club Solutions* magazine, "There is no question that business is booming for Pilates. Since 2001, participation has virtually exploded, rising by more than 500%, according to the Sporting Goods Manufacturers Association (SGMA). And, last year, 16% of all IHRSA facilities reported that they were now offering Pilates programming."

THE BOTTOM LINE

In order to increase revenue, prime-time space must be available that appeals to members and nonmembers. Dedicating a studio to small-group progressive training programs eliminates the scheduling restraint.

Yoga and Pilates mat classes are standard items on any club class schedule that can act as feeder programs into more specific and intense programs. When specialized equipment is involved, such as Pilates Reformers, Towers, and Cadillac systems, the investment and training required are a perceived value to the consumer and the need for an additional fee is understood. The market for commercial Pilates equipment has more than quadrupled since 1999, hitting an estimated $28 to $30 million in 2004 from around $6.5 million in 1999, according to Balance Body, an equipment manufacturer. IDEA Health and Fitness Association (2006) believes that Pilates equipment is one of the top 10 types of equipment expected to show the largest increase in usage over the next year. These group programs can progressively train participants to reach specific goals in performance or in the acquisition of a specific skill.

Location

A lack of time slots available in your studio for free group exercise will limit the amount of growth you can expect to see in your program. Pilates, mind–body, or yoga studios with dedicated space and equipment are on the rise. A space that is 800 to 1,100 square feet (74-102 square meters) typically can operate as a stand-alone profit center that generates revenues from group and one-on-one specialized training. Obviously, dedicated spaces with the freedom to schedule fee programs during peak hours in the club are going to generate higher revenues. The locations for equipment-based mind–body studios are best when they are visible to the membership so the programs can develop TOMA in the members. Though visible to club traffic, the studios must be soundproof with limited visibility into the studio (preferably diffused viewing) with its own heating and air-conditioning and sound systems. Light dimmers, ceiling fans, and built-in spaces for participants' shoes and gym bags are deemed necessary by avid participants.

Equipment manufacturers and Pilates certification organizations offer sample revenue-generating program packages. Package types; reservation, makeup, and cancellation policies; and expiration dates should be similar to personal training policies.

Operations

Private one-on-one sessions and semiprivate sessions for 2, 3, or 4 students are standard studio offerings. In order to maximize participation, schedule group classes during peak hours and schedule more one-on-one and semiprivate sessions during off-peak hours. Hiring a studio coordinator who teaches the majority

Equipment Costs for Pilates Programs

Group Reformer for 4, 5, or 6 participants with the use of economical equipment like Allegro make this program a great choice for health clubs. If the program includes classes with and without equipment, then stackable or collapsible equipment is recommended. Types of equipment and props include the following:

- *Mats:* The most basic and essential Pilates apparatus used in free Pilates classes, a quality mat will have a textured nonslip surface and antiskid grip on the bottom to prevent injuries.

- *Magic circle.* A flexible isometric ring with handles that can be used as a prop in any Pilates class, this tool is used to firm the muscles of the upper arms, neck, and thighs. Magic circles cost approximately $32.

- *Reformers:* These are the most popular for group classes. Portable and stackable equipment is available. The Reformer has a gliding platform on which you can sit, kneel, stand, or lie on the front, back, or side. It is equipped with springs, straps, and pulleys and designed to promote torso stability and proper alignment. Reformers can range from $1,700 (stackable) to $3,500 (studio).

- *Towers:* These upright units can be attached to a Reformer to add more exercise variations. Tower attachments for the Allegro Reformers are $1,100.

- *Chairs:* These are commonly known as *Wunda chairs* or *stability chairs* and resemble a stool. Most exercises are performed seated on top and pressing down on the step with the feet, but it can be used lying on the floor, standing up, and lunging forward. Cost ranges from $750 to $1,300.

- *Cadillac:* Also called a *rack* or *trapeze table*, the Cadillac is a raised horizontal table with a four-post frame affixed with a variety of bars, straps, springs, and levers. Cadillacs cost from $1,300 in a wall system to $5,500.

- *Barrels:* These specialized pieces of equipment are in the shape of a barrel and enhance breathing, work the spine to correct posture, and help develop the arms and legs. Semicircle barrels cost $200, whereas high ladder barrels cost $900.

Equipment can be purchased or leased. For a fully equipped studio system, expect to pay anywhere from $25,000 to $40,000.

of classes and has a lower hourly rate for administrative and marketing duties has been a successful strategy. Since qualified and certified instructors may be a limited resource, this part-time manager may be able to grow the business and train new instructors to assume more teaching hours. One caveat: A business should not be built upon one top-notch trainer or instructor. That trainer or instructor may get sick, injured, leave the field, or worse yet, open a new business with your customers. Make sure to negotiate an exclusivity clause and some type of distance restriction for operating a similar business with your coordinator and staff and continually develop a bench of certified instructors.

THE BOTTOM LINE

Small-group training sessions make personal training more affordable than one-on-one sessions and can be held in a dedicated studio simultaneously to increase your profit per class hour.

Cost of Sales and Profitability

Typically, a certified Pilates instructor commands a higher rate than a group exercise instructor, so you may not be able to run a class with fewer than three people and remain profitable. Obviously, club managers must use their judgment to determine if the marketing benefits of running a smaller class in an attempt to build the class outweigh the initial expense. Bonus incentives based on class participation are good motivators for instructors to build their classes. Since many non-health-club users participate in mind–body studios, member and nonmember pricing is recommended. The member pricing should be significantly lower than the nonmember pricing to show the advantages of membership. Make sure not to price your nonmember rate above the standard competition of stand-alone studios, however, or you will price yourself out of the market. Introductory offers, single sessions, and packages should be priced with a similar methodology to personal training packages.

THE BOTTOM LINE

> When determining pricing, you should know what the minimum class size must be in order to remain profitable.

Advertising and Promotion

Offering a free class gives participants a taste of the product before they commit to the purchase. As in an introductory personal training session, a great experience and a motivating instructor are sure ways to close a sale. Group instructors may be uncomfortable with the selling process, but they can easily show participants the benefits of training with them. Packaging a free group class with a free massage or fitness assessment are other ways to expose customers to your product. Inviting nonmembers to an open house that features free classes and demonstrations is another marketing tactic, as are direct mail and direct community outreach. For example, your instructors can lead a warm-up at a running or cycling event and talk about the benefits of Pilates and core strength to improve overall performance.

Training and Development

Well-trained instructors are expected to know anatomy, exercise physiology, human movement, and individual specialties of the discipline. Some certifications require a weekend whereas others require months, years, or even an apprenticeship before instruction is permitted.

Mat and Equipment Certifications

Pilates certifications can be divided into two parts—mat certification and equipment (apparatus) certification. Certification programs range from a weekend to a year, with some certifications requesting apprentice hours. Costs range from $600 to $3,000. Certification companies include the following:

- Power Pilates
- Stott Pilates
- Peak Pilates
- Polestar
- Pilates Coach

Spa Services

The term *spa* has long been a point of confusion in the fitness industry. The word *spa* often describes both the wet facility, also known as the *whirlpool,* and the profit center in which relaxing and healing services such as massage and facials take place. Historically spas evolved around natural mineral or hot springs. People would travel many miles to bathe and drink the medicinal waters for their healing powers. Over the years, *spa* has come to mean a place of healing and relaxation, including day spas, mineral spas, resort spas, medical spas, and cruise spas. Many health and wellness centers are now incorporating spa services, such as massages and facials, in order to provide members with a place of relaxation and stress reduction and to provide the organization with a profit center.

Spa Industry Trends

Long thought to be for only the rich and famous, spa services are becoming an integral part of many people's lifestyles because of the relaxation and stress reduction these services provide. There are an estimated 12,100 spas throughout the United States and 2,100 in Canada. In the United States, the largest spa category is the day spa. The International Spa Association (ISPA) reports that approximately 136 million spa visits were made in the United States in 2003, with 60% of these visits occurring in day spas and 27% in resort and hotel spas. The *ISPA Consumer Trends Report* found that consumers generally want bread-and-butter services (facials, pedicures, manicures, and massages). It was also noted that consumers experiment more when at spas on vacation and expect a broader array of services. Consumer visits to spas are driven by one or more of the following:

- Indulgence (i.e., pleasure, fun, appealing to the senses)
- Escape (i.e., relief from pressures of daily life)
- Work (i.e., individual work, largely related to self-improvement on some aspect of one's emotional state or long-term spiritual and personal dispositions)

The investment in a full-fledged day spa can be significant and the scheduling component complex, so many health clubs opt for individual treatment rooms that offer bread-and-butter services. IHRSA reports that 60% of its clubs offer massages.

Menu of Services

The list of possible services a fitness or wellness center could offer its members is restricted only by the amount of space, facilities, and creativity available. Examples of skin care services include aromatherapy facials; glycolic peel facials; moisturizing facials; cleansing facials; waxing services for the lip, brow, back, bikini area, and legs; and so on. Body care services include Swedish, sports, aromatherapy, and shiatsu massage, as well as reflexology, herbal wraps, and loofah scrubs, to name a few. In addition, many salon services, such as hair care and nail care, are offered. Facilities that venture into skin care and hair care services make a larger financial and spatial commitment to the spa concept and have the opportunity to reap the financial benefits of these services. Refer to table 11.1 for descriptions of skin, body, hair, and nail care services.

Facility Requirements

Most facilities that are contemplating adding spa services will initiate their effort by offering massage services. Whether the facility offers massage only or a menu of body, skin, and salon services, the facility requirements are crucial to the success of the operation. The environment must create a sensory refuge from the hustle and bustle of everyday life.

Spa services should offer a luxury experience in a quiet and relaxing atmosphere. Carefully consider renovating existing space for spa services. Although adding services such as massage won't require a great deal of space, the location of the space is crucial. The ideal spa treatment room is located in a quiet area away from the normal traffic patterns of the club. The rooms must be relatively accessible from the locker rooms or provide convenient dressing facilities close by. The decor and lighting of the rooms and surrounding areas should be soft and indirect to create an ambiance of relaxation and stillness. Equip the treatment rooms with a sink and electrical outlets. Play relaxing music in the treatment rooms and surrounding areas. The ventilation of the treatment areas is crucial. Although the treatment room is typically kept warmer (70 to 76 degrees Fahrenheit, or 21 to 24 degrees Celsius) than the health club environment, the room must never feel stuffy or hot. The space requirement for each treatment room is approximately 120 square feet (11 square meters).

Creating a private, luxurious treatment room and surroundings will enhance relaxation, project a positive image for the facility, and encourage repeat business.

Equipment Requirements

Equipment requirements for spa services vary depending on the type of services the club offers and the personal preferences of the technicians hired to perform the services. Equipping a massage room will cost approximately $1,500 to $3,000. Additional operating supplies such as linens, oils, towels, and so on will cost approximately $500 to $1,000, depending on the volume of traffic and the quality of the supplies. Facial rooms will cost approximately $7,000 to $10,000 to equip. Operating supplies will necessitate an additional investment of $500 to $1,500. Retail sale of facial products enhances the profitability of the spa by providing revenue with little overhead. An initial investment in this retail inventory can range from $500 to several thousand dollars. You can equip nail care stations for $1,000 to $5,000, depending on the types of equipment.

The necessary equipment for each spa treatment room is listed in Spa Equipment and Operational Supply Lists on page 215. These lists are intended to be thorough, but they are not exhaustive. The preferences of the therapist you hire should determine the equipment and supplies you order. Depending on the type of treatment room, it is important to purchase the best equipment available. The equipment used in most services will dramatically affect the overall service delivery. Use a spa consultant or ask the service provider you have hired before selecting and purchasing any spa equipment.

Operations

The operation of a spa facility is much different than that of a fitness facility. The types of products needed and the services delivered differ dramatically. The club manager should consider using an experienced spa consultant or hiring experienced treatment professionals to enhance the probability for success.

Marketing

Marketing spa services within the fitness operations can enhance the professional image of the facility. Careful consideration of the marketing aspects of the spa services can improve member retention and enhance the profile of the facility within the community.

Before offering spa services, the club operator should perform a market survey to analyze the need and desire for the services to be offered; determine the target market for the services; evaluate the competition and their pricing structures; and review all local, state, and federal codes involving delivery of spa services. The increasing demand for spa services nationwide should provide the club operator with a reasonable sense of security in offering these services. Local examination of the demand for these services, however, is always warranted.

Table 11.1 Spa Service Descriptions

Service	Description
BODY THERAPIES	
Swedish massage	This classical European massage technique uses gentle manipulation of the muscles using massage oils. Used to improve circulation, ease muscle aches and tension, improve flexibility, and create relaxation. This is the most common form of massage performed in the United States.
Sports massage	Performed with or without oil, this massage uses similar strokes as the Swedish massage, yet typically with much deeper pressure. This massage enhances circulation and reduces pre-exercise muscle tightness or postexercise muscle soreness.
Aromatherapy massage	Combining the sense of smell with touch, this light, rhythmic massage uses essential oils to balance and restore energy levels. Different types of essential oils produce different results (i.e., relaxation versus stimulation).
Reflexology	This ancient Chinese technique uses pressure points, usually on the feet, but sometimes the hands and ears, to restore the flow of energy throughout the body.
Shiatsu massage	This traditional Japanese massage is typically performed on a *tatami* (floor mat) with no oil. This acupressure massage applies pressure to specific points in the body to stimulate and unblock meridians, or pathways in the body through which life energy flows.
Thalassotherapy	These treatments use the therapeutic benefits of the sea and seawater products. Seaweed and algae wraps and seawater hydrotherapy treatments are common.
Fango	*Fango* is Italian for "mud," and this service involves a highly mineralized mud mixed with oil or water and applied over the body as a heat pack to detoxify, soothe the muscles, and stimulate circulation.
Loofah scrub	A full-body scrub with a loofah sponge exfoliates the skin and stimulates circulation.
Herbal wrap	Involves a body wrap using strips of cloth that are soaked in a heated herbal solution and wrapped around the body, followed by a period of rest. Used to eliminate impurities and detoxify, as well as for relaxation.
Hydrotherapy	Includes underwater jet massage, showers, jet sprays, and mineral baths.
Salt glow	The body is rubbed with a coarse salt, sometimes in combination with fragrant oils, to remove the outer layer of dead skin and stimulate circulation.

Table 11.1

Service	Description
SKIN CARE THERAPIES	
Aromatherapy facial	Essential oils are used to moisturize, cleanse, and increase circulation to the face. Fragrant essential oils enhance relaxation.
Glycolic peel facial	Low-level glycolic acids are used to remove the outer layer of dead facial skin and cleanse and moisturize the face. Typically done in a series of 6 to 10 treatments.
Moisturizing facial	This facial is ideal for those who suffer from dry skin or who are exposed to harsh environmental conditions. Uses masks, massage, and cleansing to rehydrate the skin and enhance circulation.

Spa Equipment and Operational Supply Lists

Massage Room Equipment
Massage table
Rolling chair or stool
Hydrocollator
Roll cushions and supports
Face cradle
Towel and sheet storage cabinet
Clock
Floor and room heater

Facial Equipment
Facial bed with arm set
Three-tiered trolley with drawer
Steamer with ozone and stand
Champion Lucas spray
Galvanic machine, high-frequency machine, brush and suction machine (all in one)
Double-pot wax melter
Electric terry mitts
Heating pad
Wet sterilizer kit
Facial chair with back support
Magnifying lamp with stand
Hot towel cabinet
Paraffin wax unit
Electric terry booties
UV sterilizer (dry)

(continued)

(continued)

Manicure Equipment
Manicure table
Client chair
Manicurist's chair

Pedicure Equipment
Pedicure tub (requires water hookup and drain)
Pedicurist's chair
Pedicurist's accessory cart

Nail Care Miscellaneous Equipment
Polish dryer (hands and feet)
Paraffin wax unit (hands and feet)
Nail polish rack
Locking cabinets and drawers
Terry foot mitts
Terry hand mitts
Finger bowls
Magnifying lamps
Cotton dish for pedicure station
Large sanitizer jar

Determining the target market is an important consideration. Will services be available to members only or will the local community have access to these services? Will members receive discounts on products and services? Will you allow community members who frequent the spa to join the fitness facility at discounted prices? Several opportunities exist for creative marketing. The club operator should review what competition exists for these services, keeping in mind that many people enjoy these services only if they are convenient. Pricing should be competitive, with dues-paying members receiving discounts on services and products. Review local and state codes and regulations as they relate to the treatment room, the treatment provider, and the facility offering spa treatments.

THE BOTTOM LINE

An innovative marketing staff can use spa facilities to enhance the image of the organization, to increase member satisfaction and retention, and to aid in recruitment.

Once you have researched and made decisions concerning these areas, the marketing personnel should put together a brochure or pamphlet explaining the benefits of spa services, a brief description of the services, the rates for each service, the types of services offered, the qualifications of the treatment providers, the cancellation policy, and how to schedule an appointment. Additionally, we recommend that you create a brochure regarding the services. Many first-time spa goers are apprehensive about the services. In this brochure, answer questions regarding modesty, where to go, how to pay, and how to communicate with the therapist. Enjoyment of the service will be heightened if the client knows what to expect and can fully relax.

A final marketing concern is gift certificates. Many people have their first spa experience as a result of a gift certificate. Provide gift certificates for tournament prizes, charity donations, or new-member gifts. Gift certificates for spa services are popular gift items. There is a great likelihood that people will spend money on a spa service for someone they care about before spending the money on themselves. Positioning gift certificates for spa services, particularly during the Valentine's Day, Mother's Day, Father's Day, and Christmas holiday times, will help generate strong revenues year-round.

Staffing

The staffing of the spa facility is crucial to its success. Treatment providers must be qualified and experienced in the type of luxury service the club is marketing. Spa staff are often either hired by the facility and work as employees or are contracted as laborers who work for a percentage of the revenue. If the goal of the facility is to provide the organization with a profit position, hiring the treatment providers as staff members and paying an hourly wage plus commission are desirable. If the spa services are only an amenity to enhance the professional image of the facility and profitability is not crucial, using outside contractors is worth considering.

Typically, treatment providers hired as staff members are paid an hourly wage for the hours they are scheduled to be available plus a commission for each hour of service they provide. This commission gives the professional a vested interest in building a regular clientele. Gratuities are customary. The gratuity can be at the discretion of the client, or you can apply a service charge and include it in the service price. Competitive compensation for treatment providers ranges from $15 to $40 per hour of service. Benefits are an optional incentive that the club can offer to treatment providers who demonstrate a commitment to the profitability of the spa. Although the treatment provider may be able to earn more per hour in a private practice, the benefits of working for an organization that pays all overhead, purchases all supplies, markets aggressively for clients, and may or may not offer a benefits package cannot be overestimated.

Staff members who perform services are typically required by local and state regulations to maintain a current license or registration. Maintain proof of these licenses and registrations in the human resources files of the organization. Regular training and continuing education classes are recommended for treatment providers to stay abreast of current standards of practice in the industry. Maintaining membership in the American Massage Therapy Association (AMTA) or another governing body will help in this process.

Any facility employing more than five treatment providers should consider appointing a department head or senior treatment provider. In addition to being an experienced technician, this person should possess the business, communication, and supervisory skills for handling all scheduling, commissions and gratuity reconciliation, product and supply ordering, and hiring, training, and discipline of staff. This person should work closely with the marketing and professional staff of the club to ensure all employees understand the benefits of spa services and to assist in marketing.

Legal Considerations

As mentioned, a variety of local and state regulations exist regarding the operation of spa facilities. Treatment providers in many states must maintain current registration and licensure. Additionally, the facility or spa itself must be registered or licensed by the state. Particular treatment practices, such as those that deal with implement sterilization and cleanliness and draping or covering a client during the service, are also regulated in many states. Be sure to check with the state department of health or human services that oversees the operation of spa or salon facilities.

In addition to state registration and licensure, each therapist should be covered by a professional liability and malpractice insurance policy with a minimum coverage of $1 million dollars. Insurance is a necessity. A lawsuit filed against you or your practice can be financially devastating. This insurance policy is available to treatment professionals through membership in professional organizations such as AMTA.

Profitability

For those facilities that have waded through the maze of renovation, organization, licensure, and registration and have opened a spa facility, the potential profits are significant. Massage services typically produce 40% to 55% profit after all wages, benefits, and operational expenses are paid. Facial and nail care services typically generate 30% to 50% profit when revenues from both treatments and retail skin care product sales are considered. Maintaining a tight control on operational spending, wages, and benefits can yield a successful profit center.

Maintenance

The spa area should receive normal custodial cleaning, with special attention paid to the floors around the treatment table, doorknobs, light switches, and cabinet doors. These areas should be sterilized as part of a daily cleaning schedule. Linens should be changed following each service, including pillowcases and any draping material. These linens should be washed separately from other club linens because they may contain oils, muds, facial products, wax, and so on. The table surface should be cleaned with alcohol between each service. All implements used in a facial or nail service, such as nail nippers or facial tweezers, must be sterilized between each use. Therapists must be required to wash their hands following each service and before working on the client's face. Alcohol can be used if water is not easily available. These sanitation rules are established to prevent the transference of skin infections or communicable diseases from one client to another. Check with local and state officials for specific rules and regulations in your area.

Professional Organizations and Resources

Professional organizations exist to assist the club operator in developing spa facilities and treatments. You may contact the following organizations for assistance with local and state regulations and locating potential staff.

- American Massage Therapy Association (AMTA)
- International Spa and Fitness Association (ISPA)
- Health and human services department of your state government

Youth Programming

Youth programming is a growing industry trend. According to IHRSA's *Profiles of Success* (2006), "The percentage of the U.S. population over age six that belonged to a health club increased from 13.5% to 15.5% between 2001 and 2005. During the past five years, the number of members between six and seventeen who joined a health club increased by 58%, the most growth of any age segment." About 10.8% of the U.S. population between the ages of 12 and 17 belongs to a health club, or 2.8 million juniors. Children are the second-fastest growing population of gym members, second only to the actively aging population of adults over 55 years of age.

Today's young people are considered to be the most inactive generation in history due to reductions in physical education programs and unavailable and unsafe community recreational systems. Being overweight is a serious health concern for children and adolescents. Data from the National Health and Nutrition Examination Surveys (NHANES) (1976-1980 and 2003-2004) show that the prevalence of overweight young people is increasing. For children aged 2 to 5 years, prevalence increased from 5.0% to 13.9%; for those aged 6 to 11 years, prevalence increased from 6.5% to

18.8%; and for those aged 12 to 19 years, prevalence increased from 5.0% to 17.4%. Statistics like these will help make children's recreational and fitness programs a primary focus of government, communities, businesses, and parents.

Before implementing youth programming, you must determine if your club has a family-based membership and if the majority of the membership is family friendly. You must determine if the purpose of the programming is a true profit center or adding value for members with children. After establishing baseline criteria, you should look at the percentage of children under age 15 within a 10-minute drive time to your facility. Many parents prefer skill development and recreational programs over traditional babysitting services, and it is well known that parents are more likely to spend money on their child than on themselves.

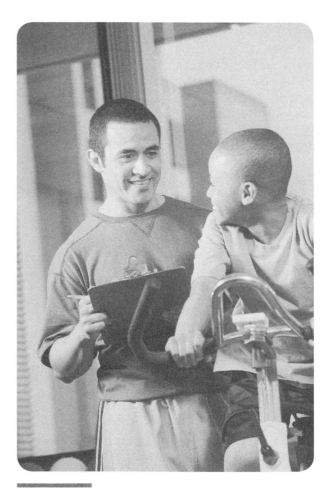

As a profit center, youth programming will be successful in those clubs that are family oriented. Parents will welcome recreational and fitness programs that provide activities for their children in a safe club setting.

© OnRequest Images/Stock This Way/Corbis

If yours is a family-oriented club and a multi-recreational facility as well, your ability to generate large profits significantly increases. Multipurpose clubs with swimming pools, basketball courts, volleyball courts and multirecreational spaces have a greater ability to generate a large amount of revenue with high profit margins. As stated previously, today's young people are considered the most inactive generation in history; this is a key indicator that youth programming in a safe club setting will be a welcome choice for a parent.

THE BOTTOM LINE

Youth programming appeals to many nonmembers and provides an opportunity to market the benefits of membership to nonmember parents.

Location

Youth programming activities or studios should be located in an area that is easily accessible to parking and strollers and handicapped access. When offering children's programs, there is a need to accommodate busy parents with multiple children of various ages. For considerations of safety, sound, and adult members, the location of your youth studio, recreational activities, and traffic pattern should be away from main areas of the club. As the programs grow, the need to add a separate registration and point-of-sale desk may arise to eliminate congestion at the front desk. Program spaces should be visible to members and create a strong impression in the parent in order to compete with stand-alone children's businesses.

Types of Programs and Scheduling

As with any new profit center, the potential for growth and the types of programs offered are directly correlated to the size and type of facility. It is recommended that you have a strong anchor program that has proven revenue results as the basis of your youth programs. A strong anchor program is typically a program that is identified as a need, like swimming lessons (a child must learn to swim to be safe around the water), summer camps for working parents, and exciting birthday party activities. Without a strong draw to the youth market, it is difficult to get the critical mass of customers necessary to build additional revenue-generating programs. Adding swimming pools and multisport areas are significant capital investments that will increase operational and facility maintenance concerns, so additional management and responsibilities should be factored into the equation. Clubs that utilize existing group exercise studios and fitness spaces have limited programming choices and time slots, which will limit the ability to drive significant profit.

Selecting a small cluster of two to three programs gives parents choices for their children. Offer packages in manageable 4- to 8-week sessions so as not to interfere with other extracurricular activities such as recreational leagues, school and church studies, and other programs.

Mommy and Me programs include water tots, tumbling, gym, and yoga. These programs fit well in group exercise studios at off-peak times. Preschool recreational programs like creative rhythm and dance, gymnastics, and sports appeal to parents, who are trying to identify their child's program preferences at an early stage. These types of programs will be successful in the morning and midafternoon. It is beneficial to use the group exercise class schedule and club usage as a filter to determine usage patterns by young mothers.

Programs for school-aged children should be offered after school until early evening and on Saturdays. Call the local school district for the school calendar, holidays, and daily school start and dismissal times before developing your schedule. Dance, gymnastics, swim lessons, sport skills, and martial arts are popular.

Programs that satisfy a need of the parents, such as swimming lessons and summer camps as an alternative to day care, are an instant win. Aquatics programs have strict licensing and safety requirements. Summer camps can be offered indoors and outdoors.

Birthday parties are a hit with everyone from preschoolers to preteens. If you have developed some core recreational programs, use them as featured elements of the party. Swim, sport, and gymnastics parties are a great fit in a health club. A complete competitive analysis of surrounding party centers is necessary before developing pricing and party options. Some businesses include cakes, food, party favors, invitations, instruction, a personal party coordinator, and more. All of these elements must be figured into the cost of sale and overall profitability.

Special events during club hours or after hours present an opportunity to open the club to the community and generate revenue. Girl and Boy Scouts, youth groups, schools, and other community groups can flow through a series of activities customized to your facility offerings.

Stand-alone sport performance centers for athletic training are on the rise, catering to the young athletes who want to improve their speed, agility, and quickness in their sport of choice. Parents are looking for ways to help their children succeed in athletic tryouts. Prime hours of operation are weekdays after school from 4 to 9 p.m. and Saturdays. Off-season training (when certain sports are not in play) are the busiest times, which include winter and summer months.

The limited usage and times of operation put the business at risk due to high overhead costs. High volume and pricing must occur in order to support a profitable structure. Club facilities with a strong membership base and available space can support this model with existing management and trainers in a more cost-effective manner. These programs can be packaged similarly to the adult personal training programs. Participants must commit to 2 to 3 days per week for a series of consecutive weeks. Measurable training results must be tracked and guaranteed with a specific amount of training in a certain time period in order for the program to prove valuable to the parent and athlete.

THE BOTTOM LINE

Define your target age market based on space accommodations. This will assist you in selecting the right programs.

Security

Security in the child care area must be of the utmost concern. In addition to medical emergencies, analyze and reanalyze the security of the children to ensure their safety. The manager and organization must ensure that only the correct parent or guardian drops off or picks up the child. The installation of security systems and cameras is warranted when access from the main desk and club management is distant.

Child Care

Child care facilities are rarely profitable as individual entities and may actually be a cost department when viewed superficially. Child care is often considered a headache to operate, yet it may mean the difference between a person joining your club or a competitive club. To combat this potential financial drain on club profitability, many leading facilities are expanding their child care offerings to include youth programming profit centers. Despite the difficulties that child care centers are experiencing, their popularity is high among members of health and fitness facilities. The increasing number of members with infants and children and the ongoing need to attract new members make child care centers a necessity for today's facilities.

KEY TERMS

active clients
bundle
conversion goals
financial pro forma

industry metrics
personal training revenue
personal training sales
profit center

REFERENCES AND RECOMMENDED READING

Agoglia, J. 2005. Money talks. *Club Industry's Fitness Business-Pro*, March 2005.

Centers for Disease Control and Prevention (CDC). 2007. Childhood overweight: Overweight prevalence. Retrieved April 23, 2007, from www.cdc.com.

Endelman, K. 2004. Pilates programs strengthen profits. *Club Solutions Magazine*, November 2004.

IDEA Health and Fitness Association. 2004. *IDEA fitness programs and equipment survey*. San Diego: IDEA.

———. 2006. *IDEA fitness programs and equipment survey*. San Diego: IDEA.

International Health, Racquet, Sportsclub Association (IHRSA). 2004. *Global Report*. Boston: IHRSA.

———. 2004. *Health club trends report*. Boston: IHRSA.

———. 2006. *Profiles of success*. Boston: IHRSA.

International Spa Association. 2005. *ISPA Consumer Trends Report*. Lexington, KY: ISPA.

Mahoney, L. 2006. The next big thing is still Pilates. *Club Business Industry Magazine*, August 2006.

McCarthy, J. 2006. *IHRSA's guide to membership retention*. Boston: IHRSA.

Sporting Goods Manufacturers Association (SGMA). 2003. *Sports participation in America*. North Palm Beach, FL: SGMA.

U.S Department of Health and Human Services. 2003-2004. *Health and Nutrition Examination Survey.*

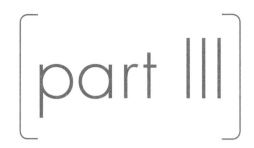

Operations and Facility Management

The operations side of running a fitness business is the last area of club management covered in this book. Do not make the mistake of misjudging the importance of the topics covered in this part's chapters. The contributors have all seen what can happen when these areas are neglected or are not thoroughly understood. The most successful clubs recognize their importance and have developed systems to ensure each area is working at its best.

In chapter 12, Mike Bates discusses the importance of financial management for the club manager. Understanding how to read financial statements and to build budgets is critical to the long-term success of any business. Managing expenses and collecting overdue accounts are two other important areas that should be closely scrutinized by the club manager interested in meeting financial objectives.

Next, in chapter 13, Anthony Abbott and Mike Greenwood describe the importance of health and safety within the fitness industry. You will learn how to identify potential hazards and to minimize their potential impact on your business. Mistakes in this area can cost millions of dollars in lawsuits and more importantly can affect the lives of members, prospective members, and staff.

Mike Greenwood and Anthony Abbott team up again in chapter 14 to cover the topic of facility maintenance. A well-kept facility and preventive maintenance schedule are cornerstones of a well-run fitness center. This chapter is full of easy-to-follow steps and guidelines to ensure that your facility and the equipment within it are running at their best.

In chapter 15, Mike Bates looks at equipment selection. From purchasing to maintaining your equipment, this chapter gives you the foundation to make informed decisions. Mike also looks at some of the trends in specialized equipment design that affects how clubs will select equipment now and in the future.

John Wolohan covers the basics of contract law in chapter 16. Employment legal issues are covered and an overview of insurance is presented. This chapter provides the information that will help you make the best decisions in the areas of legal and insurance concerns.

In the final chapter, chapter 17, Dave Hardy explains how to properly evaluate your fitness business. Stepping back and taking the time to properly evaluate your business and decide where it is going often forgotten as managers get caught up running the daily operation. This is another one of those critical skills that a fitness club manager needs to apply in order for the business to be successful.

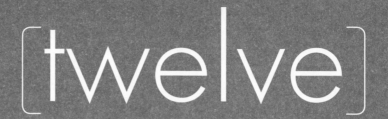

Understanding Financial Management

Mike Bates

LEARNING OBJECTIVES

After studying this chapter, the reader will be able to

- identify the key components of the income statement, balance sheet, and statement of cash flows and understand their differences;

- understand the various types of budgets and the steps involved in preparing a budget;

- recognize the importance of managing expenses; and

- appreciate the impact that taxes have on financial planning and decision making.

Tales From the Trenches

Jan was the owner of a small women's-only facility. When she opened her club she did so by borrowing money from every person she knew, along with using some personal savings that she had accumulated over the years. Her passion was fitness and helping people change their bodies, and she was good at it. After her first year in operation things seemed to be going well and she was taking a small salary out of the business. When she started to do this, she noticed that the club bank account would occasionally run low and in some instances she needed to overdraft her account to keep up with her expenses.

As she was preparing for the busy month of January, she was considering hiring new staff but did not know how many hours she could give them or how she would have enough to pay them. Up to this point Jan had relied on a friend to look after her bookkeeping, and she had not used a budget.

One of her clients was an accountant, so Jan decided to call her and schedule a meeting to discuss the financial situation of the club. When they met, the accountant was not entirely shocked that Jan didn't have a budget. She said she saw this all the time with small businesses and it was one of the main reasons why small businesses closed. The accountant explained how a budget could help forecast cash flow, expenses, and revenue. Jan was excited and couldn't believe she didn't have a budget in place already. After doing some reading on her own and meeting with the accountant again, she sat down with her bookkeeper and began to work on the budget. She was amazed by all of the information that the bookkeeper had kept, which was going to make it a lot easier to create the budget. Although it was not quite as easy as she had hoped, the final budget was soon completed.

Within 3 months of its implementation, Jan noticed some parts of the budget that were not as accurate as they could be, so she made a note to correct them on the next budget. Besides a few areas that needed to be changed, Jan found the budgeting process to be quite helpful. It allowed her to view the business from a new perspective, it allowed her to control expenses by letting staff know that the club had only budgeted for a certain amount of money in specific areas, and it allowed her to see when would be the best times to hire staff based on the cash flow. She felt she had better control over her business and had a clearer picture of where she was going in the future.

In the past, fitness club managers and owners had a passion for helping people exercise but may not have had a thorough understanding of the various business functions of running a fitness club. This has changed in recent years, and now some of the most important functions a manager oversees are the financial reporting, analyzing, and budgeting for the club. Some of these functions are done daily or weekly, and at the very least they are done monthly.

A manager needs to be able to answer the following questions:

- Is the business generating enough cash flow to pay its bills?

- Does the business have strong systems in place to collect on overdue accounts?

- Are we properly budgeting staff hours based on the ups and downs of the business?

- What are some of the benchmarks that the best clubs in the business use to determine their success?

- How can I use these benchmarks in my club?

- Do staff know the procedures for purchasing supplies?

- Do staff know the sales goals for the upcoming month?

- Is the nonprofit status (if applicable) of the organization being properly maintained?

- Will the club have enough money in 6 months to lease five new treadmills?

Whether operating a single club, multiclub chain, city recreation center, or nonprofit center, the financial principles in this chapter are critical to long-term success. An assortment of accounting terms is used throughout this chapter; see Accounting Terminology on page 225 to become familiar with the definitions of these terms.

Accounting Terminology

accounting—The recording, classifying, summarizing, and interpreting of financial data.

accounts payable—The money that your company owes to another individual or company.

accounts receivable—Individuals or companies that owe you money.

assets—Properties of value owned by a business or individual.

balance sheet—A financial statement that reveals the assets, liabilities, and owner's equity in a firm as of a specific date.

book value—The value of an asset as it appears on the balance sheet.

budget—A financial plan indicating expected income and expenses for a specific amount of time, which can be used as a means of exercising financial control.

capital—Money, goods, land, or equipment used to produce other goods or services.

equity—The money value of a property or of an interest in a property in excess of claims or liens against it.

fixed assets—The land, plant, equipment, and other physical productive assets of a firm that are expected to have a useful life in excess of 1 year.

fixed costs—Costs that must be incurred regardless of the level of production.

generally accepted accounting procedures (GAAP)—A common set of accounting principles and standards (set by policy boards) that companies use to compile their financial statements.

gross profit—The profit earned on sales after deducting the cost of the goods sold but before deducting other business expenses.

income statement—A financial statement revealing the summary of the income or loss resulting from the business transactions for the preceding period.

ledger—Individual account books that keep a running balance of the status of each account.

liability—Debt owed to others and the equity of creditors in business firms.

market value—The highest amount that a buyer would be willing to pay for a product or service.

net income—The earnings of a company after allowing for all legitimate business expenses, including taxes.

operating expenses—Expenses incurred from the production operations of the business.

profit—Excess of sales income after deducting all related expenses.

variable costs—Costs whose total magnitude varies directly with the level of production.

Cash Versus Accrual Accounting

Managers need to determine whether they will use cash or accrual accounting when recording revenues and expenses. **Cash accounting** involves recording business transactions only when the business receives or pays cash. In a cash-based system, you record the revenue when it is received, regardless of when goods are sold or services rendered. When you sell merchandise or render services in one month and collect cash the following month, cash-based accounting recognizes the revenue only when you receive the cash. Similarly, accounting for expenses means that when you make a cash payment, you record the amount as an expense. For example, if a utility bill is incurred in June (because that was the month that you actually used the electricity, water, or gas) but not paid until July, the expense is not recorded until the month in which it is paid.

Accrual accounting records transactions when they occur rather than when cash is received or paid. In this type of accounting, you record revenues when you earn them whether or not you have received cash, and you record expenses when they occur as opposed to when you pay them. Therefore, as in the example of the utility bill, you would record the bill in June rather than in July.

There are advantages and disadvantages to both systems. Although a cash-based system is simple to implement, it is difficult to determine an accurate net worth because unpaid revenue and expenses are not reflected. Also, organizations that offer prepaid annual memberships will appear financially solvent when cash is received, but if funds are not properly managed in the remaining 11 months of the year, a cash shortage could occur. For example, if a member prepays a year's membership for $900, the cash-based system recognizes all $900 in the month in which the cash is received. In the accrual system, $75 ($900 divided by 12 months) is recognized each month as member revenue.

Although it is not uncommon for a club to adopt a mix of the cash and accrual methods, the preferred system for commercial health and fitness settings is accrual-based accounting because it provides a more accurate understanding of operations. There are three reasons why accrual accounting is preferred among club operators (Grantham 1998):

1. Accrual accounting allows for better cash management because all prepaid memberships received are recorded as 1/12 of the dues for each month of the year.

2. Accrual accounting provides a more realistic picture of the financial status of the business by including all unpaid expenses and unpaid revenues that are due.

3. You can report the net worth of a club with accrual accounting but not with a cash-based system. This is especially important if a club is attempting to obtain a loan or solicit investors.

A well-organized accounting system entails several functions, all designed to record, track, protect, and analyze the financial transactions of a business. A series of checks and balances should always be in place to account for every transaction that goes in and out of the organization. In addition, the process by which you accumulate financial information to prepare financial statements is integral to the accounting system. Fried (2004) says that the purpose of any accounting system is to provide information for the following purposes:

1. Making decisions concerning the use of limited resources, including the identification of crucial decisions and determination of objectives and goals

2. Effectively directing and controlling human and material resources

3. Maintaining and reporting on the custodianship of resources

4. Contributing to the overall effectiveness of the organization

THE BOTTOM LINE

Most fitness clubs use accrual accounting and record revenue when the money was actually earned.

Financial Statements

The purpose of financial statements is to provide a financial summary of the current status of the fitness organization. Generally, an in-house or outside accountant prepares financial statements from the accounting records of the company and completes them in a timely and accurate fashion. Preparing financial statements depends on an organized bookkeeping system that tracks every transaction from its inception until it becomes part of the financial statement. Comparing industry trends, budget analysis, internal controls, and short- and long-term planning are all internal uses of these statements. External uses include financial information for refinancing, renovating, or expanding a facility or debt within the organization.

Balance Sheet

The **balance sheet** shows a company's assets, liabilities, and owner's equity at a specific point in time. For example, on October 31, 2007, Club ABC had the following balance sheet (figure 12.1).

The balance sheet is divided in half, with assets on the left and liabilities and owner's equity on the right. The basic formula that all balance sheets follow is

assets = liabilities + owner's equity.

For a balance sheet to be accurate, this formula must always hold true. Another way of looking at the formula is to express it as a function of owner's equity:

owner's equity = assets − liabilities.

Assets are anything a business owns that has monetary value. In the previous example, the cash invested, land, exercise equipment, office equipment, inventory, and building are all assets. Assets are divided into two main categories: current assets

XYZ Company
Balance sheet
October 31, 2007

Assets

Current assets

Cash		185,236	
Inventory		85,693	
Total current assets			270,929

Fixed assets

Equipment	1,256,756		
Furniture and fixtures	356,458		
	1,613,214		
Less: accumulated depreciation	563,254	1,049,960	
Land		650,000	
Total fixed assets			1,699,960

Other assets

Loan fees	56,000		
Security deposits	7,500		
Total other assets		63,500	
Total assets			2,034,389

Liabilities and stockholder's equity

Current liabilities

Accounts payable		75,896	
Current portion of long-term debt		2,584	
Payroll taxes		6,589	
Total current liabilities			85,069

Long-term debt

Note payable—bank		953,450	
Less: current portion		2,584	
Total long-term debt			950,866

Stockholder's equity

Capital stock		1,000	
Additional paid-in-capital		25,000	
Current period profit (loss)		254,875	
Retained earnings		717,579	
Total stockholder's equity			998,454
Total liabilities and stockholder's equity			2,034,389

Figure 12.1 A typical balance sheet for a fitness club.

and fixed assets. An accountant assumes current assets—cash, accounts receivable, inventory, and prepaid expenses—to be either cash or converted into cash within 1 year. Fixed assets—the land, building, office furniture, and fitness equipment—are the more long-lived resources owned by the business. With the exception of land, these assets are valued at book value minus depreciation.

Liquidity refers to the ease and quickness with which assets can be converted into cash. The entries shown under current assets are considered the most liquid, whereas the entries shown under the fixed assets are the least liquid.

Liabilities are amounts owed to creditors. Like assets, liabilities are divided into two categories: current liabilities and long-term liabilities. Current liabilities consist of notes payable, accounts payable, and accruals (such as wages or taxes payable) that are due within 1 year. Long-term liabilities are obligations to be paid beyond 1 year. A common example of a long-term liability in the health and fitness industry involves repaying a loan note for new outdoor tennis courts.

Owner's equity (or net worth) represents the owner's claims on the assets of the business. This is a residual claim because owners receive only what remains after all claims, including taxes, have been paid. It is important to understand that the amount of owner's equity is not the market value of the business. As is the case with any investment, what the business is worth on the open market (the amount a buyer is willing to pay for the business) is determined by placing a value on the future cash flow it is expected to produce. Owner's equity as shown on the balance sheet reflects the book value of the business, not the market value.

To best analyze the financial condition of a club, an owner or manager must have information about its assets, liabilities, and owner's equity. A balance sheet is a snapshot of an organization's financial status on a given date. Consequently, changes in balance sheets between two statement dates provide important information about the financial health of a club. Understanding the nature and implication of changes in financial statement accounts can help provide answers to questions such as the following:

- How much did the funds in accounts receivable and inventory increase or decrease relative to the change in member sales for the period?
- Has the amount of debt financing increased to unsatisfactory levels since the last statement date?

- Are accounts payable rising to a level of concern?
- Has the club maintained a satisfactory level of cash flow from operations?

Income Statement

The **income statement,** or the statement of profit and loss, reflects the financial results of the business operations over a specific time (month, quarter, or year). It summarizes the transactions that produced revenue for the time frame and the operating expenses and taxes the business incurred in generating this revenue. See figure 12.2 for an example.

The two major financial categories on an income statement are revenues and expenses. Revenues are earned through selling products or providing a service. In the health and fitness industry, revenues are generated primarily through membership sales, racket sport programs, fitness programs, profit centers, and miscellaneous income (e.g., guest fees, locker rentals, towel fees). To fully understand the concept of revenue, note the following two points:

1. Although you may think the value produced by the sale of a new club membership is cash received, an accountant measures the membership by either a cash sale or a credit sale. To an accountant, a credit sale means something of value: a claim on the new member for the amount of the membership sale. This claim appears as an asset and is classified as accounts receivable. Accounts receivable have a definite value to the club, but they are not cash and may never become cash.

2. In preparing an income statement, an accountant recognizes a credit sale as revenue in the time frame in which the credit sale was made. This means that the revenue figures on the income statement for a given time frame include all credit sales made during that time, even though cash from those transactions may not be received until later. There could be a significant difference between the membership sales revenue shown on the income statement and the actual amount of cash received during that time.

Comprehending these concepts is essential to interpreting an income statement and becoming familiar with cash flow.

Expenses represent the costs incurred for generating revenue and operating a fitness facility. Typically, in the health and fitness industry expenses are broken down into operating expenses and fixed

XYZ Company
Income statement
For the period ended December 31, 2007

Acct no.	Description	Year to date 2008	%	2007	%
	Revenue				
4010	Joining fees	145968	4.5	131371	4.5
4020	Membership dues	2415984	74.7	2174386	74.7
	Total membership fees	2561952	79.2	2305757	79.2
4100	Random court time	68745	2.1	61871	2.1
4110	Leagues	125698	0.0	113128	3.9
4120	Tennis instruction	254994	7.9	229495	7.9
	Total tennis revenue	449437	13.9	4044494	13.9
4155	Personal training	128952	4.0	116057	4.0
4172	Group swim instruction	8523	0.3	7671	0.3
	Total fitness revenue	137475	4.2	123728	4.2
4965	Dividends and interest	85694	2.6	77125	2.5
4990	Miscellaneous	547	0.0	492	0.0
	Total administrative	86241	2.7	77617	2.7
	Total revenue	3235105	100.0	2911596	100.0
	Expenses				
6110	Wages—tennis	350558	10.8	315502	10.8
6340	Wages—fitness	330563	10.2	297507	10.2
7140	Wages—accounting	75894	2.3	68305	2.3
	Total payroll	757015	23.4	681314	23.4
9520	Group insurance	275854	8.5	248269	8.5
9530	FICA—employer	57912	1.8	52121	1.8
9540	Federal unemployment	46935	1.5	42242	1.5
9545	State unemployment	39845	1.2	53345	1.8
	Total payroll and benefits	439974	13.6	395977	13.6
8910	Electricity	134191	4.1	120772	4.1
8920	Water	21781	0.7	19603	0.7
8930	Gas	25194	0.8	22675	0.8
	Total utilities	181166	5.6	163050	5.6
8522	Contract landscape	41142	1.3	37028	1.3
8620	Repair pool	32568	1.0	29311	1.0
8720	Supplies locker room	75105	2.3	67595	2.3
	Total maintenance	148815	4.6	133934	4.6

(continued)

Figure 12.2   Sample income statement.

Acct no.	Description	2008	%	2007	%
	Revenue				
7210	Accounting fees	50000	1.5	45000	1.5
7230	Bad debt expense	115000	3.6	103500	3.6
7820	Office supplies	35577	1.1	32019	1.1
	Total administrative	200577	6.2	180519	6.2
8120	Advertising	42897	1.3	38607	1.3
8250	Printing	25478	0.8	22930	0.8
8280	Promotions	31913	1.0	28722	1.0
	Total advertising	100288	3.1	90259	3.1
6150	Supplies tennis	31568	1.0	28411	1.0
6180	Special events tennis	24569	0.8	22112	0.8
6195	Tennis balls	27976	0.9	25178	0.9
	Total tennis	84113	2.6	75701	2.6
6450	Aerobics music	10464	0.3	9418	0.3
6480	Supplies fitness	27336	0.8	24602	0.8
6494	Nutrition	4256	0.1	3830	0.1
	Total fitness	42056	1.3	37850	1.3
	Total operating expense	1954004	60.4	1758604	60.4
7450	Insurance	737603	22.8	663843	22.8
7300	Depreciation	213517	6.6	192165	6.6
7460	Debt service	152050	4.7	136845	4.7
	Total fixed expenses	1103170	34.1	992853	34.1
	Total expenses	3057174	94.5	2751457	94.5
	Net income	177931	5.5	160139	5.5

Year to date

Figure 12.2 *(continued)*

expenses. Operating expenses are the costs associated with the normal operation of a club, such as payroll and benefits, administration, utilities, maintenance and repairs, advertising, marketing, and program and profit-center costs. Fixed expenses are costs that remain constant over a designated time. Examples of fixed expenses include rent and lease payments, interest and financing charges, real estate and personal property taxes, and depreciation. The expenses recognized in a given period are matched with revenues for that time to determine the amount of profit or loss (net income or net loss).

Statement of Cash Flows

Companies are in business to make money or at the very least to generate enough money to cover their expenses. Companies that are able to generate a positive cash flow will stay in business, whereas those that are in a negative cash flow will struggle to pay their bills and will most likely be forced to close their doors.

By *cash flows,* we are referring directly to the cash flowing into the business as well as the cash flowing out of the business. The **statement of cash flows** is a financial statement that reports changes in cash holding over a certain amount of time. To see the distinction between cash flows and other accounting measures of income, recall from the section on income statements that revenue is recorded at the time the transaction actually occurs, but this is not necessarily the time when cash is collected. This is most often the case when items are purchased on credit. Alternatively, the amount of depreciation that is reported on an income statement has no impact on the cash generated by the business because when the business reports depreciation, the monetary amount reported as depreciation is not directly paid to any vendors or employees, as would be the case with other operating expenses.

Financial Statement Analysis

Interpreting an income statement and applying the information to the operation of a club are primary responsibilities of every manager. Experienced managers take the time each month to review all revenue and expense categories and evaluate the overall business performance. Make monthly comparisons between the income statement and the projected (budgeted) income statement. Also, analyze all departments, and share the information you obtain with each department head. Either the manager or department head should investigate any significant variations between the actual and projected figures to determine the cause of the variations.

Budgeting

Now that we have an understanding of the key financial statements involved with running a business, we will apply this information to **budgeting.** All businesses rely on a budget to guide them throughout the year, and often budgets are a guide for 3 to 5 years. Budgets are based on the fiscal year, which might be the same as a regular calendar year (start on January 1 and end on December 31) or specific to when the company started (e.g., May 1-April 30). Companies can start and finish their fiscal year however they want as long as it is consistent from year to year and it encompasses all 12 months.

When preparing a budget, it is best to be conservative in your sales estimates and slightly more liberal in your expense estimations. It is much easier to deal with sales that are higher than expected and expenses that are lower than expected. Overestimating sales can put you in a position where you are not able to pay some of your expenses, and underestimating your expenses may mean that you are in a position where you have not budgeted enough money for staff wages and you may not meet your budgeted profits for the month. Often managers are given guidelines to follow when preparing a budget, such as not budgeting for more than a 4% increase in marketing expenses. If these guidelines are shared from the beginning, it will make the budgeting process run much more smoothly.

Types of Budgets

Various types of budgets have been identified in the literature and in the workplace. For our purposes, we will review the most common types within the fitness industry.

Increment-Decrement or Trend-Line Budgeting

This is probably the most popular budget used in the fitness industry. It uses the financial statements of the previous year to build the budget for the current year. It is relatively straightforward in that you use the exact numbers from the previous year and either increase or decrease them for the current year based on your knowledge of last year and your plans and goals for the coming year. The major benefit of this approach is that you are using established numbers as the starting point for your new budget. The drawback is that the numbers you are using may not be the most effective ones. For example, just because you spent $11,000 on payroll in January of the previous year does not mean you need to do the same thing the next year. That $11,000 may have been overspent and staff may not have been needed for all of this time. Or, just because you spent $2,000 on marketing in June does not mean you need to spend that same amount the following year. The results could have been poorer or better than expected. Either way, you cannot automatically assume that the numbers from the previous year were ideal.

To avoid this problem, two things need to be in place. First, it is critical that good record keeping is maintained with commentary explaining the results for a particular month or quarter. These explanations will allow the budget process for the following year to run more smoothly. Second, managers and anyone else involved in the budget process should still have to justify why they are allocating the amounts they are to specific areas. Simply rubber stamping the numbers because it's what you did last year will not result in a club performing at its best. Good managers should always be questioning the way they and their staff do things. What worked last year is not necessarily going to work this year—just ask anyone who still owns music on a vinyl record or cassette tape.

Break-Even Analysis

It is important to have a budget, but many would argue that you should also have other plans in case unexpected situations arise. In the case of a break-even analysis, a budget is developed that shows the minimum amount of revenue that must be generated in order to cover the expected costs.

Worst-Case Scenario

Another budget that can be developed is one that shows the least desirable outcome for a business. Many businesses feel it is important to know what will happen if they miss all of their sales targets and their expenses are higher than expected. If this happens, the responsible manager thus already has a plan in place to deal with it.

Zero-Based Budgeting

This approach to budgeting involves taking an in-depth look at all areas of the business and establishing a budget based on your specific goals for that year. Though you might consider what has happened in the past, it is not a major consideration when developing this type of budget. The challenge with this approach is the time it takes to accurately predict your budgeted numbers for the year.

Budget Preparation

In order to prepare a proper budget, a business needs to follow a sequential process. The steps consist of the following (Fried 2004):

1. Gathering information
2. Forecasting sales
3. Projecting profits and losses
4. Comparing against industry norms
5. Determining capital needs

Gathering Information

Some typical questions that need to be addressed at this point include the following:

- How old is the club? Newer clubs will generally see significant sales growth in their first few years. This growth will slow down after 2 or 3 years.

- What is the competition doing? Are clubs opening, expanding, or closing in your area? How will their prices and services affect you?

- What do you need to pay your staff to ensure you are able to retain them and keep them motivated?

- Where are costs for heat and water expected to go?

- Are you planning on offering any new services? What are the costs and expected revenues of these?

The starting point for any information-gathering phase is to collect information on the budgets and actual financial performance of previous years. This will give you a sense of what the club has done in the past. It may not always indicate what will happen in the future, but it is still a solid place to start. Financial statements from previous years should be accompanied by notes explaining the rationale for the numbers. This information will help you determine how relevant the actual numbers are for predicting future budgets. For example, if a club is in its second year of operation and you are looking at the employee costs for previous years, you may find that there were certain months where you did not have enough staff working and you may have been understaffed during busier months. Overstaffing may result in unnecessary overtime being paid, and understaffing may result in missed revenue opportunities.

To obtain the information that is needed to prepare a budget, managers can look to the various trade publications of the fitness industry. IHRSA has various publications that will be helpful during this phase. Some of the information that can be obtained from trade magazines includes industry benchmarks, future expectations for the industry, and new programs and products that your club may want to invest in. In addition to industry-specific publications, it is recommended that managers use data that can be obtained through the local chamber of commerce. Although these data may not be specific to your industry, they will tell you what the economic outlook is for your area, which may prove to be just as important as the industry-specific data. Other sources of data include various government groups, small-business associations, and companies that specialize in collecting and sharing business data.

Once all the information is collected, managers must examine it to figure out what it means to their business. For example, an industrywide slowdown in fitness club membership sales may not affect you if you are the only club in the area. On the other hand, a positive economic outlook for business in general may not help you if a local business that employed 2,000 people just closed. Astute managers are able to look at all of the information and determine what is relevant to them and put aside the information that isn't relevant.

Forecasting Sales

Forecasting is part art and part science. Rarely are businesses 100% accurate in their predictions of the future. Budget forecasting is based on experience, education, and assumptions. Although it is unlikely that businesses will be accurate in all of their forecasts, the alternative is to work without a budget, which would be like going on a family vacation without a map. The reality is that the more experience you have with the budgeting process, the better you will get at forecasting the future needs of your business.

To generate sales forecasts, it is always best to look at the sales data of previous years. Sales can be broken down into various elements. For our purpose here we will break them down by product line (see figure 12.3).

Projecting Profits and Losses

This is the point at which all revenue and expense items are filled in. The information you gathered in step 1 and the sales forecasts you just made are critical components in determining profits and losses. Your job as the manager is to meet certain targets that ownership has determined ahead of time. For example, an owner may ask the manager for a budget that shows a $500,000 profit while maintaining marketing at the levels of the previous year, increasing payroll no more than 7%, and spending

no more than $10,000 on equipment repairs. This is only one possible scenario; there are hundreds of possibilities. The key is to discuss the budget expectations ahead of time so that the person overseeing the budgeting process is able to move forward with all the necessary information.

Club Operating Benchmarks

Benchmarks are specific standards that fitness centers and other businesses strive to achieve. Some standards are actually determined by looking at the best companies in an industry and using their numbers as the benchmark, and other numbers are more subjective and are set by the individual business themselves. Alternatively, some benchmarks are specific to the fitness industry and some are more general. Tables 12.1 (page 234), 12.2 (page 235), and 12.3 (page 236) present some common industry benchmarks.

Elements of Budgeting

According to Rick Caro (1995a), there are four significant elements when it comes to budgeting:

1. *Guidelines and methodology.* You need a context. Many club operators have created mission and

XYZ Athletic Club annual membership projections

FYE 2008 dues projected Assets	$191,890					
FYE 2008 # members	2,675					
	Jan	Feb	Mar	Apr	May	June
# of new members	55	45	45	45	40	35
# of members lost	30	35	40	35	30	35
Net members gained	25	10	5	10	10	0
Total # of members	2,700	2,710	2,715	2,725	2,735	2,735
Attrition rate percent	13.33	15.50	17.68	15.41	13.16	15.36
Joining fees	$22,000	$18,000	$18,000	$18,000	$16,000	$14,000
Monthly dues	$1,725	$690	$345	$690	$690	$0
Dues increase						
Commissions	$6,225	$5,025	$5,025	$5,025	$4,425	$3,825
Total dues	$193,615	$194,305	$194,650	$195,340	$196,030	$196,030
Average monthly dues						

Figure 12.3 Sample sales forecast.

Table 12.1   **Five-Year Trend**

	ALL CLUBS				
	2005	2004	2003	2002	2001
Total Revenue (thousands)	$4,581.30	$4,222.00	$2,470.00	$2,753.20	$3,558.50
EBITDA as % of Revenue	16.90%	15.00%	14.70%	19.40%	24.10%
Pretax earnings as % of Revenue	8.30%	5.30%	8.20%	9.20%	11.00%
Revenue Growth	4.80%	3.20%	3.90%	2.30%	6.70%
Total Payroll as % of Revenue	44.50%	43.80%	45.10%	44.10%	40.90%
Rate of Member Retention	73.10%	71.30%	66.60%	66.40%	69.60%
Net Membership Growth	4.20%	0.50%	−0.30%	2.40%	3.90%
Revenue Growth	$962.13	$1,023.64	$979.93	$952.13	$1,044.45
Indoor Square Foot per Individual Member	16.3	21.1	21	22.5	18.6
Revenue per Indoor Square Foot	$57.22	$50.20	$47.01	$41.05	$44.62
Nondues Revenue as % of Revenue	34.80%	33.10%	33.20%	32.70%	30.90%

Reprinted, by permission, from IHRSA, 2006, *Profiles of success* (Boston, MA: IHRSA), 18.

value statements. They have at least a general 3- to 5-year plan with some concrete goals. For special annual budgeting, they need guidelines. Often you need to define an overall company goal, such as an increased bottom line of 10% over the previous year. This may force staff not to simply tweak the previous year's numbers because the goal is much more ambitious than that. Rather, you may need to operate differently, such as by creating new profit centers, significantly increasing prices, and holding steady or even decreasing expenses.

You can formally start the budget process by planning a meeting or a training session for key staff. Set deadlines, communicate goals and guidelines, and organize first drafts and reviews (the process often requires several versions before final budgets are accepted). The key is to have a final budget created and accepted before the start of the fiscal year.

2. *Two budgets with assumptions.* Create detailed departmental budgets (e.g., sales, front desk, fitness, child care) by month with specific assumptions for each line item. This way each department head can remember how a budget number was created and explain any differences that occur during the year. For example, the fitness department may have budgeted for an increase in wages during the months of January and February due to an expected increase in new memberships. The club manager

and fitness department need to make sure they are aware of the reasons for this increase and the overall expectations and limitations of this change. Senior managers should feel comfortable giving feedback on the assumptions and forecasts in the budget. Many of these people may actually know their department better than you, so it would be wise to listen to their concerns.

In the ideal situation, all budgets would be zero based and not simply a revision of the previous year's numbers. In reality, most clubs will look at the numbers of the previous year and simply increase or decrease them based on the financial performance and expected sales and upcoming expenses of the previous year. Once the budget is created, it should not be changed throughout the year unless a major, unexpected event occurs that forces you to take action. If staff members feel that they can change the budget throughout the year based on department needs, there is no point in setting goals and going through the budgeting process.

Create two separate budgets: operating and capital. It's critical to commit to a separate capital budget, which indicates your priorities and, most importantly, when large building and equipment purchases will be made. Often, the timing of renovations directly affects the operating revenues and expenses for the part of the club undergoing renovations. For example, if you are closing your

Table 12.2 **Benchmarks by Club Type**

	ALL CLUBS		MULTIPURPOSE		FITNESS ONLY		PART OF CHAIN OR MULTICLUB GROUP		INDEPENDENT	
	2004	2005	2004	2005	2004	2005	2004	2005	2004	2005
Total Revenue (thousands)	$2,476.30	$2,589.50	$3,001.60	$3,219.60	$1,516.90	$1,207.80	$6,967.50	$6,967.50	$1,972.00	$2,184.40
EBITDA as % of Revenue	—	17.30%	—	19.60%	—	15.60%	—	20.70%	—	16.90%
Pretax earnings as % of Revenue	1.60%	8.10%	5.60%	8.10%	0.50%	9.40%	5.70%	8.30%	0.80%	8.00%
Revenue Growth	—	5.90%	—	6.205	—	4.70%	—	5.40%	—	6.10%
Total Payroll as % of Revenue	42.10%	43.50%	40.70%	39.80%	43.90%	46.80%	42.80%	41.50%	40.80%	44.40%
Rate of Member Retention	69.50%	70.70%	70.70%	70.80%	68.20%	70.00%	69.10%	69.90%	69.70%	70.80%
Net Membership Growth	—	5.20%	—	3.60%	—	8.60%	—	4.90%	—	5.30%
Revenue per Individual Member	$672.39	$687.53	$643.83	$684.04	$683.33	$682.43	$735.23	$777.10	$672.39	$687.53
Indoor Square Foot per Individual Member	14.6	14.7	18.3	17.0	12.6	11.6	12.1	13.4	16.6	15.1
Revenue per Indoor Square Foot	$50.47	$54.10	$50.29	$53.60	$60.80	$65.70	$60.92	$61.44	$50.20	$47.56
Nondues Revenue as % of Revenue	—	30.80%	—	32.90%	—	24.30%	—	33.60%	—	29.20%

Note: Data reflect information from those clubs that provided complete responses for both 2004 and 2005, allowing for year-to-year comparisons.

Reprinted, by permission, from IHRSA, 2006, *Profiles of success* (Boston: IHRSA), 19.

Table 12.3 Benchmarks by Club Type

	LESS THAN 20,000 SQ. FT		20,000 TO 34,999 SQ. FT		35,000 TO 59,999 SQ. FT		60,000 SQ. FT OR MORE	
	2004	2005	2004	2005	2004	2005	2004	2005
Total Revenue (thousands)	$316.10	$341.50	$1,644.00	$1,560.10	$2,615.30	$2,437.60	$7,174.00	$7,388.00
EBITDA as % of Revenue	—	15.90%	—	20.40%	—	13.10%	—	17.70%
Pretax earnings as % of Revenue	—	10.80%	13.00%	10.40%	0.80%	−2.20%	1.10%	7.30%
Revenue Growth	—	8.10%	—	4.00%		2.30%	—	6.40%
Total Payroll as % of Revenue	38.30%	40.00%	42.80%	47.40%	38.70%	38.00%	46.30%	45.80%
Rate of Member Retention	69.20%	71.10%	67.10%	64.30%	60.40%	67.20%	73.50%	73.20%
Net Membership Growth	—	8.90%	—	6.00%	—	4.60%	—	2.90%
Revenue per Individual Member	$679.60	$731.51	$567.62	$560.40	$646.86	$664.70	$1,186.57	$1,207.64
Indoor Square Foot per Individual Member	9.4	8.9	11.6	11.1	15.5	13.7	23.3	21.4
Revenue per Indoor Square Foot	$44.40	$48.31	$59.38	$56.26	$50.29	$50.23	$50.56	$56.44
Nondues Revenue as % of Revenue	—	17.90%	—	23.60%	—	35.70%	—	41.10%

Note: Data reflect information from those clubs that provided complete responses for both 2004 and 2005, allowing for year-to-year comparisons.
Reprinted, by permission, from IHRSA, 2006, *Profiles of success* (Boston: IHRSA), 20.

racket courts and turning them into a cardio training area, it's going to affect your members who play racquetball or squash. These members may decide to cancel their membership or may require a change in their membership dues. Any capital expenses need to be closely monitored not only for their upfront cost but also their immediate impact on revenues and expenses.

3. *Staff involvement.* The best people to read trends and understand your business are those closest to each of the club areas, namely, your department heads. They should create their own department budgets to meet your predetermined guidelines. If you simply dictate these budgets to them, they'll see their role in the budget process as an academic exercise and they'll never be committed to making the bottom line.

4. *Incentives and monitoring.* Ideally, if your department heads exceed their bottom lines, they should be rewarded. This could be in the form of financial compensation or something else that you know will make the person feel special, like a day off, gift certificate, massage, and so on. Consider offering partial rewards during the course of the year, perhaps quarterly, with the majority tied to year-end results.

Income Management

In the past 10 years, industry revenue has increased 105% (International Health, Racquet, and Sportsclub Association [IHRSA] 2006). The cause of this consistent growth rate has been attributed to three factors: increasing new-member growth, lowering member attrition, and increasing average revenue derived per member. Managers have discovered that focusing on new-member sales is only a portion of the success equation. They must place additional emphasis on retaining existing members, becoming as efficient as possible with use of space, and implementing creative programming. Figure 12.4 illustrates the total revenue growth for both fitness-only and multipurpose clubs in the United States since 1993.

Membership joining or initiation fees and monthly dues continue to drive the revenue that supports commercial, community, corporate, and clinical settings. Without a strong membership base, many facilities cannot provide the necessary revenue to offset operating costs. According to industry surveys of the most successful clubs in the industry, 66% of the total revenue generated by multipurpose commercial fitness centers today comes from initiation fees and monthly dues (IHRSA 2006). The remaining 18% of nondues revenue results from racket sport programs (31%), fitness programs (6%), profit centers (7%), and other miscellaneous revenue (2%).

Although membership fees have traditionally been the backbone of industry revenues, today's fitness managers are focusing on nondues revenue as the key for future profits. Some experts believe that improving nondues revenue is one of the keys to improving attrition rates.

THE BOTTOM LINE

Health and fitness facilities that continue to rely on member dues for 80% or more of their revenue may soon find themselves at a competitive disadvantage with profit-driven clubs.

Organizations with additional sources of revenue have less need to raise membership fees and may choose to even lower the price of dues. As the industry continues to expand into all markets, the ability to be flexible with membership rates provides a strong competitive edge over dues-driven facilities. In addition, club managers have found that they can expand their target market by implementing programs and adding profit centers that attract new members from outside the regular membership. For example, some clubs have found that by renovating a racquetball or tennis court into a youth fitness center, they can attract the family market, thus expanding their revenue base. You can learn more about nondues revenue in chapter 11.

Once you have identified the income sources for a particular setting, organizing an internal system for receiving funds for services rendered is the next component of the accounting process. Identifying, tracking, and monitoring accounts receivable is a standard accounting practice used in all businesses.

Accounts Receivable

Accounts receivable refers to an amount that is owed a business, usually by one of its customers or members, as a result of the ordinary extension of credit. They are generated primarily from membership fees and dues, programming and service fees, and profit centers over a designated time frame. Being able to control the funds invested in accounts receivable is an important component of income management. In addition, the system you create for tracking accounts receivable plays a major role in establishing your credit policy. A credit policy involves decisions on how to collect, manage, and control receivables.

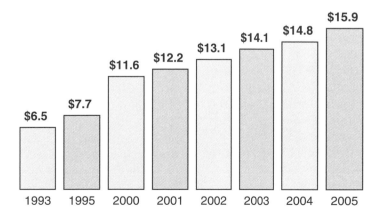

Figure 12.4 Total revenue growth of the U.S. health club industry. Revenue is shown in billions.
Reprinted, by permission, from IHRSA, 2006, *Profiles of Success* (Boston: IHRSA), 8.

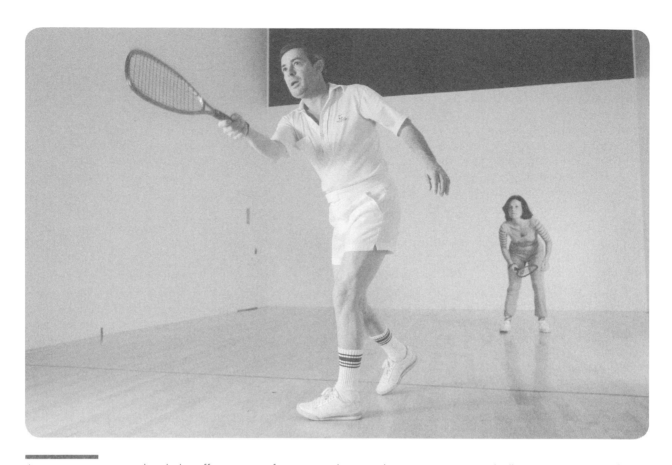

A manager concerned with the efficient use of space might consider turning a racquetball court into a youth fitness center, thereby attracting new members.

© Tim Wright/Corbis

Accounts Receivable Management

Health and fitness clubs are no different than most small businesses in that a percentage of their funds are regularly tied up in receivables created from credit sales or membership dues. A continuing problem for organizations that obtain revenue from membership and initiation fees is collecting these funds. Typically, you would mail bills before a member's anniversary date (i.e., monthly, quarterly, biannually, or annually). Cash-flow problems occur when the time that passes between sending the bills and receiving payments is extensive. Until the point of collection, an unpaid account represents a drain on financial resources. To achieve effective management of accounts receivable, it is necessary to incorporate the three following tools.

Sales Analysis

It is effective to produce a regular sales analysis that breaks down the total sales figures into components so you can evaluate the performance for each. By tracing sales revenue to the individual category, management can identify trouble spots and take action before trouble arises. Table 12.4 provides a sample sales analysis that categorizes membership types and the amount billed for each payment cycle.

Aged Trial Balance

It is important to stay apprised of the length of time individual accounts have been outstanding. You can accomplish this by generating an aged trial balance, which lists the total of all outstanding balances falling into established past due categories. Generally, the past-due categories are from 1 to 30 days, 31 to 60 days, and 61 to 90 days. From this report a manager can determine which accounts are past due and which accounts exceed established credit limits. A sample aged trial balance is shown in table 12.5.

Credit Policy

You must establish and enforce a sound collection policy and effective procedures for dealing with delinquent accounts. The policy should provide a

Table 12.4 Sample Sales Analysis

Member type	MEMBER STATUS SUMMARY								MEMBER STATUS SUMMARY		
	Active	Susp.	Term	Del.	Total	Last month	Change	Joined this month	Estimated dues	Last month dues	Change
20-Ind. annual	173	1	1	0	173	170	3	3	110	0	110
21-Family annual	362	0	0	0	364	362	0	4	0	0	0
22-Ind. midday ann.	8	0	0	0	8	7	1	1	0	0	0
23-Fam. mid. ann.	5	0	0	0	5	5	0	0	0	0	0
24-Sr. ind. annual	12	0	0	0	12	10	2	0	43	31	12
25-Sr. fam. ann.	20	0	0	0	20	20	0	0	89	89	0
26-Cor. ind. ann TE	53	0	0	0	53	54	-1	0	29	29	0
28-Yng. adult ann.	1	0	0	0	1	1	0	0	0	0	0
29-Cor. fam. ann	11	0	0	0	11	12	-1	0	0	0	0
30-Ind. semiann.	8	0	0	0	8	8	0	0	0	0	0
31-Fam. semiann.	4	0	0	—	4	4	0	0	0	0	0
40-Individual	719	10	0	1	730	715	4	21	45,511.97	45,256.97	255
41-Family	964	6	0	0	970	950	14	18	83,946.30	82,698.30	1,248
60-Midday ind.	60	1	0	0	61	52	8	5	2,100	1,820	280
61 Midday fam.	15	1	0	0	16	15	0	0	750	750	0
70-Corp. individual	39	0	0	0	39	40	-1	1	2,420	2,485	-65
71-Corp. family	40	0	0	0	40	39	1	1	3,469.20	3,377.20	92
75-Individual TE	30	0	0	0	30	29	1	0	1,881	1,816	65

(continued)

Table 12.4 (continued)

	MEMBER STATUS SUMMARY							MEMBER STATUS SUMMARY			
Member type	Active	Susp.	Term.	Del.	Total	Last month	Change	Joined this month	Estimated dues	Last month dues	Change
76-Family TE	48	0	0	0	48	48	0	1	3,601	3,606	−5
80-Nonresident	13	0	0	0	13	13	0	0	499	499	0
81-Nonres. family	20	0	0	0	20	20	0	0	801	801	0
90-Senior individual	41	0	0	0	41	42	−1	0	1,962	2,014	−52
91-Senior family	51	1	0	0	52	52	−1	0	3,321	3,394	−73
93-Leave medical	4	8	0	0	12	4	0	0	0	0	0
94-Leave other	4	15	0	0	19	4	0	0	0	0	0
95-Drop	6	1	32	267	306	6	0	0	0	0	0
96-Employee ind.	107	0	0	0	107	103	4	4	0	0	0
97-Employee fam.	26	0	0	0	26	26	0	0	275	275	0
98-Corporate	28	0	0	0	28	28	0	0	20	20	0
99-Nonpay	34	0	0	0	34	33	1	2	0	0	0
Subtotal	2,906	44	33	268	3,251	2,872	34	62	150,828.47	148,961.47	1,867
02-Family member	3,353	10	92	28	3,483	3,403	−50	68	2168	2,118	50
Totals	6,259	54	125	296	6,749	6,275	−15	130	152,996.47	151,079.47	1,917
Average dues									24.46	24.09	0.37

Table 12.5 **Sample Aged Trial Balance**

Member #	Name	Phone no.	Last payment	Current	30 days	60 days	90 days	Net due
6317	John Doe	555-3433	2/09/07	2.39	2.36	2.34	236.31	243.40
3227	Jane Doe	555-6590	11/08/07	17.76	87.81	54.53	521.12	681.22
5946	Austin Jones	555-7117	12/01/07	13.84	0.04	0	3.96	17.84
9658	Martin Smith	555-0053	4/02/07	10.54	10.54	0	1,053.64	1,074.72
6211	Becky Wilson	555-2365	6/06/07	105.17	104.15	672.65	106.21	988.18
8076	Jim Jacobs	555-6347	1/06/07	102.38	101.38	100.39	293.54	597.69
9776	Mary Walter	555-9521	1/06/07	87.81	54.53	521.12	17.76	681.22
1205	George Perkins	555-7782	5/22/07	751.17	0.03	0	3.45	754.65
3499	Samuel Johnson	555-7811	1/19/07	190.51	97.33	102.12	331.17	721.13
5674	Daniel Patrick	555-3603	5/08/07	65.89	65.03	79.88	79.91	231.71
Final total				1,347.46	523.20	1,533.03	2,647.07	5,991.76

balance between generating the pressure needed to obtain payment from delinquent accounts and not jeopardizing future business by offending members. Unfortunately, there are no industry standards or rules that guarantee an acceptable approach to collections. However, health and fitness organizations follow certain guidelines that provide a nucleus for an effective collection policy.

1. Base your collection policy on clear, effective communication between the organization and the member.
2. Establish specific procedures to follow for delinquent accounts that reach 30, 60, and 90 days.
3. Secure a collection agency to handle problem accounts that management cannot rectify.
4. Internally prevent a member with a delinquent account from using the facility.

Electronic Funds Transfer

As a means to improve the collection of accounts receivable, **electronic funds transfer (EFT)** can make payments as easy as possible for members while expediting the collection of funds for the business. This alternative billing method is the system predominately used in the health and fitness industry for collecting receivables.

EFT debits a checking, savings, or credit card account for the payment of monthly fees. Members

authorize a predetermined deduction for membership fees or other incidental charges that are automatically withdrawn from their account or credit card on an established date. You can deposit collected funds in the club account in 5 days or within a 24-hour period if necessary.

Four recommended EFT services are available to club managers:

1. *EFT provider.* A manager contracts with an EFT provider who keys in all member data from hard-copy membership forms sent by the business. The service provider updates all member files, performs the billing service, and credits the organization's account. Although this is considered a labor-saving method for personnel, it is generally an expensive form of EFT service.

2. *Software-supported EFT.* With this service, an organization is responsible for keying in all member information and bank account or credit card numbers. This information is then downloaded to the EFT provider. The EFT provider debits the members' accounts, minus the provider's service fee, and credits the account. Software-supported EFT is the most widely used service in the health and fitness industry.

3. *Bank as EFT provider.* A bank can perform all the services that an EFT provides. Although this method is the least expensive, it does not provide certain customized reports or other customer service options available through an EFT provider.

Advantages and Disadvantages of Electronic Billing

Advantages

- The cost of paper billing (e.g., monthly statements and coupon books) represents 12% of the total billing cost, whereas EFT billing ranges between 4% and 7%.
- Payments are automatically deposited into the account within a matter of days, thus securing a predictable cash flow for the facility.
- It is an easier process for members to pay monthly fees, consequently increasing member adherence.
- Administration and collection fees are reduced.

Disadvantages

- Members may have a negative perception of having fees deducted from their account each month.
- It takes time to correct clerical errors.
- Proper communication of member terminations is required so drafts can be stopped on time.

4. *Do it yourself.* Depending on the size of operation, some club operators have taken on the role of EFT provider via an internal computer system. The amount of internal administration and communication with various banks makes this option difficult to administer and more costly than hiring an EFT provider.

Expense Management

Understanding expense management is an important component of financial management. Traditionally, managers have focused on income concerns such as advertising, marketing, and new-member sales as a means to increase overall profits. The health and fitness industry has always been a market-driven business, emphasizing revenue more than controlling spending. However, over the years, managers have realized that cutting costs is more tangible and predictable than estimating member sales. Unnecessary expenditures result from not doing the following: providing proper accounting controls and security, providing regular bidding and negotiating with vendors, questioning every expense as though it were coming out of your own pocket, performing internal maintenance, and eliminating costs when necessary.

Controlling expenses starts with categorizing all costs associated with operating the business. Then divide each expense into subheadings that represent standard industry expense categories. Table 12.6 provides an expense model of a commercial fitness setting with examples of these categories. Expense categories are separated into operated department expenses (based on the specific department), undistributed operating expenses (shared among all areas of the club), and fixed charges that will not change based on traffic flow or usage.

Depreciation

A term often seen on financial statements but seldom understood is **depreciation,** the process of allocating the cost of an asset to the periods of time benefited.

Neglecting to list depreciation as an actual cash expense (although technically it is a noncash expense) could prevent allocation of the proper funds to cover the annual wear and tear of building and property. Health and fitness centers today should expect to spend funds similar in amount to the depreciation total for repairs and replacement costs for that year.

THE BOTTOM LINE

To fully comprehend depreciation, understand that the total cost of a new piece of exercise equipment or building represents an asset, which has present and future value to the business.

Table 12.6   Fitness-Only Clubs

	Mean	Median	Middle Range
Total Revenue (thousands)	$1,927.00	$1,117.40	$698.50 - 2,144.60
Membership Dues & Fees	75.50%	79.20%	66.6 - 88.0
Racket Sports	0.20%	0.00%	0.0 - 0.0
Fitness	9.70%	5.50%	0.3 - 12.2
Spa	2.40%	0.00%	0.0 - 2.4
Health Care	0.40%	0.00%	0.0 - 0.0
Pro Shop/Retail Shop	1.80%	0.50%	0.1 - 2.7
Food & Beverage	3.20%	1.40%	0.0 - 2.7
Children's Programs	2.50%	0.20%	0.0 - 1.4
Other Income	4.40%	2.00%	0.0 - 6.3
Total Revenue	100.0%	100.00%	100.0 - 100.0
OPERATED DEPARTMENTS EXPENSES			
Racket Sports	0.10%	0.00%	0.0 - 0.0
Fitness	10.80%	9.00%	0.1 - 17.0
Spa	1.70%	0.00%	0.0 - 1.5
Health Care	0.40%	0.00%	0.0 - 0.0
Pro Shop/Retail Shop	1.20%	0.50%	0.0 - 1.4
Food & Beverage	2.40%	0.80%	0.0 - 1.8
Children's Programs	1.90%	0.00%	0.0 - 1.9
Total Operated Departments Expense	18.40%	16.70%	3.2 - 33.9
Earnings Before Undistributed Operating Expenses	81.60%	83.40%	66.1 - 96.8
UNDISTRIBUTED OPERATING EXPENSES			
Member Services	6.10%	3.30%	0.0 - 6.5
Sales & Marketing	7.10%	5.70%	3.2 - 8.6
Repairs & Maintenance	3.50%	2.90%	1.4 - 5.0
Housekeeping	3.00%	2.00%	0.4 - 3.9
Utilities	6.90%	5.60%	3.9 - 8.6
General & Administrative	15.50%	9.90%	4.3 - 20.9
Total Undistributed Operating Expenses	42.00%	44.10%	23.2 - 56.2
Earnings Before Fixed Charges	39.60%	33.70%	29.5 - 52.1

Table 12.6   (continued)

	Mean	Median	Middle Range
Total Revenue Current Year (thousands)	$1,927.00	$1,117.40	$698.50 - 2,144.60
FIXED CHARGES			
Insurance	2.50%	2.30%	1.2 - 3.0
Management Fees	1.90%	0.00%	0.0 - 2.4
Real Estate/Personal Property Taxes	1.60%	0.80%	0.0 - 2.5
Rent–Land & Building	16.90%	16.00%	7.8 - 23.1
Rent–Equipment	1.60%	0.00%	0.0 - 0.4
Total Fixed Charges	24.50%	21.50%	15.0 - 29.8
Earnings Before Interest, Depreciation and Amortization, and Income Taxes	15.60%	13.10%	2.7 - 25.4
Interest Expense	4.10%	1.00%	0.0 - 3.6
Depreciation and Amortization	6.90%	5.10%	0.0 - 10.5
Income Before Income Taxes	4.50%	5.20%	-9 - 11.8
INCOME TAXES			
Current Taxes	0.50%	0.00%	0.0 - 0.0
Deferred Taxes	0.20%	0.00%	0.0 - 0.0
Total Income Taxes	0.70%	0.00%	0.0 - 0.0
Income After Taxes	3.90%	4.40%	-9 - 11.3
SUMMARY BALANCE SHEET (% TOTAL ASSETS)			
Current Assets	27.10%	12.60%	5.2 - 38.2
Noncurrent Assets	72.90%	87.40%	61.9 - 94.8
Total Assets	100.00%	100.00%	100.0 - 100.0
Current Liabilities	29.20%	17.80%	5.3 - 36.5
Long-Term Debt Net of Current Maturities	60.60%	52.70%	22.0 - 91.0
Total Liabilities	89.80%	86.20%	45.5 - 113.9
Owner's Equity	10.20%	13.80%	-13.9 - 54.5
Total Liabilities and Owner's Equity	100.00%	100.00%	100.0 - 100.0

Reprinted, by permission, from IHRSA, 2006, *Profiles of success* (Boston: IHRSA), 41-42.

Depreciation is the allocation of the cost of a long-term asset over the estimated useful life of that asset. If a fitness center purchases a new treadmill for $5,000, this machine is an asset because it represents potential value to the organization. As members use the machine, recognize an expense each accounting period for the service value received from this asset. Before you can determine depreciation, you need two important estimations:

1. *Estimate of the useful life of the asset.* The expected useful life represents how long the business plans to receive benefits from the asset. For example, the useful life for most fitness equip-

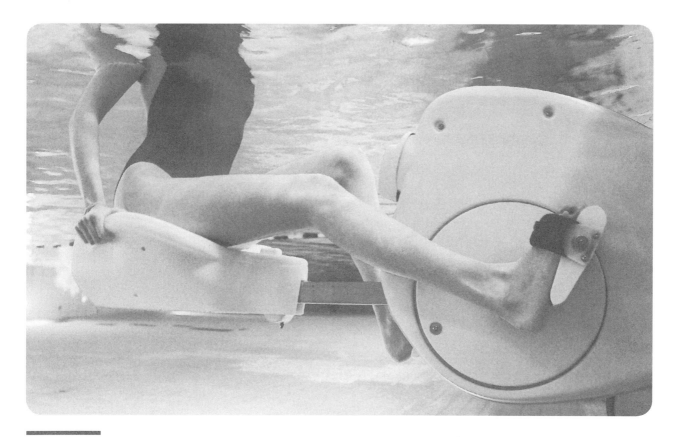

The depreciation of equipment is a noncash expense that should be reflected in the regular expense category in an income statement.
© Bongarts

ment has been estimated at 5 to 7 years. In the United States, the IRS has its own depreciation tax guidelines of recommended useful life for different categories of building and equipment assets.

2. *Estimate of expected salvage value of the asset.* The salvage value is the amount that the business can reasonably expect to receive from selling the asset at the end of its useful life. In the open market, fully depreciated fitness equipment yields 10% to 40% of original purchase prices.

Although we recommend that you have an accountant help prepare these estimates, the manager's knowledge is required to help determine them. Remember that depreciation rules change from year to year; however, the rule that was in effect when you purchased an asset is the rule that you use to determine the time frame for the write-off.

Another aspect of expense management is becoming familiar with all costs associated with operating the business. Knowing each vendor, what is being supplied, and the charge for each item is a

prerequisite for good expense control. Review and scrutinize each invoice as though you were paying it from a personal account. Take steps to ensure consistency and predictability from one month to the next. Question monthly variances, determine reasons for each variance, and take actions to minimize excessive variances.

Health and fitness professionals must understand the effect that expense management can have on business profitability. For example, if you reduced a credit card discount by 3% and projected sales for the year were $1 million, you would immediately notice a savings of $30,000. However, nobody can predict the financial outcome of the next marketing campaign or how many new members will join a facility in the next month.

THE BOTTOM LINE

Managing expenses provides a more tangible method of controlling costs than trying to generate additional revenue.

Tools for Expense Management

Learning to control the expenses of a facility should be the goal of every manager. To date, there is no comprehensive method for completely controlling the expenses of any business. However, there are industry standards and management procedures that provide a gauge for expense management. A financial profile comparing the most profitable commercial health and fitness centers with less successful operations indicates that the most successful clubs control expenses better than others. Twelve tools of expense management are listed in Checklist to Assist in Expense Management below.

THE BOTTOM LINE

By being creative and embracing change, managers can have a positive effect on the bottom line of their organization. Closely evaluating and identifying cost-saving opportunities while implementing ways to control costs are factors for ensuring higher net income for the future.

Checklist to Assist in Expense Management: Twelve Tools

The following list will provide club operators with a checklist of items to carefully monitor as they look to more effectively manage their expenses.

1. Accounting controls and security
   - Use purchase orders that include an estimated cost for the purchase and management approval.
   - Control access to cash by limiting access and using a drop safe, three-part receipt forms, and control-sheet verifications.
   - Provide physical facility security by using alarm systems, entry gates, and security cameras.
   - Provide computer security by including password protection, limited access, and room security.
   - Install management controls by preparing procedure manuals, providing a manager on duty at all times, and obtaining management's approval on large purchases.

2. Value analysis
   - Have a cost–benefit mentality. Weigh results versus costs; consider the return on investment and what the payback includes.
   - Ask key questions: Why are we purchasing this? Is this the best value for the money? What did we purchase that we didn't need?
   - Review the method of funding, such as leasing versus buying and paying cash versus borrowing from the bank.

3. Bidding
   - Bid everything—signs, insurance, office supplies, garbage removal, carpeting, construction, and so on.
   - Obtain at least three comparison bids.
   - Buy in bulk.
   - Do comparison shopping every 3 to 6 months for selected goods and services.

4. Negotiating
   - Vendors expect negotiations.
   - You can negotiate total price, payment terms, delivery date, service (e.g., guarantee, contract), guarantees, options or extra features, and training.

5. Doing it yourself
   - Use internal resources.
   - Use an in-house maintenance team for carpentry, basic heating and air conditioning, electrical and plumbing, carpet cleaning, and court floors.
   - Consider communication needs—printing, photography, and desktop publishing (e.g., newsletters, in-house flyers, forms).
6. Eliminating
   - Investigate using full-time employees for part-time work, and regularly analyze staff schedules.
   - Shift from mass media advertising to other marketing vehicles.
   - Eliminate unnecessary office supplies and unused services.
   - Eliminate unnecessary cost centers.
7. Buying used
   - Used items that you might purchase include restaurant equipment, computers, and maintenance equipment.
   - Consider name brands, appraisals, and guarantees when purchasing used equipment.
   - Locate used equipment by attending auctions and reading trade periodicals and local newspapers.
8. Contracting out
   - Reasons for contracting services include lack of expertise, internal tasks that are unprofitable, and outside resources that could improve business performance.
   - Examples of areas to contract out include restaurants, pro shops, lawn care, and heating and air-conditioning service.
   - Advantages include predictable return, reclaimed use of staff, less risk, and greater knowledge of a particular service.
9. Trading or bartering
   - Determine the value of the trade by comparing a full membership fee (initiation fees and dues) with the normal charge for the service.
   - Examples of trades include photography, printing, supplies, advertising and promotion, and architectural and legal services.
10. Substituting
    - Use lower wattage lightbulbs.
    - Use generic replacement parts.
    - Use an accountant's review statement instead of a full audit.
    - Use smaller brand name labels versus big-name labels.
11. Donating
    - Offer a free (limited) membership to charitable organizations requesting donations.
    - Offer free fitness evaluations or an invitation to a club party.
    - Avoid giving cash.
12. Using space more efficiently
    - Convert cost centers into profit centers, contract out restaurants after internal failure of running them, or convert offices to a pro shop.
    - Convert underused space to a usable (i.e., revenue-generating) function; for example, convert a lounge to a sales office or storage space to a massage room.

Adapted, by permission, from R. Caro, 1995, Management Vision, Inc. www.fitnessmanagement.com.

Tax Considerations

To understand the full nature of financial management, it is important to consider the tax environment within which a health and fitness center must operate. Taxes affect the financial planning and decision making of every business. It is essential for management to understand the tax system and its connection with financial planning and tax planning in order to successfully function in the business world today.

THE BOTTOM LINE

When a facility becomes operational, it is taxed under the three levels of government: federal, state, and local.

Because tax laws are complex and revisions are frequent, we recommend assistance from an accountant or the IRS to complete tax forms and maintain record keeping. The ever-present possibility of an IRS audit is incentive enough to keep good accounting records and receipts of all bills.

Federal Taxes

The legal form of ownership has a major impact on the way tax regulations—especially income tax regulations—apply to a business. The federal income tax assessment for sole proprietorships, partnerships, corporations, and S corporations are listed here.

Sole Proprietorship

The profits from a sole proprietorship are taxed as personal income to the owner.

- Legally, the owner and the business activity are inseparable and are taxed as though the owner is an employee.
- A sole proprietor is expected to estimate income tax each year and pay estimated quarterly taxes.

Partnership

As with the sole proprietorship, tax liability is only assessed for the earned incomes of the individual partners and not against the business.

- Partners file a separate form, noting their distributive shares of the profits.
- A report of the business must be submitted to the IRS each year. This is only an informa-

tion report; no tax payment accompanies its submission.

- As with the sole proprietorship, each partner also files an estimated tax.

Corporation

Tax reporting becomes more elaborate and complicated with this form of ownership.

- As an employee of the corporation, you report annual income and company dividends to the IRS.
- As a separate entity, the corporation must also file a return to the IRS.
- Make estimated tax payments to an authorized bank depository or to a regional Federal Reserve Bank.

S Corporation

The IRS code allows some incorporated businesses to be taxed as a sole proprietorship or partnership. The three main requirements to qualify as an S corporation are as follows:

- The company must have no more than 35 stockholders and no more than one class of stock.
- The company must be a domestic corporation and must not be affiliated with any group eligible to file consolidated tax returns.
- The corporation may not derive more than 20% of its gross receipts from royalties, rents, dividends, interest, annuities, and gains on sales of securities.

Regional and Local Taxes

The rates for state and local taxes on health and fitness facilities vary from region to region. Common among these taxes are the taxes on gross income; real estate; sales on retail goods, food, and services; and membership fees, which some regions consider an amusement or entertainment tax.

An additional local tax assessed against every for-profit facility is a property tax or, in some areas, both property and personal property taxes. City tax assessors calculate property taxes in three ways:

1. *Cost approach.* The value of the property is the selling price of the land plus the cost to construct the building and minus depreciation caused by facility wear. Regions that tax personal property also include the value of the equipment, furniture, and fixtures.

2. *Income approach.* The value of the club property is the value of its earning potential. In this approach you could use the gross income of the club or, if the facility was being rented, the rental value.

3. *Market or comparable sales approach.* The value of the club is predicated on the selling price of other land and similar businesses in the area. This approach is not used as often as the two previously mentioned because most city assessors do not have realistic information on club sales.

Every owner or manager of a for-profit health and fitness enter should monitor property tax assessments closely. On the average, 3% of gross revenues are paid annually for property taxes. For example, consider the average commercial club that grosses $1.5 million in revenues. From this amount, $45,000 would be paid in property taxes. Appeal-ing property taxes is a right afforded any owner or manager. You can obtain assistance for question-ing or appealing property taxes by contacting an accountant or by inquiring with a representative from your local city assessor's office.

THE BOTTOM LINE

In the fitness business, appealing a property tax is one of the few ways to cut costs without affecting member service, staff morale, or facil-ity upkeep.

This section on tax considerations is only a brief review of certain tax codes as they relate to the health and fitness industry. You can obtain further information on these codes from an accountant or local tax office.

KEY TERMS

accrual accounting

balance sheet

budgeting

cash accounting

depreciation

electronic funds transfer (EFT)

income statement

statement of cash flows

REFERENCES AND RECOMMENDED READINGS

Caro, R. 1995a. 35 cost-saving techniques to increase the club's bottom line. *Peak Performance,* August 1995.

———. 1995b. The latest successes in cost savings. *Peak Performance,* September 1995.

———. 2002. The latest cost-saving successes for the club industry. *Peak Performance,* May 2002.

Fried, G. 2004. *Sport finance.* Champaign, IL: Human Kinetics.

Grantham, W. et al. 1998. *Health fitness management.* Champaign, IL: Human Kinetics.

International Health, Racquet, and Sportsclub Associa-tion (IHRSA). 2006. *Profiles of success.* Boston: IHRSA.

Parkhouse, B. 2004. *The management of sport.* New York: McGraw-Hill.

Ross, S. et al. 2002. *Fundamentals of corporate finance.* New York: McGraw-Hill.

Plummer, T. 2003. *The business of fitness.* Monterey, CA: Healthy Learning.

thirteen

Addressing Health and Safety Concerns

Anthony Abbott and Mike Greenwood

LEARNING OBJECTIVES

After studying this chapter, the reader will be able to

- recognize potential safety violations and untoward events,
- identify mechanisms to limit exposure to unhealthy and dangerous stress,
- identify appropriate qualifications to ensure competency of staff, and
- develop a comprehensive emergency response plan for untoward events.

Tales From the Trenches

"Emery, Emery—report to the outdoor running track!" This directive from the public address (PA) system alerted all staff members within the facility that a code blue was in progress. *Code blue* was the name for a life-threatening emergency to which staff members had to respond immediately. By using the code word *Emery*, which stood for *emergency*, rather than *code blue*, with which most people are familiar, staff were advised of the critical incident without alarming members and creating confusion by attracting curious onlookers to the scene.

Although this incident occurred in 1979, the facility was well prepared to respond to any emergency not only throughout the building but also within the outdoor locations where physical activities took place. This capability was greatly enhanced by a buzzer system that had been installed throughout the facility and grounds. Every room within the building, the pool area, and all outdoor sites were fitted with a buzzer wired to the main office. When a life-threatening incident occurred, the staff member providing supervision had only to press a button and one of many bulbs on a light board within the main office would be illuminated, indicating exactly where the emergency was located. When the light board was activated, it was accompanied by a tone that immediately caught the attention of office personnel. Then one of the office staffers would activate the emergency medical system (EMS) while another would announce over the PA system that "Emery" was to report to that location.

Upon hearing the announcement, staff and instructors throughout the facility would report to the scene to fulfill their various roles and responsibilities as outlined in the facility emergency response plan. The emergency plan was a written document that all new employees were required to carefully read and then sign that they had read and understood the plan. All supervisors were responsible for querying new employees to ensure that they knew their roles during emergencies. Additionally, supervisors had to verify that the employees for whom they were responsible had been maintaining their first aid and CPR skills as well as keeping their certification cards current. Skill checks were conducted through both announced and unannounced emergency drills or rehearsals as well as through individual drills where fitness instructors were presented with a mannequin and told to respond to a given scenario.

In this particular incident, a member running on the outdoor track suffered a cardiac arrest. When it was determined that the member was unable to respond, the supervising instructor activated the emergency system with the buzzer and then immediately began one-person CPR. Within a minute another instructor was on the scene to assist with two-person CPR while another senior staff member was able to provide supervision and crowd control. Immediately upon activation of the EMS system, an office staff member went to the street entrance in order to expedite the emergency response by greeting and guiding the paramedics to the track area. The senior staffer on scene determined the name of the member and directed an instructor to retrieve the member's file so that its information could be made available to the paramedics upon their arrival. As soon as possible, the member's wife was notified of the incident and to which hospital her husband had been taken.

An incident report was filed along with statements from the principle responders. This became part of the after-action report that was thoroughly analyzed to identify any inappropriate or untimely responses or areas of the emergency plan that could have been improved. This in turn led to a corrective action report that outlined what type of changes needed to be incorporated in future drills and rehearsals, such as verifying the effective application of CPR and avoiding gastric inflation.

In 1979, AEDs were not available. AEDs are medical devices that dramatically improve the chances of survival for cardiac arrest victims. Of those people afflicted with a sudden cardiac arrest outside of a hospital environment, 95% die. However, due to the immediate application of effective CPR coupled with a timely response on the part of the paramedics, this member survived. At a later date, he was able to return to the facility and again use its outdoor track. The facility received numerous letters of commendation for its emergency response, and members stated that they felt more secure working out in a facility that had demonstrated concern for the health and safety of its membership through the establishment of an effective emergency plan.

Without a comprehensive and well-rehearsed emergency plan, the incident described in Tales From the Trenches could not only have undermined membership confidence in the facility but also could have led to possible litigation. Hopefully you never find yourself or your facility named as a defendant in a lawsuit. However, in a society that is becoming increasingly litigious with every passing year, fitness facility managers are finding themselves more frequently embroiled in litigation. It would appear that the current escalation of litigation is a reflection of a serious industry problem regarding member expectations versus service delivery.

It is not uncommon for a facility to advertise that the health and safety of its membership are its number one priority. If this is truly the case, it will be reflected not only in the facility's documented screening program, safety plan, and emergency procedures but also in a conscientious commitment to enact them. Unfortunately, far too often facilities lack even rudimentary screening and testing of members, staff awareness of basic safety concerns, and the ability to respond to emergencies in a timely and effective manner.

Accidents and injuries are inevitable in an environment in which people are moving at a rapid pace, pushing their physical limits, and competing against others as well as themselves. How you handle these unexpected events can literally mean the difference between life and death. Not only is the possible death of a member at stake, but also the death (financial health) of the facility if it is unprepared for such untoward events.

THE BOTTOM LINE

The prudent fitness manager knows that it is not a matter of whether an incident or medical emergency will occur but rather when it will occur.

Well-formulated safety plans and emergency procedures allow trained staff to respond with confidence rather than to react with confusion to adverse events and potential danger. This chapter evaluates the components of a well-defined **safety plan** in addition to the elements of a well-designed **emergency response plan** (see figure 13.1). It also analyzes various dangers that exist in different health and fitness programs, how to avoid them, and emergency plan modifications for these settings.

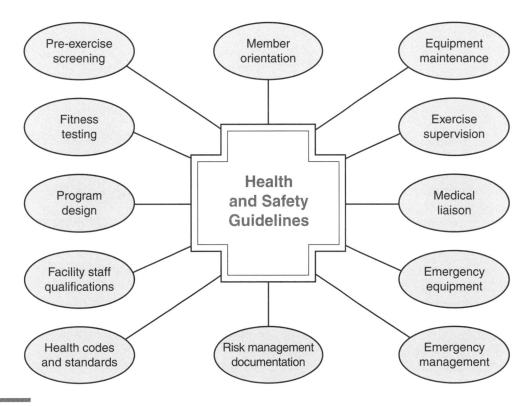

Figure 13.1 Health and safety guidelines.

Health and safety codes, industry standards, and professional guidelines are reviewed to ensure that staff members are not only suitably qualified but also properly prepared to conduct their duties. Some sample documents are provided to help protect the facility from adverse events besides potential litigation in the eventuality of a serious emergency. Additionally, the qualifications of first responders are reviewed as well as necessary emergency equipment and supply lists to ensure that all health and fitness facilities are prepared to successfully handle any exigency.

Creating a Safe Environment

A safe club environment for exercising members is a given. In spite of the fact that club management is aware of this necessity, many facilities still do not incorporate even basic health and safety practices into their daily operations. Compounding this problem are the irresponsible or ignorant actions of careless members. The best policies and procedures for ensuring member safety are often ignored by members. Only an educated and alert staff coupled with a well-planned and maintained facility can overcome the obstacles to a safe exercise environment. Ongoing training of staff and immediate correction of potentially dangerous situations, such as unsafe equipment (as addressed in the following chapter), must be a consistent practice in all facilities.

Facility

The ongoing implementation of health and safety practices enables health and fitness managers to maintain a safe club environment. This execution must start during the initial planning phase. Facility design and development techniques along with the execution of city, state, and federal health codes can build the foundation for a safe environment. With the assistance of professional consultants, evaluate the club for safety factors while the physical structure is in design stages in order to eliminate potential problems long before the first member enters the club. A well-designed facility coupled with ongoing staff training, the implementation of health codes, and the practice of industry standards and guidelines will lead to the safest possible club environment.

Signage

Health codes are unique in each city and state, so managers must determine what regulations are applicable for their specific location and type of operation. The ability to communicate and enforce such health and safety information protects members from potential injury or death as well as safeguards the business from frivolous lawsuits. Use appropriate **signage** throughout the facility to assist staff in providing this important information to facility users.

Signage should be used to provide directions, indicate points of entry and exit, issue instructional or safety information, and communicate ongoing or upcoming club events. For signage to be effective, however, it must have a clear and concise message, be easily read from a distance, and be properly located within the facility. Local, state, or federal guidelines may specify details relating to message content, design format, or placement of signage along with requirements for the posting of documents such as licenses or certifications. It is recommended that management consult the proper local authorities before designing and purchasing club signage. Additional recommendations for signage include the following:

• *Use basic terminology.* The use of layman's phraseology will be better understood by the general membership. Use terminology appropriate for the target audience.

• *Use signs that can be easily read.* Select type styles that are easily read from a distance of 10 to 15 feet (3-4.5 meters) and place the signs 5 to 7 feet (1.5-2 meters) from the ground.

• *Determine the message.* Use as few words and symbols as possible, and show this wording to different people in order to test the accuracy and effectiveness of the message.

Bloodborne Pathogens Standard

The health code relating to **bloodborne pathogens** offers a substantial challenge to the facility manager. Bloodborne viruses that are of primary concern to the health and fitness industry include HIV and hepatitis B and C. The facility manager is responsible for recognizing and understanding the threat inherent with regular fitness center operations, consequent potential dangers for exposure to staff or members with such viruses, and the necessary prevention techniques.

Managers must become familiar with the guidelines published by OSHA, which provide information on the training and record-keeping procedures related to avoiding and handling bloodborne pathogens. To adequately protect staff and members, it is important that facility managers know

- what the bloodborne pathogens are,
- what is meant by *occupational exposure* to bloodborne pathogens,
- what potential infectious materials are and how to prevent exposure to them,
- what the possible methods of transmission are and how to control them, and
- what protective equipment is required to safeguard the first responder in an emergency situation.

This information and much more are available from OSHA, which has regional offices throughout the country that can assist managers in meeting their responsibilities. Additionally, IHRSA has prepared a briefing paper for member facilities regarding the OSHA bloodborne pathogens standard. Managers should avail themselves of the information provided within this briefing paper.

In addition to bloodborne pathogens, employees and members of fitness facilities may be exposed to potentially hazardous chemical agents and toxic materials. For this reason it is essential that all employees, including independent contractors, are advised by means of posted placards, notices, and memoranda of potentially harmful materials other than bloodborne pathogens. To this end, the ACSM's most recent edition of *Health/Fitness Facility Standards and Guidelines* (2007) lists standard 5 as follows: Facilities must have in place a written system for sharing information with users and employees or independent contractors regarding the handling of potentially hazardous materials, including the handling of bodily fluids by staff in accordance with OSHA standards.

THE BOTTOM LINE

The facility manager is responsible for the existence of a written system that advises members, employees, and independent contractors about potentially hazardous materials.

Personnel

The key to the health and safety of facility members is the availability of knowledgeable and conscientious personnel capable of establishing a safe exercise environment. This requires that staff members at all levels must not only be appropriately qualified to carry out their respective duties but also sufficiently motivated to do the job to the best of their abilities.

Management

Most health and fitness facilities are managed by people lacking appropriate training and credentials. The sad fact is that, in general, managers are unqualified to oversee and direct the safe and effective operation of facilities. It is typical for managers to have a business background, which is essential for the fiscal health of the facility, but to have no exercise experience, which is essential for the physical health of the membership. Managers need not have a degree in exercise physiology, but they must have working knowledge of exercise science to understand what constitutes appropriately qualified instructors as well as safe and effective exercise programming.

As far back as 1984, a study at a 4-year college had students go into the community and survey 50 fitness facilities regarding instructor qualifications and training (Rabinoff 1984). None of the facilities stated that a college degree or certification from a credible association like the ACSM was a requirement for employment. With respect to the major criteria used in hiring a fitness instructor, only 2.4% viewed an educational degree as the most important. Appearance and previous employment as an instructor were considered the significant determinants.

The following year, another university study was conducted reflecting managers' attitudes toward instructor qualifications. This study, titled *Sport Management in the Private Sector: Selecting Qualified Managers,* was designed to investigate the professional preparation of sport and fitness facility managers (Davis 1985). The survey revealed that although many club managers had BA degrees in business, few had any formal education in exercise science. Consequently, there was little demonstrated concern for hiring qualified fitness instructors because of an inability to determine what constituted a qualified instructor.

Twenty years later, this author, who has been retained as an expert witness in over 40 fitness facility litigations of which half have been death cases, can verify that time has led to little or no improvement regarding management's understanding of the field of exercise science. Because managers are rarely well versed in this area of expertise, they are incapable of determining what is necessary to establish safe and effective fitness programming for their membership as well as unable to discern the difference between the numerous fitness instructor and personal trainer certifications. Of extreme concern is the current lack of adequate screening for new members coupled with inadequate preparation to handle emergencies.

Despite a joint position statement in 1998 by the American Heart Association (AHA) and the ACSM that addressed recommendations for cardiovascular screening, staffing, and emergency policies, the fitness industry has failed to respond accordingly (American Heart Association [AHA] 1998). In 2001, a study of fitness facilities in the state of Ohio reflected that older adults and people with occult or known heart disease are exercising at facilities that, more often than not, lack adequate cardiovascular screening and emergency procedures (McInnis et al. 2001).

In addition to this lack of training in exercise science, it is not uncommon for management to fail to employ good administrative procedures. The inability to provide leadership, professional supervision, and suitable staff development plagues most health and fitness facilities. The typical high turnover of personnel within fitness facilities is a reflection of staff disappointment with not only salary but also management. A well-run operation promotes an atmosphere leading to employee contentment and job satisfaction. The mark of a truly successful facility is not only membership retention but staff retention as well.

It is common knowledge that too many facilities are sales oriented rather than service oriented. A large percentage of facilities even rely on client failure for their financial success. Many facilities have so many inactive members that if 10% of their total membership showed up 3 days a week for an hour of exercise, they would violate every ordinance in the book for overcrowding. Obviously, the facility that fails to prioritize its members' success must also fail to provide a safe training environment.

Fitness Staff

Not only do most managers lack appropriate training and skills, but also their fitness staff. Many health care professionals and fitness authorities are deeply concerned about the qualifications, or rather, lack of qualifications, on the part of fitness instructors and personal trainers. Physical education and exercise science professions have been bypassed in the growth of the fitness industry, and as a result, quality instruction and training have been generally ignored. In an effort to keep their overhead down, facility owners and managers frequently hire minimum-wage instructors while dismissing college-educated physical education and exercise science majors as overqualified. It would appear that many facility entrepreneurs have jumped on the fitness bandwagon for financial gain at the expense of their members' health and safety.

Certification

The same entrepreneurial fever and greed that have led to the hiring of untrained staff within the fitness industry have also led to inadequate fitness instructor and personal trainer **certifications.** A survey conducted by the National Board of Fitness Examiners (NBFE) determined that there are more than 75 national certification programs; these certifications coupled with those being offered by college and university divisions of continuing education would probably account for over a couple of hundred certification programs available to the public. The lead author, who has taken over thirty certification exams and conducted research related to the knowledge base of commercial fitness instructors, has determined that most of these national programs are offered by self-appointed fitness authorities who have either limited training in exercise science themselves or an inability to develop a meaningful exam process. It must be remembered that a certificate is no more valuable than the training behind it as well as the standards used for awarding such a credential.

Becoming a competent fitness instructor or personal trainer requires an in-depth knowledge of human anatomy, physiology, kinesiology, and exercise science combined with practical training and experience. This cannot be achieved through weekend cram courses and certification programs during which students are primed for specific questions to which they regurgitate the answers on examination. Although these pseudoprofessional associations often forward candidates study materials in advance, there is never sufficient time for practical training and testing to ensure candidates are capable of safe and effective exercise programming.

In order to develop the knowledge, skills, and abilities of a competent fitness instructor or personal trainer, one must undergo formal instruction in exercise science through an accredited university or a credible vocational school that provides comprehensive theoretical education and extensive practical training taught by degreed exercise physiologists with field experience. Upon completion of academic instruction coupled with substantial practical training in the areas of health assessment, fitness testing, performance evaluation, program design, and client supervision, serious and knowledgeable students will seek certification through nonprofit, professional associations like the ACSM or NSCA. Graduates of an athletic training program from an accredited university usually seek certification through the National Athletic Trainers' Association (NATA).

Research conducted in 1988 revealed that when facility instructors were administered a nationally validated survey test examining knowledge in exercise science, those instructors with ACSM certification scored significantly higher than those who possessed other certifications, excluding NSCA (Abbott 1989). This study also found that formal education, not experience, was the most significant factor correlating with a sound knowledge base, including an understanding of exercise safety. More recent research has supported this observation by concluding that formal education in exercise science coupled with certification from either the ACSM or NSCA were strong predictors of a personal trainer's exercise science knowledge, whereas years of experience were not related to such knowledge (Malek et al. 2002).

It is worthy of note that the NSCA offered the first personal trainer certification in the fitness industry that was accredited by the National Commission for Certifying Agencies (NCCA), the certifying arm of the National Organization for Competency Assurance (NOCA). To date, the NSCA is the only fitness-certifying body accredited by the International Organization for Standardization (ISO) and recognized by the National Skill Standards Board (NSSB).

Accreditation

The last few years have seen the fitness industry trying to determine the credibility of different personal trainer certifications. This has become important to managers who have recognized the financial value of offering personal training to facility members. IHRSA, the professional trade association of the fitness industry, has recently recommended that its member clubs hire only personal trainers who have accredited certifications. At the time of this writing, IHRSA has only recognized the NCCA as an appropriate accrediting body.

Unfortunately, not all accredited certifications effectively discriminate between those recipients who have the knowledge, skills, and ability to be competent fitness instructors and personal trainers versus those who may pose a risk to the general public. **Accreditation** relies upon the ability of a credentialing organization to assess a practitioner's job description and then test that person's knowledge in specific areas related to job responsibility. This requires role delineation, task analysis, item development, psychometric review, and securely proctored exams.

When the credentialing organization demonstrates that it has followed the proper steps in examination development, it has increased the likelihood that it will develop a valid and reliable exam. However, to create a valid and reliable examination that discriminates between truly qualified and unqualified candidates, exam questions must not only be directed at identified content areas but also must be presented at an appropriate level of difficulty.

To be a valid indicator of competency, exam questions must possess a sufficiently high degree of difficulty to challenge an individual's depth of knowledge. Unfortunately, most accredited certifications are awarded based upon exams that only scratch the surface of important content areas because questions are cursory and simplistic. The majority of accredited personal trainer certification exams are primarily composed of recall questions with limited numbers of application and analysis questions. The ability to identify people who are proficient in exercise science requires that exams be also based upon the behavioral objectives and high standards promoted by truly professional associations like the ACSM and NSCA.

Litigation

In years past, people injured at fitness facilities would accept the blame and rarely hold others responsible. The injured would attribute their strained muscles and tendons, sprained ligaments, and low back pain to just being out of shape and therefore would feel embarrassed to bring their injuries to anyone's attention other than their doctor's (Alter 1983).

Today, however, the public is beginning to hold health facilities, fitness instructors, and personal trainers accountable for unsafe instruction and inadequate supervision. Consequently, there has been an upsurge in the number of personal injury lawsuits against facilities, instructors, and trainers along with a concurrent rise in liability insurance. Even with the obvious deterrent of waivers and releases, the public appears more willing to take their grievances to court.

To lessen the possibility of **litigation,** facility personnel must be capable of thoroughly screening potential members, providing suitable fitness tests, evaluating health assessments and **fitness profiles,** designing appropriate exercise programs, and supervising such member activities. Additionally, staff should constantly be aware of potentially dangerous situations and be empowered with the responsibility as well as accountability to immediately correct such hazardous conditions.

When health and fitness facilities become thoroughly prepared and truly committed to providing the most effective exercise programs and the safest training environments, then this industry will be recognized and applauded by the allied health care field. However, to achieve such recognition and success, managers of facilities will have to adhere to the well-documented Steps to Success (see figure 13.2). Screening members through **health risk appraisals** will determine if they are ready for the stress of exercise or whether **medical clearance** is needed. Testing members' physical fitness with a battery of tests and establishing a fitness profile will better enable trainers to assess their clients' current capacities for exercise. Evaluating health appraisals along with fitness profiles allows trainers to get an even better picture of the members' capability to exercise safely and what type of programs would be best suited for them. Programming based upon appraisals, profiles, and members' goals permits trainers to design the most effective and safest programs that meet members' needs. Supervision ensures that members' programs are being conducted effectively and safely while providing the necessary motivation. These steps will effectively attenuate the potential for litigation.

The failure of management to mandate proficiency in basic life support and to ensure a timely response in emergencies has also led to increased litigation. Certification and mastery of CPR and AED use along with first aid must not only be a prerequisite for hiring but also an integral part of ongoing staff training. Highly qualified personnel who are not hesitant to implement and enforce safety standards as well as to recognize and activate emergency procedures with the appropriate equipment are the key to safety in an exercise setting.

Screening Before Activity

The primary purpose of screening members before permitting them to engage in physical activity is to determine whether they ought to have a physical exam, including a clinical stress test, and whether they need medical clearance. **Preactivity screening** is the procedure by which a facility can identify those members who are at an increased risk for experiencing exercise-related cardiovascular incidents as well as musculoskeletal problems. The present **standard of care** dictates that screening procedures be practiced without exception.

THE BOTTOM LINE

Preactivity screening is a recognized standard that must be practiced by all fitness facilities. To ignore or treat this activity in a cavalier manner demonstrates a reckless disregard for member safety and exposes the facility to litigation.

Implementation of an exercise program is part of a wellness continuum that the facility makes available to its members. Any exercise programming should be initiated with a screening process that provides knowledge of a member's past and present health history as well as lifestyle considerations. Before an exercise program is undertaken, it is prudent to complete a health risk appraisal or **medical history questionnaire** to determine if there are any medical contraindications to exercise that could necessitate a physician's clearance prior to any exercise testing and fitness programming.

Contraindications of primary concern are

- cardiovascular disease (heart attack, stroke, hypertension, aneurysm, claudication, and severe mitral valve prolapse),

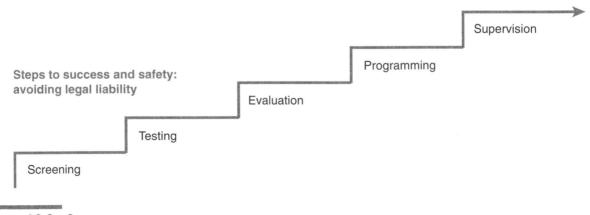

Steps to success and safety: avoiding legal liability

Supervision

Programming

Evaluation

Testing

Screening

Figure 13.2 Steps to success.

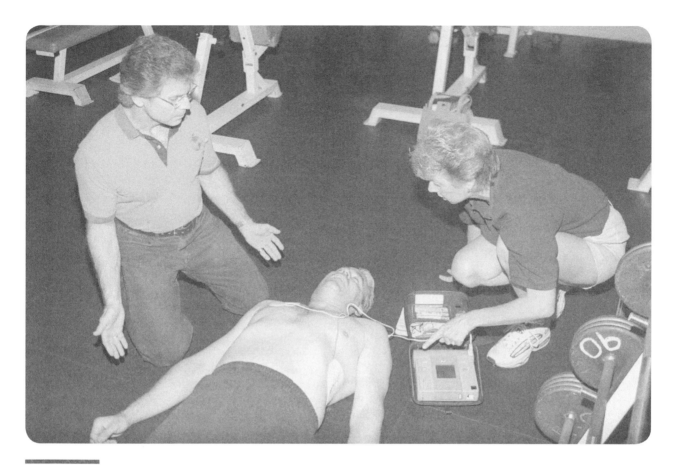

Managers who require staff to be trained in the use of an automated external defibrillator (AED) are protecting the lives of the club's members and also reducing the risk of litigation.

Photo courtesy of Anthony Abbott

- pulmonary disease (bronchitis, emphysema, and asthma),

- metabolic disease (diabetes mellitus, thyroid disorders, liver and renal complications),

- musculoskeletal problems (fractures, sprains, strains, herniations, arthritis, and structural limitations), and

- any other condition placing the exerciser at higher than normal risk.

The fitness instructor or personal trainer involved with the screening process should become familiar with the ramifications of these diseases related to exercise.

Health Appraisal

The health appraisal allows the trainer to better assess the suitability of exercise for members. Therefore, it minimizes the risk of injury, disability, or even death while lessening the potential for litigation against the facility. It also establishes the

appropriateness of the next step in this health and fitness continuum: the fitness assessment. During the health appraisal, it is typical to acquire demographic information, complete a medical history, and administer a lifestyle questionnaire. All this information contributes to the goal of member screening, which is to classify the member in one of the following categories:

- People who should be excluded from exercise due to medical contraindications

- People with known disease conditions that require referral to a medically supervised exercise program

- People with known disease, symptoms, or risk factors that require further medical evaluation and clearance before starting an exercise program

- People with special needs for safe and effective exercise programming

- People who may begin traditional exercise programs

Demographics

Typically, this section includes general information such as name, address, phone numbers, e-mail address, age, gender, height, weight, ethnicity, marital status, nearest relative, family physician, specialty physicians, education, occupation, and other data deemed pertinent. This information is expanded upon with the medical history, lifestyle questionnaire, and any other available information, such as that found within physical exam reports and laboratory test results, which may be provided to the trainer in order to generate a more complete picture of the member.

Medical History

This section allows the trainer to better assess the health and well-being of the member. There are numerous medical history questionnaires on the market that vary in length and comprehensiveness. It is recommended that facilities consider using health risk appraisals or health history questionnaires such as those found in *ACSM's Health/Fitness Facility Standards and Guidelines* (2007). In general, appraisals and questionnaires include the following subjects:

- Does the member ever experience discomfort, shortness of breath, or chest pain with moderate exercise? Does the member have any known heart disorders? Is there any family history of heart disease?

- Does the member experience severe dizziness, limb numbness, or any leg cramping (claudication) with exertion? Does the member have any history of high blood pressure or vascular problems such as stroke?

- Does the member have any musculoskeletal restrictions or arthritic conditions that are aggravated with exercise? If so, what are the limitations, and has a physician ever told the member to avoid certain physical activities? Are there any physical limitations due to operations?

- Does the member have any diagnosed metabolic diseases such as diabetes mellitus, a thyroid condition, or liver or kidney complications? If so, to what extent? Is diabetes classified as type I or type II? Is it a hypothyroid or hyperthyroid condition? Is the kidney dysfunction nondebilitating or end-stage renal disease?

- Does the member have any form of chronic obstructive pulmonary disease (COPD)? Does the member suffer from chronic bronchitis or emphysema? Does the member have reactive airway disease (asthma) or exercise-induced asthma? Does moderate exercise bring on labored breathing (dyspnea)?

- Does the member currently take any medications (prescription as well as over the counter)? If so, why are they being taken, how long have they been taken, how much is being taken, and who prescribed them?

- Finally, does the member know of any physical condition or illness that might prevent participation in an exercise program? Have any such conditions or illnesses limited physical activity in the past?

If the answer is *yes* to any of the aforementioned questions, then exercise testing and programming may have to be postponed and medical clearance may be necessary. The trainer is responsible for administering a comprehensive medical history to uncover any possible dangers in exercise testing and programming. Additionally, the trainer must be aware of exercise-related complications when dealing with these physical conditions and must be able to adjust programs accordingly.

The medical history form should conclude with a statement in which members swear that the information provided is true and correct to the best of their knowledge and that they recognize that this health assessment is not the equivalent of a medical evaluation or diagnosis. The form should then be signed by the member as well as a witness other than the trainer administering the medical history.

Lifestyle Questionnaire

The **lifestyle questionnaire** provides even more useful information related to the member's risk factors. Factors such as alcohol consumption, caffeine intake, tobacco use, legal and illegal drug use, nutritional habits, sleep patterns, stress and tension, driving record, recreational interests, physical activities, exercise likes and dislikes, and many other lifestyle considerations help paint a picture of the member's mental and physical health. This information along with the health history questionnaire, physical exam report, and lab test results may reflect heightened risk for heart attack, stroke, cancer, and other diseases, as well as unnecessary accidents.

Although it is impossible to change certain risk factors such as age, family history, and some illnesses, many other factors may be altered as the trainer addresses concerns of the health risk appraisal. More than 50% of chronic degenerative diseases are lifestyle related. Consequently, people can make a major impact on their health through lifestyle modification. According to the AHA, the four major risk factors for coronary heart disease are smoking, high blood pressure, elevated cholesterol, and physical inactivity. In most cases, these major risk factors can be readily modified through smoking cessation, reduced intake of dietary fat, and regular exercise. Available literature indicates that such behavior modification will have a significant impact not only on life extension but also life enrichment.

Physical Exam

Ideally, everyone should have a physical or medical exam before participating in fitness testing or an exercise program. For this reason, it is recommended that trainers encourage all members to have a physical exam, including laboratory tests. When exam reports and lab results are accessible to the trainer, there is that much more information to assist with the development of a safe and effective exercise program.

According to the ACSM, a physical exam that includes a diagnostic **clinical stress test** is an essential screening component for older adults contemplating vigorous exercise. By ACSM standards, older adults are men aged 45 years or older and women aged 55 years or older, and vigorous exercise would constitute intensities above 60% of $\dot{V}O_2$max. Understandably, people at increased risk for cardiovascular events as well as those with signs or symptoms of coronary heart disease and those with known cardiac, pulmonary, or metabolic disease should also have complete physical exams with a clinical stress test before engaging in vigorous exercise.

Many members will object to spending money for a physical exam and laboratory tests, so facilities may initially decide to work with some members without the benefit of this information. Whether this is the case or not, it is recommended that the trainer use information from medical histories and lifestyle questionnaires in order to classify members as to the degree of risk in exercise testing and program participation. Through the ACSM **risk stratification** process, members can be classified as low risk, moderate risk, and high risk. At this point, the trainer can make the decision to either continue with fitness testing or insist upon medical clearance from the member's physician.

The risk stratification process is thoroughly outlined in the seventh edition of *ACSM's Guidelines for Exercise Testing and Prescription* (2005). It is recommended that facilities adopt these guidelines. Additionally, the trainer should become familiar with the third edition of *ACSM's Health/Fitness Facility Standards and Guidelines* (2007) as well as the 1998 joint position statement by the ACSM and AHA titled *Recommendations for Cardiovascular Screening, Staffing, and Emergency Policies at Health/Fitness Facilities* (AHA 1998).

Unfortunately, many facilities solely rely on the **Physical Activity Readiness Questionnaire (PAR-Q)** as a screening device without understanding its limitations. Frequently trainers assume that no reported *yes* answers to this questionnaire gives the member a clean bill of health and, therefore, provides clearance for exercise programs. It must be stressed that the PAR-Q is a minimum standard for entry into a low- to moderate-intensity exercise program and should not be the screening device of choice for facilities.

Laboratory Tests

Although it may not be feasible to obtain all test results from every physical exam, their availability can be most useful in the screening process; therefore, the trainer should make every effort to secure this kind of information. Of greatest importance is the blood profile, including analysis of the following variables: fasting blood glucose, fasting triglycerides, total cholesterol, LDL cholesterol, HDL cholesterol, and ratio of total cholesterol to HDL. Classification of these blood variables can be found within *ACSM's Guidelines for Exercise Testing and Prescription*, and from such classification scales the trainer is able to better assess the member's health. It should also be noted that many physicians are looking more seriously at other variables, such as C-reactive protein as a marker of systemic inflammation and high blood concentrations of homocysteine, that appear related to occlusive heart disease.

The preactivity screening process is a vital step in the health and fitness continuum. It enables trainers to begin on a safer footing as they prepare to test and create a program for the facility member. Additionally, it establishes a baseline of health parameters that serve as markers for monitoring future progress. As such, it becomes invaluable as a motivational tool. It should never be overlooked or bypassed.

Good managers understand both the physiological and psychological value of comprehensive health risk appraisals. They must also understand that if trainers are to be viewed as true allied health professionals and facilities are to be recognized as safe training environments, then thorough preactivity screening is a must.

At a minimum, a health history questionnaire coupled with a blood pressure assessment should be employed as screening devices.

Considering that high blood pressure is a major risk factor for heart disease, stroke, and kidney failure; that approximately one-third of Americans have hypertension; and that one-third of hypertensives are unaware of having this silent killer, it stands to reason that facilities must administer blood pressure testing as part of the screening process. However, management must ensure that trainers do not go beyond their scope of practice when screening members and taking blood pressure. Screening with blood pressure assessment only enables trainers to suspect the need for a medical diagnosis or to determine if medical clearance is necessary.

It is essential that management not allow personnel involved with preactivity screening to make medical diagnoses or prescribe treatment from the data collected on health history questionnaires. Allowing them to go beyond the scope of practice in this way could lead to potential litigation related to the unauthorized practice of medicine. All states have statutes that authorize certain licensed health care professionals to diagnose and treat people. A violation of these statutes by unauthorized individuals such as facility trainers could result in criminal prosecution. Although trainers may feel that a particular diagnosis is likely (e.g., a member has hypertension), they may not make medical diagnoses or prescribe treatment. Managers must make sure trainers understand that they are suspecticians, not diagnosticians.

Management must establish a systematic approach to ascertain that the information in health risk appraisals or health history questionnaires is accurate, current, and readily available in case of an emergency. By including this form in the introductory process of membership, the club ensures that documents on all members are available and that review of the documents for potential risk is concluded before finalizing the membership agreement.

THE BOTTOM LINE

Require completion of a health history questionnaire before finalizing any membership agreement.

The information contained in the health history questionnaire is valuable only if it can be retrieved.

A poor filing system renders the information useless and places the facility in a less than optimal legal position. Maintain the information in a computer database and keep a hard copy on file. Ensure that only authorized employees have access to the information and that the data are readily available in the event of an emergency. Set a standard that all health history questionnaires, lifestyle questionnaires, physical exam reports, laboratory test results, and any other personal health information be maintained at all times either in the individual's membership file or in a confidential filing system maintained by the fitness director. Implement a process for regularly reviewing the information to ensure data are complete and current.

Medical Clearance

In the **medical management model** (see figure 13.3), results of the preactivity screening are examined to see if the participant is apparently healthy, at above-average risk for disease, or at high risk. The ACSM uses a risk classification scale that categorizes facility members into one of three strata:

- Low risk—Men younger than 45 years of age and women younger than 55 years of age who are asymptomatic and have no more than one positive risk factor as outlined in *ACSM's Guidelines for Exercise Testing and Prescription* (2007)

- Moderate risk—Men older than 45 years and women older than 55 years or those who meet the threshold for two or more risk factors

- High risk—People who have one or more signs and symptoms as listed in *ACSM's Guidelines for Exercise Testing and Prescription* or have known cardiovascular, pulmonary, or metabolic disease

Screening personnel should refer to the *ACSM's Guidelines for Exercise Testing and Prescription, Seventh Edition*, for more detailed information regarding risk stratification as it relates to coronary artery disease risk factor thresholds and major signs or symptoms suggestive of cardiovascular, pulmonary, or metabolic disease. It is recommended that facilities adopt these classification guidelines along with other guidelines found within the third edition of *ACSM's Health/Fitness Facility Standards and Guidelines*.

People deemed high risk or any person identified through screening to have potential health problems should see a physician and obtain medical

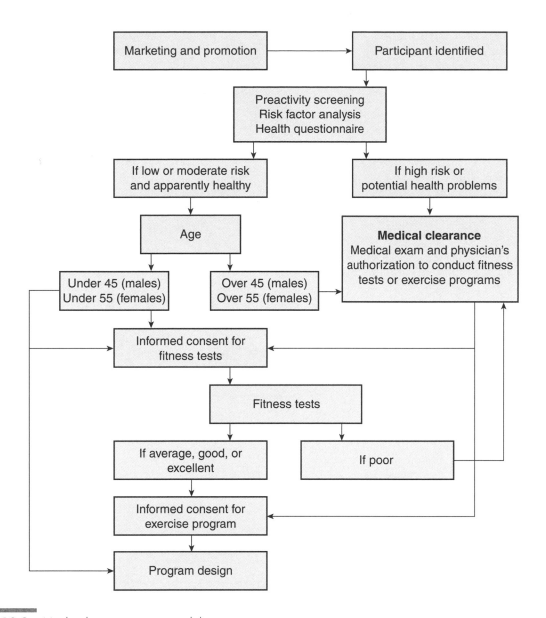

Figure 13.3 Medical management model.

Adapted from R.W. Patton et al., 1989, *Developing and managing health/fitness facilities* (Champaign, IL: Human Kinetics), 209. By permission of R.W. Patton.

clearance before undertaking further fitness testing or exercise programming. *ACSM's Health/Fitness Facility Standards and Guidelines* provides examples of **assumption of risk** and physician release forms for participation in physical activity programs.

Every facility should have a medical director or consultant who provides medical clearance for members or directs such individuals to their personal physician for medical clearance. With a medical director and a legal counsel, fitness management should establish a detailed process and written policy for identifying high-risk individuals and those with potential health concerns and exactly how medical clearance will be obtained.

Screening of Guests

A constant challenge facing fitness managers is the registration and screening procedures for guests and prospective members using the facility. Management must prepare and staff must practice the process of registration and **guest screening,** which provides facility personnel with a level of confidence that every guest is apparently healthy or at low risk. Additionally, this process must guarantee that the guest knowingly assumes all risks related to physical activity within the facility (i.e., an assumption of risk statement). Furthermore, the staff must provide the guest with an orientation of the activity areas and equipment while stressing safety considerations.

The registration and screening procedure should include basic personal information in the event of an incident or emergency. It can also serve as a sales tool to identify prospective members. Facilities frequently use a two-part guest registration and screening procedure. The first part is the registration form (see Guest Registration form below), which includes the guest's name, address, phone number, and emergency contact, as well as an assumption of risk statement. The second part is the health screening form, which is a PAR-Q that is also to be signed.

Managers must work with their legal counsel to determine a registration and screening procedure, to identify appropriate information that must be gathered, and to create the assumption of risk statement in order to minimize the possibility of untoward incidents and consequent liability. Regardless of whether the guest is accompanied by an existing member, participating in a special event, or spon-

sored through a cooperative arrangement with a local hotel, business, or organization, the manager must recognize that the standard of care regarding preactivity screening is still in effect.

THE BOTTOM LINE

All guests must undergo a screening process and should be advised to limit their exercise to a low to moderate intensity.

Administering Physical Fitness Assessments

Many health and fitness facilities routinely perform physical fitness assessments to determine level of physical fitness as it pertains to disease prevention and health promotion. Proper procedures to identify and test only appropriate individuals are as important as preactivity screening. People undergo

---

Guest Registration

Please complete the Physical Activity Readiness Questionnaire (PAR-Q) and the information below prior to initiating activity.

Name: _____   Date: _____

Address: _____

_____

Telephone: (Home) _____ (Work) _____

Emergency contact: (Name) _____(Telephone) _____

Have you visited ABC Club before? _____ Yes _____ No   If yes, when? _____

I understand and acknowledge that there are inherent risks associated with exercise and use of exercise equipment and facilities, such as those available at ABC Club, and I agree that all exercise and activities that I engage in at ABC Club will be done at my own risk. I will limit my physical activity to that of low to moderate intensity, which will be explained to me by a fitness instructor. I waive my right to any claims against ABC Club (or any affiliated agent) that may arise out of any activity, event, use of ABC Club equipment or facilities, or my presence on the premises, including personal injury, theft, and all property damage, even if caused by the negligence of any of these persons. However, I am not waiving any claims to the extent it may be based upon gross negligence or willful misconduct.

Signature: _____

From M. Bates, 2008, *Health Fitness Management*, 2nd ed. (Champaign, IL: Human Kinetics).

voluntary fitness-related physical assessments for several reasons. ACSM has identified the following purposes for fitness testing:

- Provide data that are helpful in developing a program design.
- Collect baseline and follow-up data that allow for the evaluation of progress by the participant.
- Motivate the participant by establishing reasonable and attainable fitness goals.
- Educate the participant about concepts of physical fitness and individual fitness.
- Stratify risk and limit potential for litigation.

Regardless of the individual reasons for a fitness assessment, it is imperative that the examiner be well trained and qualified to safely administer all components of the assessment. The test technician must be able to determine the most appropriate testing protocols for all individuals based on their age, physical condition, health status, and current physical activity level. Any trainer administering fitness assessments should have a degree in exercise science or be certified by the ACSM, NSCA, or another reputable credentialing body that conforms to similar standards as espoused by these two professional associations.

As indicated previously, the facility should initiate a member's program with a comprehensive health risk appraisal, including a medical history and lifestyle questionnaire, perhaps along with a review of physical exam reports such as blood profiles and even a clinical stress test. Once members have been thoroughly screened and cleared for exercise programming, the next step is the physical fitness assessment. Similar to preactivity screening, management must develop, adopt, and adhere to specific pretest procedures as well as a reasonable and prudent testing format.

This initial education of members regarding their health status and fitness profile is important not only from the standpoint of program design but also from the perspective of providing members with greater confidence in their efforts to take charge of their health and fitness. As with so many areas of life, the more knowledge you have about a given endeavor, the more confident you will be and, therefore, the more likely to achieve success. The adage, "The educated consumer is the best consumer," certainly holds true for club members.

The ability to provide follow-up fitness testing for members will even further enhance their chances of achieving success. Follow-up assessments enable the trainer to provide members with definitive data about how they are progressing with their health and fitness programming. This positive feedback reinforces their efforts and allows them a taste of success, which is essential in maintaining motivation for ongoing training. Remember, success breeds success.

Before the Assessments

Before members arrive for testing, they should be given written instructions regarding how to prepare for the tests. Explicit instructions are necessary to ensure testing validity and accuracy. In addition to not smoking within 3 hours of testing, members should be instructed not to ingest food, alcohol, or caffeine within this time frame. It is also important that members wear appropriate attire, be well rested, and not have exercised within the past 12 hours.

The testing environment is critical for test validity and reliability, especially concerning constancy of environment for accurate follow-up testing. It is recommended that room temperature be set between 70 and 74 degrees Fahrenheit (21-23 degrees Celsius) and that humidity be controlled at approximately 60%. Equally important are comfortable surroundings wherein anxiety can be minimized; privacy, therefore, is of utmost importance. Regarding privacy, a cautionary note would be to avoid any situations in which staff could be accused of making sexual advances; a third party acting as an assistant can help deter such allegations. Additionally, testing procedures should be thoroughly explained, and any tendency to rush through the battery of tests should be avoided.

During pretest instructions, all members should be required to read and sign an **informed consent** for exercise testing. For legal purposes, it is recommended that informed consents have specific content areas to be shared with members about to undertake fitness testing. Typically, these content areas are

1. purpose and explanation of the test,
2. attendant risks and discomforts,
3. responsibilities of the participant,
4. benefits to be expected,
5. inquiries about testing procedures,
6. use of testing data and confidentiality, and
7. freedom of consent to engage in testing.

In addition to this written document, examiners should discuss each content area with the member and ascertain that there are no questions that have not been answered satisfactorily.

The trainer should carefully review this information before proceeding with the assessment. Should either the member or the trainer feel that testing is not appropriate, or should the member request to stop at any point during testing, the fitness assessment must be discontinued. For a detailed discussion regarding health-related fitness testing and appropriate informed consent forms for exercise testing, consult both the *ACSM's Guidelines for Exercise Testing and Prescription, Seventh Edition*, and *ACSM's Health/Fitness Facility Standards and Guidelines, Third Edition*.

Before initiating the actual physical fitness tests, preliminary testing should be done regarding resting heart rate, blood pressure, and lung function. Most trainers are unfamiliar with spirometers and therefore fail to include lung function testing as part of their assessment. Consequently, trainers miss an invaluable opportunity to screen members for COPD such as emphysema so that those who perform poorly may be referred to physicians for further evaluation and diagnostic workup.

Again, when trainers do a lung function analysis, they do so not as diagnosticians but rather as suspecticians. Trainers should never diagnose a member as having high blood pressure or a lung function disability because such a diagnosis is beyond their scope of practice. Trainers only screen members for the purpose of determining their suitability for exercise, and if they suspect that there is a problem, they should refer the member to an appropriate health care professional.

Assessments

The specific tests to be administered will vary from one person to another depending upon the screening process and determination of the member's health status. Typically, tests fall within the five components of physical fitness, which are cardiorespiratory endurance, muscular strength, muscular endurance, flexibility, and body composition. Some facilities may go beyond physical fitness testing and even provide physical performance tests to those who are more athletically inclined, testing such components as agility, balance, coordination, power, quickness, and speed.

If all components of physical fitness are to be evaluated during the same session, then the organization and sequencing of the tests are important. The test order should be structured so that the resting measurement of body-fat percentage precedes the active measurements. Otherwise, the accuracy of both skinfold testing and bioelectrical impedance analysis (BIA) can be adversely affected as a result of peripheral blood flow to the skin surface and possible dehydration caused by cardiorespiratory endurance testing.

Cardiorespiratory endurance testing should precede muscular testing in order to avoid the misleading effects that muscular testing could have on heart rate response during submaximal work. The testing of muscular strength should precede that of muscular endurance because single maximal efforts are less likely to interfere with endurance activities whereas endurance testing can have a significant impact on subsequent strength testing. Flexibility can most safely and effectively be measured after the member has thoroughly warmed up, which certainly would be the case after the other tests have been completed.

Body Composition

Although body composition testing with BIA has gained in popularity, it has some significant drawbacks in comparison to skinfold testing performed by appropriately trained technicians. Of particular concern is the fact that BIA tends to overestimate body fat in lean athletes. Variations in hydration may also adversely affect body-fat predictions.

Although testing with near-infrared interactance (NII) is used by many facilities and is a simple, quick, and noninvasive method of body composition analysis, it too has significant drawbacks. The standard of error remains excessively high; therefore, this method is not considered comparable to skinfold testing, BIA, and even body-fat calculations based upon girth or circumference measurements.

Skinfold testing remains the most widely applied field technique for determining percentage of body fat. In addition to the lesser expense of calipers, skinfold testing allows the client to see exactly where decreases in total body fat are occurring. When performing skinfold testing, however, it is essential that trainers not only use acceptable technique but also match their clients with suitable protocols. Although skinfold testing is not perfectly accurate, its real value lies in the ability to effectively monitor change.

Hydrostatic weighing has been recognized as the gold standard in body-fat testing, but it poses many obstacles for the average fitness facility. Equipment cost, space requirements, maintenance requisites, time needed, and subject anxiety (holding one's breath underwater after exhalation) all make this procedure of testing expensive, awkward, and bothersome. However, a more recent body-fat testing procedure called *plethsymography,* which relies upon air displacement, has proven equally accurate and reliable as well as more convenient. It is extremely expensive and usually beyond the budget of most facilities, but with effective marketing it could become an additional source of revenue.

Cardiorespiratory Endurance

Cardiorespiratory endurance testing is usually conducted by means of step tests, ergometer tests, or treadmill tests. Additionally, many trainers have used field tests to assess cardiorespiratory fitness. When analyzing these tests, the trainer must take into consideration the various advantages and disadvantages of each test and how they relate to the capabilities and health status of the member.

Although treadmill testing is appropriate for most populations, the majority of trainers do not have access to calibrated treadmills dedicated to fitness assessment. For this reason, along with the fact that heart rate and blood pressure monitoring can be more difficult on the treadmill, many trainers prefer to do ergometer tests. In many facilities, however, due to the expense of ergometers and treadmills, limited space considerations, and greater training requirements for examiners, only step tests are administered.

Many trainers rely on the traditional 3-minute step test on a 12-inch (30-centimeter) bench. After 24 lifts per minute, a recovery heart rate is taken while the subject remains seated. The obvious concern with this test is that it exposes the member to an immediate 7.4 metabolic equivalent (MET) level, which may be overly demanding for those who are seriously deconditioned. The potential danger is that the trainer could be literally administering a maximal stress test without the safety net that is available in clinical settings.

There are safer ways to administer a step test than the traditional 3-minute test. The knowledgeable trainer may administer a progressively graded exercise test (GXT) while monitoring both heart rate and blood pressure and subsequently ensuring an appropriate cool-down. Recorded heart rates for known workloads can be applied to formulas that will predict aerobic capacity or cardiorespiratory endurance.

In order to get a handle on aerobic capacity, many trainers require members to undergo field tests such as the Cooper 12-minute test and the 1.5-mile (2.5-kilometer) test for time. Although these tests can be valid predictors of cardiorespira-tory endurance, a serious concern is the tendency for subjects to overextend themselves, thereby increasing the possibility of a cardiovascular complication. For this reason, the Rockport Fitness Walking Test has gained widespread popularity because subjects are less likely to overdo it and endanger themselves.

Muscular Strength and Endurance

Numerous muscular strength and endurance tests can be found within the fitness testing literature. Again, the tests should be chosen based upon an evaluation of the member's health status, capabilities, goals, and anticipated program design. The caveat is to recognize that due to resistance to peripheral blood flow, muscular testing can place greater demands on the cardiovascular system, especially as it relates to transient blood pressure elevation.

Muscular strength can be measured by dynamometers, tensiometers, digital strength meters, and 1-repetition maximum (1RM) tests. When using static strength tests, it is advised that the member take about a second to ease into a maximal contraction and then maintain the maximal effort for no more than a couple of seconds. Although many athletes can do actual 1RM lifts with minimal risk, it is recommended that the general public avoid such lifts. Instead, they should perform multiple lifts to failure, from which the 1RM can be predicted.

Muscular endurance can be measured using traditional resistance exercise equipment such as a bench press, leg press, and so on. Additionally, many muscular endurance tests can be completed using only body weight, as in a push-up or timed curl-up. Although static endurance tests are rarely administered, there are valid tests in which members can be evaluated for their ability to maintain a constant force against a dynamometer, tensiometer, or digital strength meter for increasing periods of time.

Flexibility

Flexibility, or range of motion (ROM), is a component of physical fitness that is normally evaluated to a limited extent. Most often trainers do little more than administer the traditional sit-and-reach test. Keeping in mind the concept of specificity of exercise, it should be remembered that this traditional test measures only low back and hamstring flexibility and is not an overall indicator of flexibility. Multiple static as well as dynamic ROM tests exist, thus enabling the trainer to acquire a more complete picture of the member's flexibility.

However, the value of flexibility assessments is being seriously questioned in light of the fact that research has documented that stretching per se has little if no impact upon injury prevention and sport performance. Flexibility remains an important component of fitness, but it may be better assessed through more functional approaches rather than traditional stretching tests.

Again, there is a vast menu of cardiorespiratory, muscular, and flexibility tests that can be administered, and the professional trainer should become familiar with this array of tests in order to provide members with the most appropriate testing medium for their needs. Numerous books on fitness testing are available, and such literature should be available within the facility's testing center. If examiners have not taken a course on how to administer fitness tests, they should be required to undergo training with local universities or vocational schools in order to learn these valuable skills and avoid some of the pitfalls that compromise testing safety.

In summary, fitness testing is essential not only for safe and effective program design but also for establishing a baseline against which future progress will be measured. This type of feedback reinforces member behavior and maintains motivation. Probably one of the greatest reasons for membership attrition is the failure of facility managers to recognize the importance of comprehensive fitness assessments as a necessary component of exercise programming. Fitness testing should not only be strongly encouraged but perhaps even required as part of the screening process.

THE BOTTOM LINE

The failure to provide and even require fitness testing during the screening process not only lessens members' chances of achieving their fitness goals, it also may increase the chances of injuries or cardiovascular complications, which may lead to litigation.

Continued Screening Through Testing Evaluation

Trainers must evaluate the data from the fitness tests along with the health appraisal and be prepared to share such information with the facility member. Typically, initial evaluation of data for each test is based upon classification scales for gender and age. However, the trainer must be careful not to get locked in to just comparing members with the normative data available. To evaluate members strictly upon this basis is to overlook the important principle of individual differences. Failing to recognize such differences violates the basic premise of understanding member needs in order to design tailor-made programs that improve the chances of success without risk of injury.

The trainer accepts the responsibility of being proficient in the science of exercise programming and therefore being knowledgeable about the appropriate stresses to be applied to the member. Suitable stress that will bring about positive physiological changes (training effects) without negative physiological consequences (injury) can most effectively be determined if the trainer has access to the information found within the health appraisal and the fitness assessment.

Sometimes, there is a tendency for trainers to impersonalize the fitness testing profile. In this age of technology, many trainers hand members a computer printout of testing results. Members are then instructed to read this printed profile in order to see how they performed in comparison to normative data. For many people, this type of approach to a fitness evaluation is a turnoff. The trainer must remember that although there are advantages in employing technology within the testing and evaluative process, the personal touch cannot be sacrificed. The competent trainer knows how to marry high tech with high touch.

When analyzing and evaluating testing data with a member, it is essential to conduct the process in a professional setting and in a motivational manner. In the privacy of an office or similar sanctum, the trainer establishes a relationship that reflects the air of confidentiality that must exist between trainer and member. The testing and evaluation room should not be cold and sterile like a doctor's office but rather warm and friendly (e.g., soft pastels versus white walls).

Members must see themselves and the trainer as working together in achieving program goals. They must not view the evaluation as a necessary embarrassment where they are chastised for a lack of health and fitness. Rather, they must view the evaluative process as one in which they have the opportunity to get a better handle on their current capabilities and future potentialities. They must see this as an educational opportunity as well as a platform from which they will be launched into a program ensuring future success. The evaluative process should be a positive and motivational experience that sets the stage for the next step: program design.

Designing Safe Exercise Programs

Although the term *exercise prescription* is frequently found within textbooks and scientific literature, it may not be the most appropriate wording when dealing with the average facility member. The term *prescription* has clinical overtones, and people associate this word with sick individuals in need of medical assistance. Because the term *exercise prescription* may discourage some members, management should instead promote the concept of **program design** within the context of the preventive setting. Additionally, avoiding the word *prescription* may make a disgruntled member less likely to pursue litigation.

Program design typically has five components: exercise mode, intensity, duration, frequency, and progression. These five components can be applied not only to aerobic training but also to muscular strength and endurance training as well as flexibility activities. The challenge for personnel is to ensure that these components of program design are based upon the information gleaned from the health appraisal and fitness assessment.

When trying to determine the best mode of aerobic activity for a given member, trainers must be careful not to interject their own personal bias. The cardinal rule in choosing an activity is whether it meets two criteria. First, is the activity appropriate for the person regarding muscular strength and endurance, metabolic requirements, and skills? Second, is the activity one that the person is likely to enjoy? Choose a physical activity that is both appropriate and enjoyable. Note that the term *physical activity* may also be better received than the word *exercise,* which is frequently associated with sweat, discomfort, and obligation.

Safe program design for new members with low fitness levels would be reflected in their involvement with continuous rather than discontinuous physical activities. Continuous activities allow for stable state heart rates whereas discontinuous activities require fluctuating heart rates as a result of varying exercise intensities. Discontinuous activities require better stabilization of joints due to rapid changes of direction and lateral movements such as those found in exercise dance, step classes, martial arts, basketball, racquetball, and so on. Because beginners may want to get involved with these types of programs, such activities then become a goal to be pursued. Once an acceptable level of cardiorespiratory and muscular conditioning is achieved, the member advances to this preferred activity.

From a safety standpoint, managers and staff must recognize that strengthening of the muscles, tendons, ligaments, and skeletal structure is necessary to undergo the rigors of most group aerobic activities. Sometimes muscular strength training is ignored in deference to aerobic conditioning, in which case the aerobic activity may have to be eventually curtailed because of inadequate joint stabilization and consequent injury. Strength training is equally important in the initial phases of conditioning and sometimes may even take priority over the aerobic training program.

When considering the initiation of aerobic conditioning, staff must appreciate the physiological concerns of bone resorption and remodeling as well as musculoskeletal weakness. Too often beginners jump into a program, doing too much too soon. There is a tendency to try to get fit overnight by engaging in an activity every day and thereby overdoing it. Although the cardiorespiratory system rapidly responds to the stress of exercise, the musculoskeletal system is slower to react. Due to initial bone resorption from new stresses upon the body, the skeletal system is temporarily weakened and thus is more susceptible to injuries such as hairline fractures. The skeletal structure needs adequate time to undergo remodeling, which will eventually enable bones to endure even greater forces. Likewise, muscles, tendons, and ligaments need gradual and progressive exposure to stress in order to avoid muscle tears, tendon strains, and ligament sprains. Consequently, it is considered advisable that beginners not engage in aerobic activity more than three times a week with at least one day of rest between each session.

Due to the standard deviation in maximal attainable heart rate (MAHR), prudent trainers do not rely on target heart rate (THR) as the sole means of determining exercise intensity. The talk test and rating of perceived exertion (RPE) must also be used to verify that members are not overstressing themselves. Members have to learn not only how to control the intensity of their physical activity but also how to determine the duration and frequency appropriate for their capacity for exercise stress. Additionally, since the instrument panels of aerobic equipment may provide feedback related to METs, it is important that staff be knowledgeable of this concept and be capable of conveying the value of such information.

As discussed, the last component of program design is exercise progression. When planning progression, the trainer must consider factors such as the member's functional capacity, age, and medical and health status, in addition to activity preferences and goals. Progression planning is normally divided into three stages: the initial, improvement, and maintenance stages. The initial stage is nonaggressive to maximize program safety and compliance and tries to minimize discomfort and muscle soreness as well as any possibility of injury. Usually the stage lasts 4 to 6 weeks depending upon member adaptation and receptiveness to escalating program demand.

Typically a more rapid rate of progression is seen during the improvement stage. Intensities will work well into the moderate and even vigorous ranges with duration as high as 30 to 40 minutes, and frequency will progress from 3 to 5 sessions per week. Again, these increases will be dictated by member adaptation and motivation. Normally the improvement stage will last for 4 to 5 months. Inevitably, there will come a time when, in order to make any further improvements, the member's efforts and time requirements will become excessively demanding. At that point, the trainer looks to the maintenance of the member's physical fitness by implementing variety within ongoing aerobic programs and other enjoyable physical pursuits to ensure adherence to the active lifestyle.

Regarding program design for strength training, the number of sets to be assigned has always been an area of confusion and controversy; however, it is generally agreed that the beginner does not need to do more than a single set of a given exercise. The ACSM has a position statement in which the recommendation for the general public is to do muscular training 2 to 3 times per week, with 8 to 10 exercises at a load allowing for 8 to 15 repetitions and only 1 set of each exercise (Feigenbaum and Pollock 1999). Granted, research has documented the additional benefits of multiple sets; however, the increased time required by multiple sets may lead to a further commitment that the members feel they cannot afford. Trainers must question whether multiple sets are to be promoted with everyone since a single set can achieve good results whereas multiple sets may discourage members who are seeking expediency in fitness programming. Another possible concern with multiple-set training is safety since it can lead to excessive overload and potential injury.

Regarding program design and flexibility training, it bears repeating that according to research, stretching per se has little if no effect on injury prevention and sport performance. Additionally, it appears that the people most susceptible to injury are those who are the least flexible as well as the most flexible. Couple this with the fact that there are many potentially unsafe postures found in programs such as yoga, it is incumbent upon management to have a staff member who is extremely well versed in kinesiology and biomechanics in order to analyze programs and ensure that contraindicated exercises are being avoided. As stated earlier, staff should consider the advantages of achieving healthy ROM through functional approaches rather than some of the contorted but traditional stretching exercises found with many group programs.

THE BOTTOM LINE

The fitness director should be an exercise physiologist with strong credentials in kinesiology and biomechanics for overseeing the soundness of all exercise programming.

Management and staff must determine that exercise programs are soundly based upon health appraisals, fitness profiles, and members' goals. Trainers must have not only thorough knowledge of anatomy, physiology, kinesiology, and exercise science but also good social skills, enabling them to communicate effectively with members and motivate them to take charge of their health. The ability to personalize program design and to ascertain member success is both a science and an art.

Providing Safety Orientation

Ideally all members should undergo fitness assessments and be provided a program design to meet their unique needs. However, some facilities may only offer this more extensive service as an additional expense. Therefore, managers assume the responsibility to ensure that all members receive a comprehensive orientation related to safety and effectiveness in exercise programming.

During the orientation, members should be advised about the concept and advantages of personal training, including fitness profiling, which will enhance the chances of success. Additionally, other program offerings and their benefits can be outlined with appropriate cautionary notes regarding fitness preparedness for some of the more demanding activities. Beginning carefully and progressing gradually must be the theme throughout the orientation.

Areas to be addressed during the orientation should include appropriate exercise clothing and footwear as they relate not only to safety but also to facility standards. A walkthrough of the facility reviewing both aerobic and resistance equipment should be available, with an emphasis on equipment operation and safety concerns. Body mechanics should be discussed regarding skeletal alignment, safe ROMs, and back protection during lifting, stooping, and exercise with more challenging equipment.

The ability to control aerobic exercise intensity must be learned by all members through both explanation and application of principles using the target zone, Karvonen formula, talk test, and RPE. Members must become acquainted with how to safely monitor and adjust their heart rate during exercise as well as how to recognize the symptoms of overexertion. A concern of vital importance is that members appreciate the dangers of inadequate warm-up and cool-down, especially the concept of **blood pooling** and how it may lead to fainting and cardiac arrest. In light of blood pooling and possible cardiac complications, members must be strongly cautioned about leaving class to take water breaks and departing class before the cool-down. Members need to be advised that staff have the responsibility to ensure that all members have an adequate warm-up, work at appropriate intensity levels, and complete their workout with an effective cool-down.

Safe and unsafe breathing patterns must be addressed to avoid such problems as hyperventilation, which may lead to fainting, as well as the Valsalva maneuver, which can cause syncope along with blood pressure irregularities and hernias. Members must be cautioned that during exercise there is to be no gum, candy, or anything else within the mouth since this could lead to an obstructed airway. This is a safety policy that the staff must enforce and the members must respect.

Members must be advised as to the difference between muscular fatigue that comes from overload during strength training versus joint pain that results from unsafe activities and unhealthy ROMs. Additionally, members should be instructed as to the signs and symptoms of heart attack and how to respond. Along this line, they also need to be instructed how to respond to specific crises such as fire, power outage, weather emergencies, bomb threats, and so on.

The orientation should conclude with the distribution of a handout that reviews the essential information that was discussed. The handout may be divided into general fitness information and then the primary safety precautions. Again, there ought to be an emphasis on beginning carefully, progressing gradually, avoiding competition, and most importantly, having fun!

Supervising Members During Exercise

Supervision refers to observing and directing activities in order to ensure their success. More specifically, it refers to the actions of management and staff required to bring about both safe and effective exercise programming. In reality, supervision must begin with the first contact with members, continue throughout their physical activities within the club setting, and end only with the termination of their membership.

The ability to relate well to members, communicate effectively, motivate sufficiently, and move to action appropriately is the hallmark of the professional staff member. This means being able to deal with all types of personalities in compelling members to achieve success. Consequently, management must seek out personnel who not only understand the science of exercise but also the art of influencing human behavior. Social skills coupled with a sincere concern for others, an appropriate knowledge base, exercise expertise, and a conscientious commitment to the job provide the essentials for a well-supervised facility.

Additionally, supervision as it relates to facility management obviously entails the commitment to having adequate numbers of qualified personnel overseeing all the physical activities within the exercise setting to ensure effectiveness of training and member safety. During personal training, this would mean constant attentiveness to a client's exercise regimen and the ability to promptly recognize ineffective or unsafe movements requiring correction. During group classes, this would require an observant instructor and assistant instructor prepared to monitor several members at once in order to rapidly intervene and remediate such concerns as an unsafe dance step pattern, exercise intensity, ROM, and so on.

General floor supervision requires at least one qualified trainer capable of answering any member questions, instructing beginners on equipment operation, providing guidance as needed, and responding to any potential emergency situations. Staff must be aware of potentially unsafe activities and alert to their impending use. Safe floor monitoring also requires that all areas are readily visible to staff personnel on duty and that there are no blind spots in which a member could become endangered without being observed.

Locations where supervision is frequently lacking include locker rooms and wet areas. All too often, members develop cardiovascular complications in the locker room, and the only people likely to be present, if any, are other members; therefore, a locker room attendant should be available at all times—an attendant who can be providing housekeeping chores while simultaneously monitoring members. It is not uncommon to witness sauna, steam, and whirlpool rooms completely unattended. There are numerous anecdotal reports of people being discovered dead in sauna and steam rooms or drowned in whirlpools. Not only should these areas be under constant surveillance, but they should also have signs warning of potential dangers, especially to high-risk members, such as those with heart disease, diabetes, and high blood pressure. In addition to limiting exposure time, there are numerous cautionary notes to be posted on signage, such as "Do not use alone," "Do not use after vigorous exercise," "Do not exercise within," "Wait an hour after eating," and "Do not use while under the influence of alcohol, anticoagulants, antihistamines, vasoconstrictors, vasodilators, stimulants, narcotics, or tranquilizers."

Finally, members should be educated that the only benefit to saunas, steam rooms, and whirlpools lies in the ability to provide relaxation. No permanent weight loss can be achieved, and any weight reduction is temporary water loss that will be replaced after eating and drinking. Besides having no real health benefit, wet areas generate unsanitary conditions and usually turn out to be a maintenance headache. They often become a financial burden and also pose one of the highest risks to safety in facility operations.

THE BOTTOM LINE

Wet areas become not only an unnecessary expense and maintenance nightmare for management but also a potential area for litigation.

As stated, supervision begins with the first contact and ends with membership termination. Therefore, faulty supervision is charged to the facility that fails to screen members for risk factors before undertaking an exercise program; fails to provide a fitness profile determining members' capacity for exercise; fails to design an exercise program befitting members' level of health and fitness; fails to educate members about safety concerns relating to exercise; and fails to supervise activities. To compound these shortcomings, faulty supervision is epitomized by the lack of a well-rehearsed

emergency plan that can be executed by qualified personnel in a timely manner.

Managing Emergencies

While in your office and working on next year's budget, a hurried and excited message comes blaring across the PA system. "Code blue, code blue, code blue. Report to the aerobics center!" As a manager, these words will get your heart racing as if you were one of the members on the exercise floor. Immediately you know what has happened—a member is down, and your emergency response system is going to be put to the test.

Regarding safety requirements and **emergency management** for fitness facilities, a comprehensive emergency response plan is of paramount importance and, therefore, a standard to which all facilities must adhere. As stated in the NSCA executive summary on professional standards and guidelines, "Strength and conditioning professionals must develop a written, venue-specific emergency response plan to deal with injuries and reasonably foreseeable untoward events within each facility" (National Strength and Conditioning Association [NSCA] 2001). Similar to this NSCA standard, both the ACSM and IHRSA share a standard that states, "A club/facility must be able to respond in a timely manner to any reasonably foreseeable emergency event that threatens the health and safety of club/facility users. Toward this end, a club/facility must have an appropriate emergency plan that can be executed by qualified personnel in a timely manner" (American College of Sports Medicine [ACSM] 1997).

Some of the typical facility emergencies to be anticipated are heat-related illnesses, physical injuries, and heart attacks. The emergency plan is designed to ensure that minor problems do not escalate to major incidents and that major incidents do not intensify to fatal events. Heat exhaustion dealt with promptly and effectively can forestall a heatstroke, a severe laceration with appropriate administration of first aid can prevent blood loss, a myocardial infarction responded to with emergency cardiac care can avert a cardiac arrest, and a sudden cardiac arrest responded to with timely and effective CPR coupled with a swift application of an AED can convert the victim to a lifesaving rhythm, leading to a full recovery with no neurological damage.

Emergencies entail not only these accidents and injuries but also crises such as fires, floods, tornadoes, earthquakes, hurricanes, severe storms, bomb threats, and even terrorist activities. Crises could also include sexual harassment, intoxicated clients, hazardous spills, thievery, unruly behavior, parking lot accidents, and other health concerns or life-threatening events. Fire evacuation plans, severe weather contingencies, and even procedures for handling and ejecting disruptive patrons are important considerations with which the staff might have to deal.

How to Develop an Emergency Plan

Where do you begin when developing such an important procedure as the emergency plan? If the facility is located in a large development such as a resort, office tower, or shopping complex, contact the building supervisor or the security department to review existing emergency plans that can be modified to meet the resources of the facility. Managers of freestanding facilities large or small should contact city offices that deal with emergencies, such as police and fire departments, advisory physicians, and legal counsel, as well as local safety consulting firms. Although this chapter presents issues to be considered during the development of an emergency plan and although you may have access to other facilities' plans, it must be emphasized that no single plan will accommodate all facilities.

All facility personnel should be involved in developing the emergency plan to ensure that it is appropriate not only for each activity area but also nonactivity areas as well. The input of staff members will both lead to a more effective plan and allow staff to thoroughly buy into a plan that they helped develop. Instruct all facility personnel that they must be well versed in the procedural deployment of the emergency plan, and remind them that their failure to act in a reasonable and prudent manner can result in a serious injury, unnecessary death, and potential litigation.

Emergency plans must be detailed, but not overly complicated. The plan should be logical and written in concise terms that are easily understood by staff as well as members. Modify emergency procedures to fit both the type of emergency and the location of the emergency. For example, the response to a life-threatening medical emergency will differ from that for a fire evacuation. A medical emergency on the fitness floor should be handled differently than one in the swimming pool or child care center.

Emergency plans need not be memorized in their entirety. However, every staff member should memorize the code or phone number that sets the plan in motion. Beyond that, post specific emer-

gency plans next to every telephone in each area of the club for quick reference. The staff member in charge of risk management should carefully review the completed emergency plan with local fire and police departments as well as EMS and maintain contact with these city resources during planning of training sessions and practice drills so that these departments and resources are made aware of specific facility needs.

Components of the Emergency Plan

A well-conceived and comprehensive plan must be written, and all personnel involved should sign off on the fact that they have read it and that they understand and agree to comply with all actions outlined. This plan should include the posting of emergency procedures that highlight the sequence of events to be followed and list emergency agencies and their phone numbers. These sheets can be posted at convenient and strategic locations throughout the facility, thereby permitting periodic review by staff. Knowledge of agencies and numbers is worthless, however, if phones are not readily available and rapidly operable. Whether a large multiplex or a small facility, the requirements of an emergency action plan remain the same.

Emergency plans must guarantee the fastest available access to on-site first responders, EMS, and advanced care facilities. To this end, a good plan outlines specific roles for staff members such as who should recognize an untoward event, activate EMS (phoning 9-1-1), alert staff to the incident, attend to the victim, secure first aid equipment, assist the principal caregiver, verify EMS personnel are en route, take charge of crowd control, guide EMS to the scene and, most importantly, take responsibility for the coordination of the overall effort. Other duties to be assigned are for staff to notify the victim's family, secure the victim's clothing and valuables, record the incident, write up the after-action report, and follow through with remedial actions for any duties that were not handled expeditiously and correctly.

From the initial recognition of the emergency to the final report, there are numerous steps that must be followed to maximize the health and safety of the membership. Each step needs to be analyzed with regard to the uniqueness of the facility, qualifications of staff, type of membership profile, and physical and financial resources available. For example, in alerting staff to a potential cardiac arrest such as with the earlier scenario of a code blue, would it be most advantageous to announce to the entire membership that an emergency was in progress? Perhaps not; it might be wiser to have a code word that would alert staff only in order to avoid curious onlookers who would only create more confusion (see Tales From the Trenches at the beginning of the chapter). On the other hand, would the facility want to enlist the help of members possessing medical skills?

The following list of plan components assists in developing or refining an emergency plan that meets the unique needs of a given facility. It is recommended that these components be listed on a 2-page emergency sheet. The front page simply outlines the vital procedures a first responder should initiate and follow, and the detailed information and directions are located on the back page for quick reference by the manager on duty or assisting staff members.

- *Activation code.* Activating the emergency plan is the most essential component. Once a potential emergency has been identified, select a method to discretely notify staff and management. This can be accomplished by announcing a code over a PA system, sending a code over a group paging system, or setting a prearranged sequence of telephone calls in motion. Direct staff members to immediately proceed to the location of the incident.

- *Telephone numbers.* Make sure several telephone numbers are readily accessible. Although most cities in the United States use the 9-1-1 emergency system, some cities may not have this service or the plan may direct staff to call an in-house emergency department that then activates EMS. Keep numbers for emergency assistance, poison control, the general manager, and other management personnel posted by every telephone. Because telephones are known to break down, there should be a backup communication system, such as cellular phones or radios.

- *Location of nearest telephone.* If there is not a telephone in an activity area, specify the exact location of the nearest phone and how to get there.

- *Location identification and accessibility.* Post a plan with detailed instructions regarding the location of the emergency in reference to other club areas, such as the main entrance. The printed location on the emergency plan should direct EMS personnel to the closest building entry. In many larger facilities, you can contact an internal department such as security or an operator. These internal departments have the responsibility to call 9-1-1,

meet EMS as they enter the property, and direct them to the emergency site.

- *Locked doors or gates.* If the possibility exists that a door or gate will prevent the prompt entry of EMS, note the location of the door or gate and the location of the key.

- *Location of emergency supplies.* Provide the location of the nearest first aid kit, emergency oxygen, AED, first responder bloodborne pathogen kit, and bloodborne cleanup kit.

- *Information to share.* When calling for assistance, be prepared to relay who you are, where you are (post the club address on the emergency plan), the number you are calling from, the type of emergency, what has happened, how many people need assistance, their gender and approximate ages, and what is currently being done to assist them, and then ask for estimated time of arrival of emergency support. Direct staff members to stay calm and to stay on the line until emergency assistance tells you to hang up.

- *Directions for personnel responsibilities.* The plan should designate the first responder to direct the incident until a manager arrives and can assume responsibility. The first responder should stay with the injured party, leaving only to activate the emergency plan or call for assistance. The first responder or manager should then delegate a staff member to call 9-1-1 or another predetermined resource and to provide the information as listed in the previous directions for information to share. The manager should delegate additional staff members to assist with the rescue, assume responsibilities for crowd control, retrieve any health information that may be on file, meet and direct EMS to the scene, and record the names of people who are present and may have witnessed the incident.

- *Call for member assistance.* Many medical emergency plans include a call for any medically trained members (i.e., doctors, nurses, or paramedics who may be in the facility) to proceed to the location of the incident for assistance.

- *Incident and accident reports.* Immediately following the removal of the victim by emergency personnel, the manager on duty should direct the staff to go to a quiet place and to write down everything they can remember about the incident and the care provided, including timelines, names of witnesses, care administered, and any outstanding concerns. During this time, the manager on duty should complete an incident or accident report; a sample form appears on page 275.

Incident and Accident Report

Date of incident/accident: _____ Time of incident: _____ a.m./p.m.

Injured member/guest: _____ Age: _____

Membership number: _____

Address: _____

_____

Telephone (Home): _____ (Work) _____

Location of incident: _____

_____

Describe in full how incident occurred and what actions were taken by staff. (Write everything you can remember no matter how insignificant it may seem.)

_____

_____

_____

Describe the injury in detail and indicate the body part(s) affected:

_____

Did any medically trained members (doctors, nurses) assist?

_____

Staff members present: _____

Witnesses: _____

_____

Was the emergency plan activated? _____ Was EMS called? _____

Was the individual taken to the hospital _____ Yes _____ No

If yes, what hospital? _____

If no, did he/she refuse medical attention? _____

Was the family notified? _____ Who? _____

On the back of this page, please document any observations or comments regarding this incident you feel important.

Signed by: _____ Date: _____ Time: _____

MOD/dept. head: _____ Date: _____

Follow-up notes:

Contact made by: _____ Date: _____

Condition of member: _____

From M. Bates, 2008, *Health Fitness Management*, 2nd ed. (Champaign, IL: Human Kinetics).

> A backup communications system should be available at all times in case phone lines go down.

Equipment

The proper handling of untoward events will often require special emergency equipment, so a first aid kit or multiple kits, depending upon the size of the facility, must be available. It is crucial that kits be properly marked, identifiable, accessible, and easily transportable as well as stocked according to foreseeable events and the skills of responders. Kits must be checked at least once a month to verify that contents match the enclosed recommended list of supplies. Equipment and supplies must be used according to manufacturer's instructions and recognized professional guidelines, and when using these materials, it is imperative that precautions for preventing disease transmission be followed as outlined by the Centers for Disease Control (CDC) and OSHA.

Safety supplies are essential to effectively respond to an emergency. Well-stocked first aid kits provide the necessary items and materials in the event of a minor cut or more serious injury. First responder kits provide the staff with all the OSHA requirements as well as suggested protective barriers necessary to respond to a medical emergency in which there is the potential for contamination. Biohazard cleanup kits conveniently package all the personal protective devices and necessary cleanup supplies to reduce the risk of secondary contamination following an accident in which possible infectious conditions exist.

For suspected **myocardial infarction (MI)** or **sudden cardiac arrest (SCA),** trainers may use a crash bag that contains latex gloves, goggles, resuscitation mask, blood pressure unit, and, most importantly, an AED. Accompanying the crash bag would be an emergency oxygen canister that can be attached to a nonrebreather mask for MI and resuscitation mask for SCA.

Additionally, flashlights and sharps containers should be kept in all first aid kits as well as designated areas throughout the club. Flashlights can assist during a medical emergency in which vision may be difficult as well as during power outages. OSHA requires **sharps containers** for the proper disposal of any sharp items that may potentially cause a biohazard risk. Sharps containers prevent the accidental incision or puncture of a staff member by securing sharp items in a solid waste container. OSHA requires proper disposal of full sharps containers or any biohazard waste.

Additional equipment suggestions include the following:

- Designate a cell phone to use in the event of an emergency. This phone allows the manager to make phone calls while moving throughout the club.
- Consider having all trainers carry a resuscitation mask with inflatable cushion in a soft pack on their belts to ensure the immediate availability of a barrier device.

Training Staff

Facility trainers should be certified in both first aid and CPR, including the use of an AED. Additionally, it is recommended that trainers be capable of providing emergency oxygen. Although precautionary measures, these are essential safety considerations, and a staff that lack these credentials and skills reflect professional irresponsibility. Informal surveys show that although trainers are typically certified in CPR, most do not have certification in first aid. Of those with CPR, most are certified in only adult CPR without training in AEDs. Few facilities have emergency oxygen available. It would appear that the commitment of the average fitness facility to the safety of its members is sadly lacking.

There are obvious reasons why facility staff should be capable of providing first aid. From minor cuts to major lacerations, simple contusions to severe concussions, heat cramps to heatstroke, mild hypoglycemia to insulin shock, staff members ought to be able to respond to these emergencies. Notwithstanding the importance of such emergencies, it would seem appropriate to address the most serious concern likely to confront management—a cardiovascular complication such as a severe MI or SCA. The crucial question for the general manager is whether the facility staff are prepared to make the difference between life and death.

Maintaining adequate health and safety certifications among staff members is a crucial responsibility of the manager. Ideally, all facility staff, including maintenance personnel, should be required to have CPR certification as a prerequisite for employment. Trainers should have the more advanced certification with AED. Staff supervising child care facilities should have pediatric CPR as well as adult CPR certification. Although this requirement poses a challenge for facilities that experience high turnover rates, setting a requirement that all personnel be CPR certified places staff on notice that emergency response is a high priority. Certifying long-term staff members or managers as CPR instructors is an easy way to offer continuing education classes not only for facility personnel but for members as well.

Although not all facility personnel need to have first aid certification, there should be a sufficient number of trainers certified to ensure that at least two are on duty at all times. Ideally, the facility would always have on duty one certified first responder who has undergone the requisite 60 hours of training. As with CPR, certifying long-term staff and supervisors as first aid instructors enables in-house continuing education for staff and members alike. If emergency oxygen is going to be available, then a sufficient number of trainers need to be certified so that appropriate administration will always be available.

Managers must educate new and existing staff about their personal responsibilities in the event of an emergency. This training, which should be a priority of the supervising manager, begins with employee orientation and never ceases. The training must encompass all types of emergencies including medical, fire, aquatic, and disaster. Emergencies can occur in any location within the facility—a group exercise class, the aerobics room, the weight training area, the swimming pool, a racquetball court, a locker room, a restaurant, the child care center, and so on. Therefore, training must consist of not only reviewing written documents but also conducting hands-on drills in which staff members respond to a variety of emergency scenarios in different settings.

Practicing the Plan

Emergency and crisis plans must be practiced and rehearsed with regularity. Ideally, mock emergencies should be conducted at least quarterly if not more often, and some of these rehearsals should be unannounced. Responsible critiques and remedial actions of such rehearsals will only improve the plan. The emergency response plan, including rehearsals, should be evaluated by facility risk managers, legal advisers, and medical providers to ensure that timely and effective procedures are being followed as well as modified when needed. It is recommended that facilities enlist a medical liaison to keep the emergency plan updated and to periodically evaluate the skills and ability of all personnel, including independent contractors such as personal trainers.

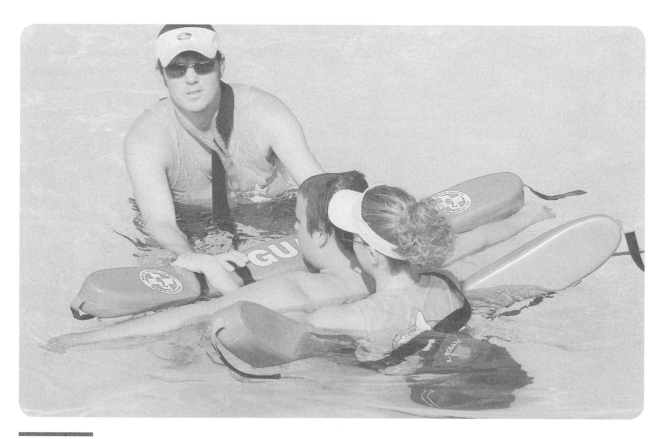

Rehearsals of the club's emergency and crisis plans must be conducted regularly.

Rehearsals allow for the practical implementation of what has been reviewed and studied within the comprehensive emergency plan. The number of rehearsals will depend upon the size of the facility, the number of staff and their level of training, the number and variety of exercise environments, the types of potential emergencies, and the emergency equipment available. Nevertheless, rehearsals become almost meaningless unless management ensures that all personnel participate in drills multiple times throughout the year. Training aids such as first aid materials, emergency oxygen, resuscitation masks, and mannequins need to be available to heighten realism.

Qualified emergency professionals must be appointed to monitor all rehearsals with an eye on corrections. A critical review of rehearsals needs to be conducted as soon as possible in the form of an after-action report. Recommendations are made as to how staff may improve their overall emergency response, their individual actions, and their timing. Afterward, documentation of remedial action should be verified and filed along with the after-action report.

THE BOTTOM LINE

Every drill or rehearsal should be monitored by appropriately trained emergency personnel who can submit an after-action report to management.

However, just practicing the emergency response system is not enough to ensure a successful outcome in real life. The system can only be fine-tuned when inappropriate actions are observed, noted to management, and then corrected through remediation. After each drill, therefore, debriefings should be conducted to address shortcomings, and discussions should be initiated as to how best to correct these deficiencies. Involve building management, maintenance personnel, and local city resources (fire, police, EMS) in all emergency drills. These trained professionals may offer additional information or ideas that will better prepare the staff for future responses. Evaluating an emergency response plays an important role in the ongoing training of staff and should never be overlooked.

Medical Emergency Plan for Cardiovascular Complications

Medical complications due to exercise are a reality, and of greatest concern are cardiovascular complications. It has been well documented that the occurrence of coronary incidents increases with vigorous exercise in comparison to everyday, spontaneous occurrences. For those free of coronary artery disease, the relative risk of exercise is extremely low, but this risk is dramatically increased for those with the disease. Unfortunately, occult coronary artery disease is prevalent among older, sedentary people, many of whom are now availing themselves of fitness facility services. In fact, it is estimated that the largest segment of the population currently joining fitness facilities is the over-50 age group.

Use of Oxygen

As previously indicated, cardiovascular complications within the fitness facility typically take the form of an MI or SCA. In either case, facility staff must respond with emergency cardiac care. Such care requires appropriate training and equipment. When a mild to moderate MI is suspected (e.g., tightness of the chest, radiating pain), EMS activation by calling 9-1-1 is essential. In addition to making the member as comfortable and calm as possible, the trainer should immediately administer emergency oxygen.

Emergency oxygen is vital because low oxygen levels to the heart are likely to lead to cardiac arrest where blood circulation ceases. In addition to activation of EMS, supplemental oxygen is probably the most important step that can be taken in treating the suspected MI. In addition, any victim of a potentially life-threatening illness or injury should receive emergency medical oxygen (American Red Cross 1993). It has been estimated that oxygen administration may double a person's chances of survival. Management need not worry whether oxygen may be harmful during a medical emergency; the administration of oxygen will only enhance the likelihood of a positive outcome. All emergency medical literature reflects that the immediate use of supplemental oxygen is crucial for victims of sudden, life-threatening illness or injury.

Although it is true that oxygen is a drug when given in concentrations beyond that found in the air we breathe, such as when used for medical treatment, the U.S. Food and Drug Administration (FDA), the regulating agency for medical gases, has exempted the prescriptive requirement for emergency oxygen. In order to qualify as nonprescriptive emergency oxygen, the delivery system must provide a minimum flow rate of 6 liters per minute for a minimum of 15 minutes. As stated by the FDA, anyone properly trained in oxygen administration can provide this emergency drug. Not only should staff rescuers be familiar with the instructional materials and directions of an oxygen delivery system, they also should undergo formal training. Such training is available by a number of organizations such as the American Red Cross and can be accomplished in just a few hours. When trainers fail to provide emergency oxygen, it could mean missing an invaluable opportunity to save a life.

Oxygen administration is also important with SCA when CPR is required. By attaching the oxygen delivery system to a resuscitation mask, the rescuer can provide the victim with an oxygen concentration well above that of normal air. This procedure will buy the victim more time while awaiting lifesaving defibrillation or drug administration.

Use of Automated External Defibrillator

When SCA occurs within the fitness facility, the prognosis is poor unless an AED is available. In the United States, SCA strikes between 350,000 and 450,000 people each year outside of the hospital environment, and more than 95% die. Rapid defibrillation is the only definitive treatment. Due to the unavoidable response time of EMS personnel, defibrillation by paramedics is usually too late to provide successful resuscitation. Once blood stops circulating, as with ventricular fibrillation or pulseless ventricular tachycardia, every minute without defibrillation decreases the chances of survival by approximately 10%. The only solution to this dilemma is to have an AED on the premises that can be immediately applied to the victim.

AEDs have been effectively used for over 10 years and are credited with saving thousands of lives. As a result of their proven success, the U.S. Congress passed the Cardiac Arrest Survival Act in 2000, legislation that directed the Department of Health and Human Services to develop guidelines for placing AEDs in federal buildings nationwide. This bill also established a Good Samaritan provision that protects people from liability in those states that had not already enacted such laws regarding AEDs (Abbott 2000). Presently, all states have a Good Samaritan law protecting lay rescuers.

With the publication of a 2002 joint position statement, the ACSM and the AHA urged health and fitness clubs to implement AED programs. The ACSM and AHA recommended that AEDs be part of an emergency response plan within all facilities that have memberships of 2,500 or more, have special programs for the elderly, serve members with known medical conditions, or are in locations where EMS response time (recognition of the cardiac arrest until delivery of the first shock) is likely to exceed 5 minutes (AHA 2002).

It should be noted that the third edition of *ACSM's Health/Fitness Facility Standards and Guidelines* (2007) has published 21 standards, of which the seventh states, "Facilities must have as part of their written emergency response system a public access defibrillation (PAD) program." In chapter 4 ("Risk Management and Emergency Policies"), two full pages are devoted to this standard, which include steps for implementing a PAD program, such as, "A facility must have at least one employee on duty at all times who is currently trained and certified in BCLS (basic cardiac life support) and administration of an AED."

In addition to all states having enacted a Good Samaritan law, several states and the District of Columbia have also passed legislation requiring that fitness facilities have emergency plans that include AED deployment. In states that have yet to mandate AED programs within facilities, many municipalities have legislated this type of emergency preparedness.

AEDs are safe, simple, reliable, and relatively inexpensive. Considering that the cost of an AED is comparable to that of a piece of gym equipment ($2,000), it is inexcusable that not all facilities have them as part of their emergency response equipment. With the availability of AED instruction through the AHA, American Red Cross, National Safety Council, and equipment manufacturers, the cost of training is also reasonable. Likewise, emergency oxygen systems can be picked up for a few hundred dollars, and, as with AEDs, the training is neither overly time consuming nor expensive. Emergency oxygen coupled with an AED provides a winning combination that will greatly improve the chances of survival during a cardiovascular complication.

Some lawyers will argue that the use of AEDs and oxygen may increase the exposure of fitness facilities to litigation by holding to a higher standard of care. There is little merit to this argument, especially considering the 2002 joint position statement by the AHA and ACSM. Regarding liability, *Best's Review*, a leading insurance industry publication, stated in the August 2002 issue, "The need for defibrillators outweighs potential liability." Additionally, the article indicated that a failure to provide an emergency response with an AED to an SCA becomes a liability concern. The only important question to ask is, "Will the availability of oxygen and AEDs save lives?" The answer to this question is a resounding "Yes!"

When it comes to delivering emergency cardiac care, we should look to professional organizations that specialize in this field, primarily the AHA. As far back as 1997, the AHA's *Basic Life Support Manual for Healthcare Providers* stated that "because of the intrinsic simplicity of AEDs, a markedly expanded range of persons can now be trained to provide early defibrillation, including . . . supervisory personnel at exercise facilities" (AHA 1997). The AHA's newest guidelines reflect an even stronger commitment to public access defibrillation through the use of AEDs, which have been hailed as the most exciting breakthrough in CPR since the advent of mouth-to-mouth rescue breathing. It is the goal of the AHA that victims of SCA be defibrillated within 5 minutes of onset. For this reason, the AHA recommends that AEDs be placed in locations where there is a reasonable probability of one SCA occurring every 5 years. Certainly fitness facilities fall within this category.

THE BOTTOM LINE

In order to provide the gift of life as well as health to facility members, staff must be able to respond with the ready availability of AEDs and oxygen. This emergency equipment is essential if we are to give the victims of MI and SCA a fighting chance.

Plans for Other Emergencies

Although medical emergencies are more likely to occur and threaten the safety of members, there exist a number of other potential emergencies that management must take into consideration. An out-of-control facility fire could become disastrous and lead to multiple injuries and deaths, as could unheeded weather warnings. Natural disasters catch facilities unaware and can wreak death and destruction, and the threat of terrorism poses potential harm to all kinds of buildings and structures. A poorly supervised aquatics area could result in an unnecessary drowning; likewise, a poorly supervised child care area could result in a physical injury or a choking death. Thus, the management team must plan for a variety of potential emergencies.

Fire and Evacuation Plan

During any emergency situation, the health and safety of members and guests are the highest priority. The ability to calmly and systematically notify members of an emergency that requires immediate evacuation of the building is extremely important.

Management must establish a fire and evacuation plan that specifies procedures to effectively and efficiently clear the building. As with the medical emergency plan, obtain assistance in preparing this procedure by contacting on-site security personnel, building managers, or local departments such as fire and police. Review and practice your completed fire and evacuation plan in cooperation with these local emergency services.

Aquatic Emergencies

A medical emergency in aquatic facilities requires special considerations. Trained and certified water safety instructors or lifeguards typically handle aquatic emergencies until emergency personnel arrive. In addition to emergency plan procedures, specific aquatic guidelines include the following:

- If the victim is unconscious, suspect a neck injury.

- In the case of a possible neck injury, do not remove the victim from the water. Ensure all vital signs are stable. Stabilize the victim's head and body and await the arrival of emergency personnel. Use only the tools and techniques in which you are thoroughly trained and well practiced.

- In the case of possible drowning, remove the victim from the pool. Turn victim on the side to allow water to drain. Check vital signs and begin rescue breathing or CPR as necessary.

- If using an AED, make sure that the victim's chest is dry and that the victim is not in a puddle of water.

Emergencies Involving Children

The child care center in every facility should emphasize safety as a part of its daily operations. Even carefully supervised children will have accidents. Establish and practice safety procedures in the child care area. The following are some guidelines to ensure a safe play environment:

- Obtain the medical history of all children.

- Obtain a signed parental directive and emergency medical authorization form. (Seek advice of legal counsel in preparing this form.)

- Set rules requiring the parent or guardian to remain on property at all times.

- Create a safe play environment by covering all electrical outlets, removing or padding

Aquatic emergency equipment and guidelines are required at all public pools. Check with local and state regulatory agencies for a complete listing of required aquatic safety and emergency equipment as well as guidelines for use. Examples of emergency equipment and safety guidelines include the following:

AED	First responder kits
Backboard	Resuscitation mask
First aid kit	Life rings and buoys
Megaphone	Safety and pool rules signs
Cervical collar	Clear depth markers on pool sides
Shepherd's crook	Pool gates secured and locked when pool is closed
Emergency oxygen	

all sharp corners, installing padded carpet to protect against falls, and purchasing only child-safe toys and equipment.

- Ensure that no items small enough to constitute a choking hazard are within children's reach.
- Maintain strict rules to ensure direct staff supervision at all times.
- Make sure a first aid kit is available.
- Ensure personnel are first aid and CPR certified.
- Practice emergency procedures monthly.
- If an AED is available, make sure it has pediatric pads.
- Conduct weekly safety inspections of indoor and outdoor play areas.

Disaster Plan

Disasters can come in many forms: earthquakes, hurricanes, tornadoes, fires, floods, tsunamis, and terrorist acts. All disasters endanger lives, create a costly disruption, and may cause financial ruin for the facility. As with many medical emergencies, these problems are difficult or impossible to prevent. However, being prepared may ensure the safety of members, control the extent of damage, and minimize potential liability. Management can lessen the impact of a disaster by establishing sound emergency and evacuation procedures that are practiced, by securing complete insurance coverage that is reevaluated annually, by developing a solid risk-management program, and by maintaining strong communication channels with members, local business associates, and reciprocal clubs.

Weather Emergencies

Weather emergencies often strike with minimal warning. The geographic region where the facility is located will assist in determining the types of weather that may pose a threat. Preparation of emergency procedures when facing a tornado, hurricane, or flood will minimize liability and control damage. Points to consider when preparing a weather plan include the following:

- Weather advisory television channels, radio stations, or telephone numbers
- An outdoor activity (playgrounds, pools, athletic fields) evacuation plan
- A communication plan and script to follow
- A predetermined evacuation zone or shelter and procedures to transport members to this area
- Definitions of commonly used watch and warning systems in the community
- Specific actions to be taken by members depending on the type of threatening weather

Bomb Threat

Although most bomb threats turn out to be false alarms, they should nevertheless be taken seriously. Specific procedures and questions for gathering information from the caller should be readily available to all staff taking incoming calls. Prompt but calming evacuation procedures must be instituted with the intent of getting members as far away as possible from the building. Have the receptionist recall and record the content of the threatening message for law enforcement personnel.

Non-Life-Threatening Emergencies

Nuisance emergencies, such as power outages or accidental activation of the fire sprinkler system, can create havoc in a facility. The facility manager or chief engineer should train staff how to respond quickly and effectively when faced with such emergencies.

Power Outage   Power outages occur frequently in many locales. However, for those facilities in which an electrical disruption is not routine, this loss of power can frighten members and cause panic if the staff do not respond in a confident manner. Ensuring members' safety is the highest priority while handling this type of emergency. The following points may be helpful in creating a power-outage response plan:

- Ensure that no one has been hurt as a result of the sudden stoppage of equipment.

- Confidently communicate that someone is looking into the problem.

- Confidently request that all members remain where they are until emergency generator lighting or flashlights are available to assist them in moving around the club.

- The director of maintenance or chief engineer should clearly label all breaker boxes in the electrical room so that trained personnel can locate a breaker that has switched off, resulting in an isolated power outage.

- In the event of a complete power outage, ask members and staff to wait patiently for a few minutes to see if power is restored. If it is not restored quickly, ensure emergency lighting is working in all areas and assist members in exiting the building.

- Once power is restored, check the calibration on all exercise equipment, reset time clocks and cash registers, reboot computers, and so on.

Accidental Activation of Sprinkler System   Accidental activation of the fire sprinkler system can result in severe water damage to the facility. Flooding of a facility can ruin expensive wood flooring, such as a group exercise floor or racquetball court, as well as electrical equipment. Additionally, failure to have a rapid and thorough water extraction after such an incident can lead to mold and mildew, which can cause health concerns and in turn can lead to costly indoor environmental restoration or bacterial-growth remediation. To prevent the accidental activation of the fire sprinkler system, incorporate the

following suggestions into a regular maintenance checklist:

- Ensure all sprinkler heads are recessed or protected. Most accidental activations occur when an exposed sprinkler head is knocked off or bumped loose. This can be prevented by ensuring that if heads are not recessed, then the exposed structure is covered by a cage.

- The maintenance director should train enough key personnel so that someone is always on duty who knows exactly how to shut down the system.

Risk Management Documentation

Documentation is an important component of risk management. Maintaining complete records, including medical histories, lifestyle questionnaires, informed consents (testing as well as programming), fitness profiles, physician releases, assumptions of risk, parental consents, maintenance checklists, after-action reports, remedial action reports, equipment checklists, restocking dates, and safety surveys, is invaluable in the event of an accident or litigation. Some of these forms have been presented throughout this text; others may be found within referenced literature. General Manager's Safety Overview and Checklist on page 283 provides a basic checklist that can be modified to incorporate the unique issues of a facility. It is recommended that any forms be reviewed by legal counsel and a medical director.

Maintenance Records and Safety Checklists

Regular maintenance inspections are important in preventing accidents and incidents. Maintenance inspections of flooring, exercise equipment, wet areas, mechanical equipment, and facility grounds will assist in identifying potential accident sites and injury situations. More extensive information is presented in following chapters regarding proper selection, installation, and maintenance of exercise equipment. It is recommended that management prepare an equipment history card along with a maintenance checklist for each piece of equipment within the facility. The following chapter includes a sample form as well as general facility and mechanical information with appropriate checklists. Proper

General Manager's Safety Overview and Checklist

Task	Initials
Membership director:	
1. All new members complete health history questionnaire. Forms forwarded to fitness director for review.	_____
2. PAR-Q and guest registration completed on all guests.	_____
3. All reviewed health history and related forms filed properly.	_____
Fitness director:	
1. All health history questionnaires reviewed by FD. Medical clearance forms requested where necessary.	_____
2. Equipment maintenance review and checklist complete.	_____
3. Maintenance requests written as necessary.	_____
4. CPR/AED and first aid certifications current on all fitness staff.	_____
5. Emergency plan posted by all phones.	_____
6. Monthly emergency plan practice session complete.	_____
7. Aquatic emergency supplies in proper location.	_____
Maintenance director/chief engineer:	
1. Mechanical system review and checklist complete.	_____
2. Fire warning system tested monthly.	_____
3. First aid and first responder kits fully stocked.	_____
4. AEDs and emergency oxygen fully charged.	_____
5. Monthly test of emergency public address system complete.	_____
6. Weekly safety review and checklist of grounds complete.	_____
7. All sprinkler heads protected (recessed or cages).	_____
Child care director:	
1. CPR certifications current on all child care staff.	_____
2. Outdoor equipment safety review and checklist complete.	_____
3. Parental consent forms current.	_____
4. Monthly emergency evacuation practice complete.	_____
To be reviewed at weekly department head meetings.	

From M. Bates, 2008, *Health Fitness Management*, 2nd ed. (Champaign, IL: Human Kinetics).

maintenance of all club equipment and facilities provides a safer environment for the member. Proper documentation of regular maintenance practices provides the facility with a means of defense in the event of legal action.

Manager's Safety Checklist

Health and safety concerns within a facility can demand an excessive amount of time if they are not managed properly. Therefore, managers must insist upon the awareness and action of all departmental supervisors and staff in this effort to offer a safe environment. Appointing specific people who can be held accountable for known health and safety concerns will assist in this important task. A weekly review of completed and incomplete tasks as well as issues demanding proactive measures will enable the busiest general manager to be aware of existing and potential health and safety concerns within the facility. A reference checklist for review by the general manager can simplify this task.

KEY TERMS

accreditation

assumption of risk

blood pooling

bloodborne pathogens

certification

clinical stress test

emergency management

emergency response plan

fitness profile

guest screening

health risk appraisal

informed consent

lifestyle questionnaire

litigation

medical clearance

medical history questionnaire

medical management model

myocardial infarction (MI)

Physical Activity Readiness Questionnaire (PAR-Q)

preactivity screening

program design

risk stratification

safety plan

sharps containers

signage

standard of care

sudden cardiac arrest (SCA)

REFERENCES AND RECOMMENDED READINGS

Abbott, A. 1989. Exercise science knowledge base of commercial fitness instructors in the State of Florida. Research study presented at the ACSM annual conference, 1990.

———. 2000. Code blue—member down. *Personal Fitness Professional Magazine*, November 2000.

Alter, J. 1983. *Surviving exercise*. Boston: Houghton Mifflin.

American College of Sports Medicine (ACSM). 1997. *ACSM's health/fitness facility standards and guidelines*. 2nd ed. Champaign, IL: Human Kinetics.

———. 2000. *ACSM's guidelines for exercise testing and prescription*. 6th ed. Philadelphia: Lippincott Williams & Wilkins.

———. 2005. *ACSM's guidelines for exercise testing and prescription*. 7th ed. Philadelphia: Lippincott Williams & Wilkins.

———. 2007. *ACSM's health/fitness facility standards and guidelines*. 3rd ed. Champaign, IL: Human Kinetics.

American Heart Association (AHA). 1997. *Basic life support for healthcare providers*. Dallas: AHA.

———. 1998. *Recommendations for cardiovascular screening, staffing and emergency policies at health/fitness facilities*. Dallas: AHA.

———. 2002. Automated external defibrillators in health/fitness facilities, AHA/ACSM scientific statement. *Circulation* 105:1147-1150.

American Red Cross. 1993. *Oxygen administration*. St. Louis: Mosby Lifeline.

Arria, S. National Board of Fitness Examiners (NBFE). Santa Barbara, CA.

Baechle, T., and R. Earle, eds. 2000. *Essentials of strength training and conditioning*. 2nd ed. Champaign, IL: Human Kinetics.

Best's Review Magazine/Journal, August 2002, A.M. Best Company, Inc., Oldwick, NJ.

Black, H. 1991. *Black's Law Dictionary*. 6th ed. St. Paul: West.

Cotten, D., and M. Cotten. 1997. *Legal aspects of waivers in sport, recreation and fitness activities.* Canton, OH: PRC.

Cotten, D., et al. 2001. *Law for recreation and sport managers.* 2nd ed. Dubuque, IA: Kendall/Hunt.

Davis, K.A. 1985. *Sport management in the private sector.* Unpublished manuscript, Rice University, Houston.

Feigenbaum, M., and M. Pollock. 1999. Prescription of resistance training for health and disease. *ACSM's Medicine and Science in Sports and Exercise* 31(1):38-45.

International Health, Racquet, and Sportsclub Association (IHRSA). 1998. *Standards facilitation guide.* 2nd ed. Boston: IHRSA.

Malek, M., et al. 2002. Importance of health science education for personal fitness trainers. *NSCA Journal of Strength and Conditioning Research* 16(1):19-24.

McInnis, K., et al. 2001. Low compliance with national standards for cardiovascular emergency preparedness at health clubs. *Chest* 120:283-288.

National Strength and Conditioning Association (NSCA). 2001. Strength and conditioning professional standards and guidelines, executive summary. Supplement to *Strength and Conditioning Journal,* November 2001.

Rabinoff, M.A. 1984. *Fitness club evaluations.* Unpublished manuscript, Metropolitan State College, Denver.

Sharkey, B. 1984. *Physiology of exercise.* Champaign, IL: Human Kinetics.

[fourteen]

Maintaining Your Facility

Mike Greenwood and Anthony Abbott

LEARNING OBJECTIVES

After studying this chapter, the reader will be able to

- understand the four areas of maintenance management,
- undertake a needs assessment,
- identify goals and objectives for a facility maintenance program,
- know when to use in-house personnel and when to use outside contractors,
- understand the importance of monitoring inventory levels and controlling inventory costs, and
- evaluate a maintenance program.

Tales From the Trenches

Over the years Beth became accustomed to regular repair bills within her fitness facility. She considered it part of the cost of doing business. When something broke down she would call a local repair person and have it fixed. Although she did not like the high fees this person charged, she did not have time to think about any other alternatives. She had much bigger projects to handle, like increasing membership numbers and dealing with two new competitors in the area.

One day, a longtime member asked if he could speak with Beth. He had recently noticed that some of the cables on the strength training equipment were becoming frayed. Beth thanked Juan and said she would have someone look at it right away. She called in her usual maintenance person and told him about the situation, and 3 days later the problem was taken care of. A couple weeks went by and another member knocked on Beth's office door and mentioned that the tiles in the bathroom were getting mildew stains on them. Once again, Beth said she would get someone on it, but this time she wondered to herself how she would find out about these things if the members did not let her know, and what other problems might exist that the members might not be letting her know about.

She had recently read an article about the silent customers who just stop using a business because they are unhappy with something but never let that business know about their unhappiness. She did not want this to happen at her business. It was also obvious that she was putting herself and her business in a litigious situation by not checking the equipment regularly. Her members could easily injure themselves due to a lack of preventive maintenance and regular facility checks.

Beth called a meeting of her department heads the next day. The department heads understood her concerns, and as a group, they came up with a list of areas and pieces of equipment that needed to be checked regularly. Once this list was complete, they came up with a separate list of things that needed to be checked for cleanliness or maintenance improvements. With these lists in hand, Beth delegated the tasks of checking specific areas to the most relevant department heads and gave them specific expectations with respect to how often each area should be checked and how the check should be recorded and reported.

During the initial period of implementation, many concerns were reported and many problems were addressed. Although this was a stressful period initially, the regular checks eventually led to fewer problems and less money being spent on quick fixes. Beth regularly talked with her department heads to make sure the checklists were being followed and stressed the importance of preventive and ongoing maintenance to her staff. In the long run, these actions led to a much more efficient fitness center.

Establishing a maintenance program for a health and fitness organization is a vital but extremely challenging task. Realizing the positive impact that a safe, clean, well-maintained facility has on prospective members and current member renewals; taking the necessary time to identify maintenance needs; developing and implementing a plan; and regularly evaluating the plan are essential not only for the success of an organization but in some circumstances its survival. In today's competitive market, operators must place a high priority on such areas as client safety, housekeeping, preventive maintenance, general maintenance, equipment repairs, and renovation improvements.

This chapter addresses the organizational steps involved in creating a facility maintenance program for the corporate, clinical, community, and commercial health and fitness sectors. We discuss a four-step strategic plan that incorporates a needs assessment, program planning, implementation, and evaluation. The chapter also discusses the various labor options available in different fitness settings, and it concludes with how to organize and initiate a preventive maintenance program. The intent of the chapter is to present a guide for fitness professionals to follow in organizing and implementing a well-designed maintenance management program.

The importance of keeping a safe, clean, and well-maintained facility cannot be emphasized enough. Today's consumer is more aware of the areas to examine and evaluate when choosing a facility. Checklists established as guidelines for rating health and fitness settings now classify facility convenience as number one, followed by maintenance and equipment upkeep, qualified staff, program variety, and organizational management. In short, in the eyes of a prospective member, having a clean facility ranks second in value when considering the purchase of a health and fitness membership.

Maintaining a safe, clean, well-kept facility is equally important to existing members. The results of annual member surveys have shown that facility cleanliness ranks at the top in the areas members like most about a facility.

The proper maintenance of a health and fitness facility is easy to define and evaluate. However, achieving an acceptable, consistent level of maintenance is difficult. Generally, if everything is working properly and cleanliness is up to par, members are happy, and a facility manager should feel a sense of pride and accomplishment. Unfortunately, the dynamics of the health and fitness industry do not always provide this luxury, and it does not occur without a concerted effort.

THE BOTTOM LINE

Often facility managers become jugglers, weighing the options of maintenance, repair, and replacement costs against profit, budget, and staffing priorities.

We can define facility maintenance management as the set of work-ordered activities that, when properly managed, allow for continued operation of a facility. These activities include decisions, work orders, and actions taken by maintenance employees. The coordinated effort among management, employees, and other members of the maintenance team can make or break a facility.

Four Areas of Maintenance Management

When discussing maintenance management, there are four areas managers should focus on to ensure successful facility operation:

1. *Safety.* All equipment in the facility must always be in top working order. Club operators cannot afford to take risks when their members' safety is involved. Fitness facility professionals should strictly observe and evaluate areas of potential liability (i.e., wet areas, weight rooms, swimming pools, day care, restaurants). **Preven-**

tive maintenance is the preferred method for enhancing member safety. Waiting until after an accident occurs to address a problem is not only too late and too expensive but also unethical. Furthermore, manufacturer's manuals for equipment should be catalogued and made available in an equipment or maintenance library for easy access to all staff members. This process allows staff to become familiar with operating procedures for all equipment, information viewed on instrument panels, and any specific safety concerns. Instructor staff should be required to become familiar with equipment manuals and sign a form indicating that they have read, understood, and will comply with specific manufacturers' operating instructions.

2. *Quality.* The difference between quality facilities and lesser facilities is noticeable. Consider all features of the facility from the ground up—floor surface; carpet; mirrors; **heating, ventilation, and air-conditioning (HVAC)** equipment; wall surfaces; lighting; and so on. Facilities must not only look good, they must also be durable enough to withstand the test of time. The old adage, "You get what you pay for," is true where facility quality is concerned.

3. *Cleanliness.* The daily maintenance of a club must be thorough and consistent. A facility maintenance program should take into account such things as after-hours cleaning, locker-room maintenance, prime-time cleaning, special events, parties, and outdoor maintenance. Each area has unique needs for workers, maintenance regimens, and supplies. The goal of any maintenance program should be to transform qualitative care into quantitative care; in other words, be specific about the desired maintenance needs and communicate those needs to the proper staff members.

4. *Amenities.* The extras involved in serving members' needs are considered amenities. These items include such things as towels, swimsuit plastic bags, hangers in lockers, and personal toiletries (e.g., shampoo, conditioner, shaving cream, deodorant, body lotion, hair spray). Understanding your members' needs will determine the level of amenities and the most cost-effective way to provide them. Members' perception of quality is often dictated by the details. A smart operator never downplays the importance of the little things. Often these differences provide the subtle touches necessary to separate an organization from its competition.

Continual review of these four areas ensures that you always maintain a level of excellence.

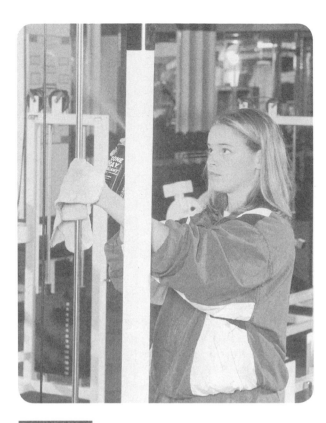

Daily maintenance should include the routine cleaning of equipment in order to provide a safe and sanitary workout environment for club members.

Determining Maintenance Needs

Establishing and refining an organized facility maintenance program should be a goal of every manager. Because few fitness facilities have a similar design, the scope of maintenance needs varies. The facility requirements for a full-service, multirecreational fitness facility differ significantly from those of a corporate club in an office building. Facilities encompassing 10,000 square feet (929 square meters) do not have the same maintenance needs as facilities of 75,000 square feet (6,968 square meters). For example, operators of large multipurpose facilities allocate approximately 7% of their total expenses for maintenance and repairs, whereas smaller facilities budget half of that amount. Larger facilities generally have both indoor and outdoor maintenance considerations, whereas smaller facilities have predominately indoor needs. Due to the increased size, larger facilities use both contract and in-house employees, whereas smaller facilities incorporate primarily in-house personnel.

Although there are many differences related to such size variances, you can apply the same process for determining the required maintenance in any setting, whether it be commercial, corporate, community, or clinical.

Developing a maintenance management program must start with a **strategic plan.** Everyone agrees that a maintenance program is necessary, but to what degree will you implement the program? How much money will it cost? Will you use additional personnel or **contract labor?** Should maintenance be performed after hours or only during the workday? These are questions that you must address during the early stages of organizing a maintenance program. Consider insurance risks, workforce, payroll, supplies, and facility scheduling. A sound strategic plan provides the direction to follow once you have established the profile of the organization.

Fried (2005), Ray (2000), and Patton, Grantham, Gerson, and Gettman (1989) have reinforced that an effective strategic management plan is a four-step, iterative process that involves

1. assessing needs and interests,
2. planning the program,
3. implementing the program, and
4. evaluating the program to ensure that goals are being met.

The cycling or **iterative process** is what makes this plan so effective. For example, as you implement and evaluate a maintenance program in the third and fourth stages, you collect information on how to improve for future planning. This cycling allows you to use information obtained from an initial program to design a new and improved model of maintenance. The manager then continues through the four stages of the follow-up program. The four-stage management process is illustrated in figure 14.1.

Performing a Needs Assessment

The first stage in developing a facility maintenance program is to perform a **needs assessment** to evaluate the facility. You need a clear understanding of the size and scope of the organization in order to adequately assess maintenance needs. Greenwood and Greenwood (2000) recommend developing a professional multidisciplinary team whose members represent relevant areas of expertise to assist in strategizing and implementing viable questions and answers to identify specific facility assessment needs. This team could include the following

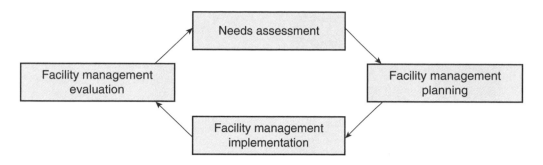

Figure 14.1 Four-stage management process.

experts: fitness facility administrator, architect and contractor with credible fitness facility experience, legal consultant, staff members, and select club members who represent various client populations (i.e., age groups, genders, fitness levels).

Obviously, the needs assessment should revolve around program goals and objectives for the populations that are served as well as the future direction of the industry. Following are practical examples of pertinent questions that can be included in a facility needs analysis, which should be derived from qualified professionals representing the multidisciplinary team.

Perform a comprehensive facility evaluation that obtains answers to the following questions:

- What is the overall size of the facility and grounds?
  - Determine the size of the facility by measuring each room and activity area in order to obtain total square footage or by referring to construction plans.
  - If outdoor maintenance is required, establish the acreage or square footage of the grounds and determine the specific uses for the area.
  - Note whether the facility is enclosed in one building or separated into multiple complexes.
- What are the hours of operation?
  - List the number of days per week the facility is open and the operating hours.
  - How is holiday scheduling handled?
  - Identify the best times of the day to perform maintenance.
  - What times of day do you consider prime or peak membership usage times?
- What is the operating budget for maintenance?

- The setting (i.e., corporate, commercial, clinical, or community) generally dictates the availability of funds.
  - If performing in-house maintenance, consider payroll, payroll taxes, supplies, and capital costs (equipment).
  - If contracting an outside service, obtain bids and determine a monthly charge for the service.
  - Weigh the costs of including a mix of contract labor and in-house personnel.
- How many members are you serving daily?
  - What is the average number of members who use the facility daily?
  - Which days of the week are the busiest?
  - Are weekends a slower time for usage than weekdays or vice versa?
- What is the availability of staff?
  - Are in-house staff available to perform maintenance needs?
  - How will you divide the daytime and evening maintenance shifts?
  - Can maintenance tasks coincide with other job responsibilities?
  - Is contracting for outside services a possibility, and if so, how will maintenance responsibilities be divided?
- What are the mechanical aspects of the facility? Become familiar with the following areas:
  - Pools—mechanical areas (e.g., filters, heaters, pumps, chlorinators)
  - Spas—mechanical areas (e.g., filters, heaters, pumps, chlorinators)
  - HVAC systems
  - Boilers—steam rooms

- Water control systems and shutoff valves
- Electrical panel placement, as well as grounded electrical outlets
- Lighting systems throughout the facility
- Security and energy management systems
- Emergency sprinkler systems
- Provisions for people with disabilities

Whether using in-house personnel or contracting with an outside cleaning service, the next step in the needs assessment is to establish itemized cleaning and maintenance specifications for each room and activity area. Outline a detailed description of the nightly, daily, and weekly tasks for the complex. Give additional consideration to special-use areas that require specific maintenance and cleaning treatments. For example, the various cabinet finishes and floor surfaces in a locker room, such as carpet, tile, and marble, all have certain requirements for proper cleaning. Address each area before contract labor or in-house employees begin a regular maintenance schedule. Supervisor Work Assignment on page 293 provides a sample cleaning task and checklist.

After compiling a cleaning task list, if you are considering in-house maintenance, develop a list of supplies, vendors, and equipment (e.g., carpet cleaners, pool vacuum systems, automatic scrubbers). This step allows operators to become familiar with the various types of chemicals available, how they should be applied, and their corresponding interactions with other chemicals. Managers will also be introduced to working with vendors and the supply and cost side of the business.

After completing the needs assessment, perform data analysis to define where the organization is currently and where it wants to be in the future. The answers you obtain from the needs assessment provide a road map to follow while implementing the program. The analysis provides answers to such questions as the following: Is the facility large enough to justify the cost of contracting for maintenance services or should in-house personnel be used? Does the number of members served daily support both a daytime and evening housekeeping crew? Does the number of mechanical and electrical systems validate the need for a full-time operations manager? Is the operating budget large enough to support the maintenance needs of the organization?

During the needs assessment, managers must keep in mind that every facility is unique. Factors such as the existing facility layout, equipment placement, wall partitions and barriers, types of furniture and fixtures, and local and state regulatory statutes are some areas to consider when establishing a maintenance program. These factors play an important role in determining which direction to follow when assessing the various cleaning and maintenance options available.

Planning the Facility Maintenance Program

Maintenance planning uses the information derived from the needs assessment and applies that data toward the management plan. Understanding the scope of cleaning and maintenance requirements for the facility plan allows management the opportunity to choose a format best suited for the club. Without incorporating the needs assessment, it is difficult to establish goals and objectives for the maintenance division. Maintenance goals vary considerably depending on the intended use of the facility. See Maintenance Goals and Objectives on page 294.

The goal statement defines the direction for the maintenance effort and should indicate the intensity of effort required. For example, if a goal states that the locker rooms are to consistently meet the maintenance standards established by management, then this should be emphasized to the people responsible for cleaning that area. For goals to be effective, they must be enforced with specific objectives. These objectives should address the various components of the entire maintenance program.

Components of daily maintenance include activities that maintain and restore the function of the facility. This category is divided into the following categories: housekeeping, general maintenance, preventive maintenance, repair, replacement, improvement, and utilities. Place each maintenance task in one of these categories. Although the names of these categories are likely to vary from setting to setting, the basic elements are present in every facility maintenance program.

Housekeeping

Housekeeping comprises the daily tasks—basic cleaning, emptying trash receptacles, replacing towels and toilet paper, sweeping, mopping, and dusting—that make the facility presentable and functional. Facility staff members can be trained to perform basic daily cleaning tasks, and select **contract maintenance** companies can be employed

Supervisor Work Assignment

General duties: Supervisors are responsible for seeing that all shift personnel are in proper uniform and that the uniforms are clean and worn neatly. Also, supervisors will review daily the accuracy and integrity of staff time cards.

Position	Duties	Freq/time
Laundry	1. All equipment is clean and operating properly.	[ ] Hourly
	2. Load each washer to no more than 3/4 full.	[ ] Hourly
	3. Load each dryer to bottom of dryer window.	[ ] Hourly
	4. Towels are folded and stacked with round ends together.	[ ] Hourly
	5. Room is clean and neat.	[ ] Hourly
	6. Lint traps are cleaned.	[ ] Hourly
	7. Washers and dryers are never left unattended during operation.	[ ] Every 2 hours
Locker rooms	1. Shelves are stacked with clean towels.	[ ] Hourly
	2. Soiled towels are in bins for return to the laundry.	[ ] Every 1/2 hr
	3. Vanity toiletries have been stocked; sink tops, bowls, and drains have been cleaned.	[ ] Every 1/2 hr
	4. Soap/shampoo dispensers have been cleaned and filled and are working.	[ ] Hourly
	5. All mirrors have been cleaned; lightbulbs are working.	[ ] Every 2 hours
	6. Large and small wastebaskets are not filled more than 2/3 full.	[ ] Hourly
	7. Carpets have been swept or vacuumed.	[ ] As needed.
	8. Saunas and whirlpools have clean towels, papers, cups, etc. Check for proper temperature.	[ ] Hourly
	9. All hair dryers are clean and working.	[ ] Hourly
Housekeeping	1. Large and small wastebaskets in lounge and bar have been emptied.	[ ] Hourly
	2. Vacuum club manager's and accountant's offices; trash has been emptied.	[ ] Before 9 a.m.
	3. Exterior property is free of all trash.	[ ] Before 9 a.m. and 4 p.m.
	4. Public bathrooms are clean and neat; supplies have been filled.	[ ] Hourly
	5. Fourth floor locker rooms are maintained (cf. steps 1-6 in L/R).	[ ] Hourly
	6. All vinyl floor surfaces are spot cleaned as needed.	[ ] Hourly
	7. Lounge area is free of paper, cups; carpet is spot cleaned as needed.	[ ] Hourly
	8. Stairways and walls are spot cleaned as needed.	[ ] Hourly
	9. Nursery trash has been emptied and toilet cleaned.	[ ] Before end of shift

From M. Bates, 2008, *Health Fitness Management*, 2nd ed. (Champaign, IL: Human Kinetics).

(based on financial availability) to handle more extensive maintenance responsibilities before or after hours of operation. It is critical for facility administrators to evaluate the credibility of the contract maintenance companies they wish to employ. A sample objective for a common housekeeping function is as follows:

Ensure that all locker-room facilities are cleaned at least once every 20 minutes. Fitness equipment should be cleaned and sanitized at least 4 to 5 times within operating hours and thoroughly maintained after operating hours in order to prepare for the demands of the next business day.

General Maintenance

General maintenance might also be referred to as *infrequent housekeeping*. It often requires trained personnel to use specialized equipment. Typical general maintenance activities include steam-cleaning carpets, painting walls, stripping and sealing wood floors, cleaning and waxing tile floors, changing filters on HVAC equipment, and sweeping parking lots. General maintenance improves and preserves the appearance of a facility and is performed at regular intervals based on seasonal considerations

and aesthetic preferences. An objective for general maintenance is the following:

Promptly respond to and repair any discrepancies or deficiencies in facility operations.

Preventive Maintenance

Preventive maintenance comprises a major portion of the maintenance effort in a health and fitness facility. These tasks are intended to ensure the continuous operation of all areas within the facility, with primary emphasis placed on safety awareness, operational functionality, and the interdependent implementation of each factor. Preventive maintenance programs are performed at regular intervals, usually by skilled employees.

THE BOTTOM LINE

The difference between preventive maintenance and general maintenance is that the preventive maintenance tasks are established by the manufacturer's recommendations and should be followed to maintain the life of the equipment, whereas general maintenance improves and preserves the facility.

When preventive maintenance is neglected, dramatic, costly, and potentially dangerous failures often occur. For this reason, a formal preventive maintenance program should be a high priority. A preventive maintenance objective is the following:

Establish a program of routine inspection and service of exercise equipment to prevent premature failures. Always have a backup plan to avoid unnecessary breakdowns and repair delays.

Repairs

Repair work involves restoring to operation some component or piece of equipment after it has failed. Unfortunately, failures do not occur at convenient times and must be dealt with immediately, usually at the expense of other scheduled maintenance. In establishing objectives for repairs, it is often necessary to set priorities based on the importance of need for repair. These priorities set the maximum time required to complete repairs. As problems occur, they are classified by priority and workload. Repairs that are not immediately required (low priority) are often reclassified for future scheduling. Staff members should place professionally created "out of order" signs on equipment down for repair. Ideally, if equipment is going to be inoperative for a few days, it should be taken off the floor for safety compliance and effective repair.

Excessive downtimes of equipment and facility operations can be avoided with an ounce of prevention strategy. Planning and thinking ahead of challenges via the previously mentioned needs analysis can solve many problems before they occur.

One method that has proven effective is setting aside two budgets, one for simple repairs and another for extensive repairs. This budgeting technique can prove vital since monetary concerns are often a major cause for untimely repairs. Further, it is imperative to consider the quality and functionality of equipment and facilities regarding viable manufacturer warranty and service options to help control and minimize repair challenges. This approach can also help avoid displeased members who can become easily frustrated with defective planning and repair issues associated with maintaining a fitness facility. A typical objective for repair work is the following:

Complete 90% of all repair work within a designated time (i.e., within 1-3 weeks of notification, depending on the nature of the repair). There is no substitute for quality facil-

ity products and the warranty and service options associated with your equipment.

Replacement

As an element of facility management, replacement is confined to a program of planned replacement of facility components. It may include such things as air-conditioning compressors, furnaces or water heaters, or steam-room generators. Replacement is performed when the equipment has reached the end of its useful life—when it can no longer perform due to internal damage or its repair is no longer cost effective.

Although replacing a piece of equipment is generally inevitable, it is not without a variety of options. Accordingly, a replacement program should be based on the costs of the equipment, installation, and maintenance. Considering these factors, maintenance managers have an opportunity to analyze the impact of using a different model that is perhaps more expensive initially but requires less repair or energy to operate and is not replaced as often. The replacement objective for a facility is the following:

Establish a program of planned replacement that replaces failing equipment with new or rebuilt components.

It is always beneficial to stock common replacement parts (i.e., cables, pulleys, belts) to avoid long and frustrating out-of-order delays. Extensive repair delays that are easily correctable and not alleviated in a reasonable time frame can lead to unhappy customers and ultimately a reduction in memberships. You don't want to lose clients in such a competitive and challenging industry for factors that can be easily controlled.

Improvements

Improvement projects enhance the operation of a facility and can possibly reduce the operating costs. These projects may include installing an energy management system to conserve electricity, upgrading an existing pool filter system to improve water clarity, or providing security cameras for members' safety. When the budget allows, many professionals recommend enhancing the aesthetic quality of a facility by incorporating techniques such as improved lighting, windows with greater scenic views, and mirrors strategically placed for appearance and training functionality, as well as remodeling lobbies for positive initial impressions.

Many fitness facilities have also enhanced their programs by providing professional personal training assistance, fitness evaluations and prescriptions, child care areas, nutritional snack bars, nutritional counseling centers and weight management programs, specialized aerobic and core stabilization training rooms, and club exercise apparel in an effort to upgrade their facilities as well as provide better service to their members. Administrators may also emphasize landscaping improvements when relevant to enhance the aesthetic qualities of their facility. Each improvement has a positive impact on the overall efficiency of a facility complex if effectively implemented and maintained.

The age of the facility and the equipment already in place dictates other maintenance projects, but improvement projects are often initiated by the operations manager or general manager. Although the initial cost of an improvement project may appear high, the long-term results should always reflect a cost savings to the facility or an increased perceived value to members. An improvement objective is the following:

> After conducting a complete needs analysis and determining viable project feasibility, identify and conduct any improvement project that will pay back the initial investment in 3 years or less.

Utilities

The maintenance areas previously discussed generally require on-site labor. However, complex and extensive utility work often calls for skilled laborers from utility companies or independent electrical or plumbing contractors. Utilities work includes electrical power, water, gas, collection and disposal of sewage and other wastes, and disposal of storm water. It is highly recommended to periodically assess as many of these utility categories as possible to avoid serious facility damage and personal injuries as well as implementing current upgrades to improve the safety, maintenance schedule, and function of the facility.

Municipal utility companies usually provide utilities for health and fitness settings smaller than 34,000 square feet (3,159 square meters). In this instance, the involvement of a maintenance manager is minimal. For most small to midsize facilities, utility responsibilities are limited to verifying monthly bills and calling the utility company when service is interrupted or repairs are required.

However, in settings larger than 85,000 square feet (7,897 square meters), the involvement of a

full-time operations manager is a necessity. Some facilities have full electrical generating equipment, boilers for heat distribution, and even a small sewage treatment plant. Such systems become minifacilities within themselves, requiring attention around the clock. These systems are a large investment and contribute substantially to the operating cost of a facility. A key objective for utility maintenance is as follows:

> Regularly maintain and immediately respond to any and all utility problems in order to avoid serious consequences and to improve the safety, maintenance schedule, and function of the facility.

Value of Reputable Certifications for Staff

Maintaining a safe, clean, and well-kept facility is vital for success in the fitness industry, but it is only one piece of the puzzle. One relevant area that is often overlooked is hiring staff members who are certified by reputable professional organizations. Depending upon the certification earned, this process can have many positive benefits regarding the overall professional knowledge base of qualified staff members. Most certified fitness professionals should have the appropriate background to assist members in improving their quality of life through properly designed fitness training protocols. However, as discussed in chapter 13, it must be remembered that "certified" does not always mean "qualified"!

Many members lack the knowledge needed to derive maximum benefits from their exercise program, which creates a need for qualified fitness professionals who can design and implement safe and effective training programs for all segments of the population. Because people of all ages and abilities use physical activity to enhance and prolong their quality of life, these groups have special needs that require modified or customized workouts to maximize benefits. This suggests that owners and or administrators of health and fitness facilities should hire certified professionals who are capable of providing adequate instruction. These fitness professionals should possess the knowledge to work with many types of clients with special needs and should also understand which clients require medical clearance before any training begins.

Another benefit of hiring certified fitness professionals is the training they often have regarding facility and equipment maintenance. Specifically, according to Greenwood (2000, 2004), people who attain professional fitness certifications are often required to learn about the following areas:

- Facility layout and scheduling
- Facility design
- Equipment layout (organization, spacing, and placement)
- Staff-to-client ratios
- Maintaining, repairing, and cleaning facility equipment

Consider Staffing Alternatives

A principal function of maintenance planning is to list the primary categories of facility management and match those categories to the proper setting. In some cases, the operating manager is responsible for all facets of the facility; in others, responsibility is shared with outside vendors or contract personnel.

For example, in a corporate fitness setting, the housekeeping and repair work could be the responsibility of the landlord of the building or the corporation. In a commercial setting, the operations manager may be in charge of all the subdivisions. Despite the setting, define each maintenance category and identify responsibilities before evaluating staff options or establishing job descriptions.

Out of the needs assessment and program planning phase emerges a maintenance organization of a particular size and scope necessary to meet the goals and objectives of the facility. In 2006, IHRSA conducted an industrial survey regarding the reported range and size categories of commercial fitness facilities. For the purpose of describing the relationship between management and the maintenance organization, the following information was compiled from the survey:

- Average multipurpose facility = 96,530 square feet (8,968 square meters)
- Average large facility = 140,000 square feet (13,006 square meters)
- Average small facility = 9,611 square feet (893 square meters)
- Average of all clubs = 57,355 square feet (5,328 square meters)

Note that select professional organizations such as the ACSM recommend that facility size be determined on the following select membership considerations (Tharrett, McInnis, and Peterson 2007):

- Fitness facilities = 12 square feet (1.1 square meters) per member
- Multipurpose facilities = 27 square feet (2.5 square meters) per member

Of course, these recommended facility sizes should be based on aspects such as specific target audiences, program design options, and governing business models. Due to these flexible considerations and diverse facility structures, there is latitude in the effort to safely and effectively meet the needs of all parties involved in this process.

Large Facilities

Large health and fitness centers often have several divisions and use full-time maintenance personnel. The operations director or facility manager is generally a skilled person with a mechanical background and previous experience in facility management. The facility manager answers directly to the manager of the club and has a support staff available for both daytime and evening maintenance. This manager's overall responsibility is to coordinate the direct effort of the maintenance division. Internal personnel, often referred to as *locker-room attendants,* handle daytime housekeeping responsibilities. Primary duties of a locker-room attendant include maintaining a clean and sanitized locker room, providing general facility maintenance, and performing laundry tasks. Either a contract maintenance service or an in-house staff with a supervisor conducts evening housekeeping. In some cases, independent contract services are hired on retainer to maintain HVAC, boiler, or pool systems.

Maintenance personnel in a large setting generally have regular duties and have the workforce to perform preventive maintenance. As a result, they can prevent or quickly repair many mechanical problems. This benefit is not always available to midsize and small clubs, which may end up spending most of their days putting out fires. A sample organizational chart for a large fitness organization is shown in figure 14.2.

Midsize Facilities

Although in a midsize setting the maintenance needs are reduced, the basic elements of control and execution that apply to a large facility also exist. Overall maintenance responsibilities usually belong to a maintenance supervisor who has knowledge of various mechanical systems. The maintenance supervisor is sometimes assisted by either a part-time or full-time employee who performs minor repairs and equipment upkeep.

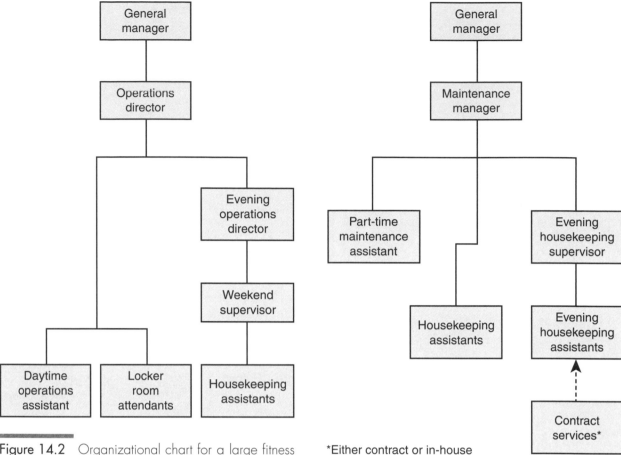

Figure 14.2 Organizational chart for a large fitness facility.

Because housekeeping is a major portion of the work, locker-room attendants or service-desk personnel are regularly scheduled to complete assigned tasks around the high-usage areas of the facility. Evening housekeeping is performed by either a contract maintenance service or an in-house crew with a supervisor. Service contractors are brought in to perform major repairs, such as plumbing, HVAC, and electrical work.

Operations in a midsize maintenance organization are less structured than those of a large organization. More time is spent on emergency responses and repairing minor equipment problems than modifying and improving the facility. Communication is a primary consideration for midsize maintenance. Consequently, key members of the maintenance staff usually carry walkie-talkies or pagers to alert staff of problems in a timely fashion. Figure 14.3 illustrates the maintenance structure of a midsize facility.

Small Facilities

In small organizations, generally only one or two people are involved in maintenance. The mainte-

*Either contract or in-house

Figure 14.3 Organizational chart for a midsize fitness facility.

nance worker, a jack-of-all-trades, works directly for the general manager and is responsible for all maintenance duties. Housekeeping is handled internally with all levels of personnel involved in the daytime cleaning. In the evening, housekeeping duties are performed by staff before closing or designated employees assigned to complete more rigorous cleaning tasks. A small facility uses contract services more than a midsize facility. In small facilities, the major system components (plumbing, HVAC, electrical) are repaired almost exclusively by service contractors. A sample organizational chart for a small club is shown in figure 14.4.

The three classes of maintenance management (large, midsize, and small) can be adapted to fit most facility needs. The reasons for choosing to conduct maintenance internally are plentiful—better control, scheduling flexibility, ability to define specific duties, and quick response to emergency maintenance tasks. However, if conditions are not favorable for hiring an internal staff, consider contracting for maintenance services.

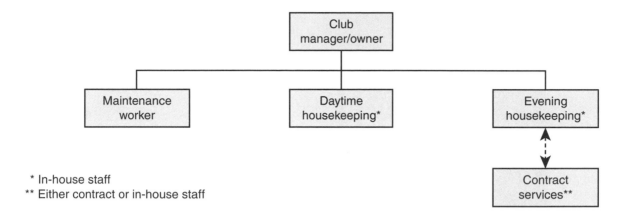

```
                    ┌──────────────────┐
                    │      Club        │
                    │  manager/owner   │
                    └────────┬─────────┘
        ┌────────────────────┼────────────────────┐
 ┌──────┴──────┐      ┌───────┴──────┐      ┌───────┴──────┐
 │ Maintenance │      │   Daytime    │      │   Evening    │
 │   worker    │      │ housekeeping*│      │ housekeeping*│
 └─────────────┘      └──────────────┘      └──────┬───────┘
                                                   ↕
                                            ┌──────┴───────┐
                                            │   Contract   │
                                            │  services**  │
                                            └──────────────┘
```

* In-house staff
** Either contract or in-house staff

Figure 14.4 Organizational chart for a small fitness facility.

Contracting for Maintenance Services

In the commercial health and fitness industry, contract maintenance usually refers to such services as evening housekeeping, general repair and preventive maintenance of equipment (both exercise and mechanical), lawn care, computer maintenance, and pool maintenance. Although these services are used as needed, rarely does a facility manager contract all maintenance work to an outside service. Consequently, it is not uncommon to have a mix of in-house and contracted services. Analyzing the needs assessment and the cost comparisons of all the options suggests the best direction to follow. There are, however, several factors that may allow an independent contractor to provide services at a lower cost than in-house employees:

- Specialization allows higher productivity.
- Expensive servicing and diagnostic equipment can be purchased.
- Spare-parts inventory can ensure quicker repair time.
- Employee benefits can be varied with greater flexibility.

Make the choice between hiring in-house employees and contracting for services based on several factors:

- *Frequency of need.* Certain maintenance actions are necessary only infrequently or seasonally. For example, the routine inspection and preventive maintenance for HVAC systems requires a skilled technician, yet few facilities have the number of HVAC systems to justify a full-time worker. You may reduce or control maintenance costs by identifying these infrequent maintenance activities and considering the cost of contracted services.

- *Inadequate in-house personnel.* Depending on the complexity of the mechanical equipment, having qualified personnel may be essential. The sophistication of some systems may require the contract services of specialists. State and local regulations may require a particular level of qualification and licensing for certain work. If in-house personnel do not possess or cannot obtain such certifications, you should contract for these services.

- *Workload and staff balancing.* A dilemma occurs when some maintenance work can be performed by in-house personnel, but there is only enough work to justify part-time employment. It may be possible to combine several of these tasks to justify the employment of a single maintenance person. Creating a full-time job by combining tasks provides the desired flexibility and responsiveness for emergency maintenance needs. However, you should cover overflow work by a contract service or through authorized overtime rather than adding a potentially underused employee to the payroll.

- *Other cost considerations.* Adding a maintenance employee to the payroll requires assuming the cost of providing benefits to an additional employee. These benefits commonly include health insurance, workers' compensation insurance, retirement plans, bonuses, paid vacations, and several other benefits. Even if there is justification to use in-house maintenance personnel, the added cost of providing full benefits may be too expensive. In the unskilled trades (housekeeping, security, child care), the cost of contracted services is often less than the total cost of wages and benefits combined.

In a corporate fitness setting, maintenance is generally contracted through a service provided by either the building landlord or the corporation. Because the facility is housed on company grounds, this maintenance arrangement is usually the only option available. Unfortunately, this method does not always ensure a well-maintained and clean atmosphere. The maintenance standards for a fitness facility are much higher than for an office building. Regular facility usage by clients throughout the day necessitates continual housekeeping and maintenance repair. Periodic cleaning by a building maintenance crew is both impractical and inefficient. Consider identifying the areas that need emphasis and renegotiating with the company for additional maintenance services.

The maintenance arrangement for a clinical setting is similar to that for a corporate facility. If the facility is on the hospital campus, the wellness or fitness center usually contracts with the hospital maintenance staff for housekeeping and general repair. Because the cleaning standards and consistent housekeeping requirements for a hospital are much higher, this system has proven to be more effective than in the corporate setting. Facilities that are off the hospital campus have the option of entering into a contractual arrangement with an outside service or hiring personnel for maintenance and housekeeping needs.

Community fitness facilities have the same options available as commercial settings. They may choose to enter a contractual arrangement with an outside cleaning service, hire their own maintenance and housekeeping personnel, or use a combination of both options. Some community settings can contract cleaning services already being used by the city to perform evening cleaning duties. During the day most community centers use a limited maintenance staff and in-house personnel to accomplish all maintenance and housekeeping needs.

If given the option, managers should have on-site, qualified maintenance staff available. There is great security in knowing that a quick response is available for any maintenance problem. However, smaller facilities might find that financial limitations dictate that fitness staff or front-desk attendants may have to assist with maintenance responsibilities. Although not preferred, if supervised and scheduled properly, this approach can accomplish the necessary housekeeping goals. This option should always be weighed against the possible negative effect on customer service and the maintenance standards established for the facility.

Implementing a Maintenance Program

Select professionals have reported that implementing any program involves five steps (Fried 2005; Patton, Corry, Gettman, and Graf 1986; Ray 2000):

1. Reviewing the planned objectives for the program
2. Reviewing the planned tasks for the staff
3. Delegating the tasks to the staff
4. Scheduling the tasks for action
5. Supervising the program implementation to ensure tasks are accomplished

This model assumes that the needs assessment has been analyzed, goals and objectives identified, and staff or contract labor hired and that the maintenance plan is ready to be implemented.

In addition to these steps, an integral part of implementing a maintenance program is to identify functions that facilitate the maintenance work. These functions assist in identifying and coordinating the daily tasks and ensure that the proper level of maintenance is being sustained. Such functions include

- work identification;
- scheduling;
- purchasing, supplies, and inventory control;
- cost controls;
- equipment and mechanical histories; and
- work tracking and monitoring.

These functions are inclusive and may not be present in every health and fitness setting. Depending on size and scope, some managers may choose to implement only a few of the functions, whereas others may fully integrate all the functions mentioned. Despite the setting, we recommend that management personnel be familiar with and understand how to implement each function if deemed necessary.

Work Identification

All maintenance work has a point of origin. Preventive maintenance, for example, is scheduled in advance to prevent equipment breakdown or to meet seasonal needs, such as switching from heat to air-conditioning. Housekeeping is a regularly scheduled activity. However, general maintenance and repair work are not scheduled until someone notices a problem and reports it to the maintenance staff. In the case of preventive maintenance and the daily rounds of equipment checks, the staff should log any problems they notice. Implement a formal reporting system to identify needed repairs. In addition to using maintenance personnel, club operators depend on staff and member input for obtaining work orders. Many facilities have found that adopting a work-order request form successfully allows staff and members to report maintenance or equipment problems. Request for Maintenance Services below is a sample work-order request form and is discussed in detail later in this chapter.

Scheduling

Because maintenance involves both planned (preventive maintenance and housekeeping) and unplanned (repairs) elements, the manager must be able to schedule maintenance accordingly. Typically, it is necessary to provide scheduled staff for the planned jobs while maintaining flexibility for unforeseen problems. Develop fixed schedules to cover such areas as preventive maintenance and housekeeping, and identify tasks with a corre-

sponding time goal for completion. Anticipate time intervals for the unexpected repair work as well. Developing historical data for the time it takes to perform various tasks is the only way to prepare a realistic schedule. Depending on the size of the facility, some managers incorporate daily time logs to track work completion. Figure 14.5 provides a sample maintenance schedule.

Purchasing, Supplies, and Inventory Control

As routine maintenance work is carried out, there is a constant need for materials and supplies to sustain the work being performed. This necessitates a system for predicting needs and purchasing and inventorying materials and supplies. Routine preventive maintenance requires a predictable type and quantity of materials. Being unpredictable, repairs may cause interruptions to facility operations if parts are not readily available.

A **purchase order system** is commonly used for ordering supplies and materials. The purpose of a purchase order system is to account for all maintenance items ordered and received. A purchase order describes what specific supplies need to be ordered, the estimated cost, what vendor you are using, bids from various vendors, who is ordering the supplies, and management authorization.

Request for Maintenance Services

Description of requested services		
Location	Work requested by	Phone
Date submitted	Request priority (please circle one)	A - Immediate attention B - Urgent attention C - Routine attention
Below portion to be completed by Maintenance Division		
Special instructions		
Date completed	Completed by	Time to complete
Remarks		
Repair costs		

From M. Bates, 2008, *Health Fitness Management*, 2nd ed. (Champaign, IL: Human Kinetics).

Tuesday evening cleaning shift
Assigned to housekeeping supervisor

Time	Facility area
6:00 p.m. - 6:30 p.m.	Clean administrative offices, tennis entry and walk, and lower hallway.
6:30 p.m. - 8:00 p.m.	Continuously walk through facility correcting problem areas; provide special attention to rear hallways, employee entrance, and rear stairways.
8:00 p.m. - 9:00 p.m.	Clean aerobic studio and transition area.
9:00 p.m. - 9:30 p.m.	Clean day care.
9:30 p.m. - 10:00 p.m.	Lunch break.
10:00 p.m. - 10:30 p.m.	Clean fitness and membership offices. **Place vacuum in pool.**
10:30 p.m. - 12:30 a.m.	Sweep designated indoor tennis courts (see schedule).
12:30 a.m. - 1:00 a.m.	Empty trash cans on all tennis courts and pick up loose trash around courts.
1:00 a.m. - 2:00 a.m.	Clean gymnasium floor, floor molding, backboards, and water fountains. Spot clean all racquetball courts, clean glass, and dust mop all wood floors. **Remove vacuum from pool.**
2:00 a.m. - 2:15 a.m.	Walk through the entire facility checking for problem areas; check and lock all entry doors; set security alarm.

Housekeeping assistant evening schedule

Time	Facility area
8:00 P.M. - 11:00 P.M.	Walk through the entire facility checking for problem areas; check and lock all entry doors; set security alarm.
11:00 P.M. - 11:30 P.M.	Break time.
11:30 P.M. - 2:30 A.M.	Clean assigned areas per housekeeping guideline.

Laundry assistant evening schedule

Time	Facility area
10:30 P.M. - 2:30 A.M.	Launder all soiled towels and member laundry. Return clean laundry to the front desk.

Figure 14.5 Sample maintenance schedule.

A sample purchase order form is shown on page 303. Each order is given a number and filled out in duplicate with a copy given to the employee who initiated the order and to the bookkeeper or accounting department. If the amount of the order is higher than a prearranged limit, approval must be obtained by management before initiating the order. When the supplies arrive, the purchase order and vendor invoice are matched before acceptance. Only a system of this nature can provide accountability against cost overruns and unnecessary supplies being ordered.

The level of inventory control depends on the size and control of the inventory. In most health and fitness settings the maintenance workforce is small, the facility systems are simple, and the numbers of renovation projects are minimal. Consequently, the facility manager or maintenance person can keep a mental inventory of supplies and spare parts. More complex facilities must have a formal system for

Purchase Order

Date: _____ Date needed: _____

Name: _____ Dept.: _____

Vendor: _____

Item	Item #	Qty	Price	Page
_____	_____	_____	_____	_____
_____	_____	_____	_____	_____
_____	_____	_____	_____	_____
_____	_____	_____	_____	_____
_____	_____	_____	_____	_____
_____	_____	_____	_____	_____

Date ordered: _____

_____

_____

For Office Use Only

Date ordered: _____ PO #: _____

Vendor #: _____ Invoice #: _____

Amount	G/L code	G/L #
_____	_____	_____
_____	_____	_____
_____	_____	_____

Obtained from general supplies: Yes _____   No _____

If yes, which ones? _____

From M. Bates, 2008, *Health Fitness Management,* 2nd ed. (Champaign, IL: Human Kinetics).

monitoring the inventory of consumables (e.g., toilet paper, Kleenex, paper towels).

You can set up this inventory manually or through a computer system. Manually, inventories are usually maintained on index cards in a file. When an order is received, the quantity of new materials is added to the index card. When products are expended, the quantity used is subtracted from the card. If you regularly update this system and there is sufficient security for the stored materials, you can rely on it to reflect the inventory status. Make one person responsible for issuing purchasing orders, maintaining the number entry, and verifying management's approval of the purchase. You can set up a computer inventory system to automatically generate purchase orders for inventory items when the stock level reaches a designated low point.

Cost Controls

Although most health and fitness organizations have an accounting system that monitors accounts payable and receivable (see chapter 12), it is ultimately the responsibility of the maintenance manager to identify and code all supplies and materials used. Without this interaction between accounting and maintenance, it would be difficult to control the cost breakdowns between divisions (i.e., fitness, tennis, day care, pro shop, restaurant). Despite the scope of the setting, maintenance managers must have a system (manual or computer) to provide feedback for the maintenance transactions that occurred during the day.

The purpose of cost accounting is to measure the ongoing and historical costs of each maintenance activity. From this measurement, the maintenance manager can make decisions to redirect or reallocate resources to reduce possible cost overruns. For example, excessive overtime costs might lead to hiring or reassigning additional full-time personnel. The maintenance manager also has the ability to frequently monitor and manage the annual budget to meet financial goals. Consequently, timely reporting of ongoing costs is essential.

Equipment and Mechanical Histories

To properly predict and adjust the maintenance program, the manager must have a thorough understanding of the particular facility and its components. Only with a total building history can you make proper decisions regarding the best course of maintenance for a given problem. Keep accurate documentation of all construction and renovation plans. Track major and recurring minor repairs.

Record periodic inspections by the health department, OSHA, and the fire department and update them for future reference. Accurate facility records enable immediate troubleshooting and repairs.

A proper equipment history should include the make and model of the equipment, date of installation, all major repairs, any preventive maintenance, and parts replaced. You can use this equipment history to predict the need for eventual replacement or rebuilding of a unit, or to diagnose an unexpected problem, which can often be traced to a recent repair. A sample form, Equipment History Card, is shown on page 305.

Work Tracking and Monitoring

In addition to monitoring the cost of all the maintenance work performed, it is important to ensure that all work is completed in a timely manner. Establish internal procedures to alert management or operations personnel of all maintenance problems. Use a corresponding system to ensure quick turnaround of all repairs and to inform the member of expected completion time. If you do not accomplish member-identified minor repairs in a reasonable amount of time, the member may decide that it is useless to report minor problems. If minor problems are not reported, they could lead to major problems. Consequently, the tracking system must be timely and complete.

THE BOTTOM LINE

Because forgotten preventive maintenance or neglected repair work can lead to costly repairs, facility downtime, or potential injury, use a system for tracking the source, assignment, and accomplishment of all work.

Most facilities use a work-request form (see page 301) to track member-identified repairs or problem areas. The form should provide space for the following information:

- What—a concise statement of the problem. There is sometimes the tendency to request specific actions or solutions rather than stating the problem.
- Where—the location of the problem. Depending on the size of the facility, this may include the name of the specific area where the problem has occurred or any other necessary information to enable the maintenance worker to locate the problem.

Equipment History Card

Equipment name		
Manufacturer		Model no.
Equipment location		Specific installation area
Date of original installation		Installed by

Equipment Repair History		
Date	Description	Repair costs

From M. Bates, 2008, *Health Fitness Management*, 2nd ed. (Champaign, IL: Human Kinetics).

- Who—the name and phone number of the member or employee making the request. The maintenance staff use this to obtain further information on the problem and to let the member know when work has been completed.
- When—the date and time that the request was made. Include follow-up information regarding when the repairs were made, who completed the repairs, and how long it took to fix. Also include estimated or actual repair costs to assist bookkeeping in tracking overall repair charges.

These forms are usually placed at strategic points (check-in desk, membership office, locker rooms) around a facility where members or employees may quickly and conveniently report any repair work needed. Once the work is completed, the work-request forms are recorded and filed for future reference.

Evaluating Facility Maintenance

The implementation phase ensures that the system established for overall maintenance care is well organized, properly staffed, and within the financial parameters authorized by management. The only way to assure this is through an internally developed set of goals and objectives as discussed previously in this chapter. By regularly reviewing and updating these goals and objectives, facility managers will always be able to assess whether the maintenance program is producing the intended results.

Once the implementation phase is initiated, the ongoing evaluation process begins. Patton and colleagues (1989) include two steps in the evaluation phase: process evaluation and outcome evaluation (see chapter 17). These evaluations involve analyzing the implementation tasks that were assigned to the staff to determine if maintenance tasks are being accomplished (process evaluation) and if objectives of the maintenance program are being met (outcome evaluation). Figure 14.6 summarizes process and outcome techniques.

THE BOTTOM LINE

Evaluating a maintenance program is different from evaluating an activity program that has a beginning and ending point. Facility maintenance is dynamic and continual and must be reviewed at regular intervals. Perform any changes or modifications to an existing maintenance program daily rather than waiting for an appropriate time.

Schedule periodic meetings with staff to review the maintenance process and address strategies to maintain or improve current procedures. Staff should maintain careful work-order records detailing when the work was completed, how long it took to complete, what materials were used, and who performed the work. Maintenance software programs are now available to tabulate work-order data and assist in inventory management.

A new and innovative program called **benchmarking** has recently been introduced into the health and fitness market. Benchmarking is the process of measuring services, supplies, and practices against competitors, similar facilities, or industry standards. Although this practice began as a means to improve worker performance and productivity in large corporations, only recently has it been introduced into the health and fitness market. Benchmarking involves reviewing the existing operation, looking at other operations, selecting the best practices, and incorporating them into the current maintenance and housekeeping operations.

Begin benchmarking by analyzing the existing facility and identifying areas to benchmark. Second, determine the methods of data collection, and, finally, identify comparative clubs or facilities. Because benchmarking is relatively new to the health and fitness business, no industry standards exist specifically for facility maintenance. However, there are national standards reported annually by *Cleaning and Maintenance Management* magazine and the Cleaning Management Institute for all types of facilities nationwide (e.g., hospitals, schools, hotels). You can use a number of categories from this survey to compare the average

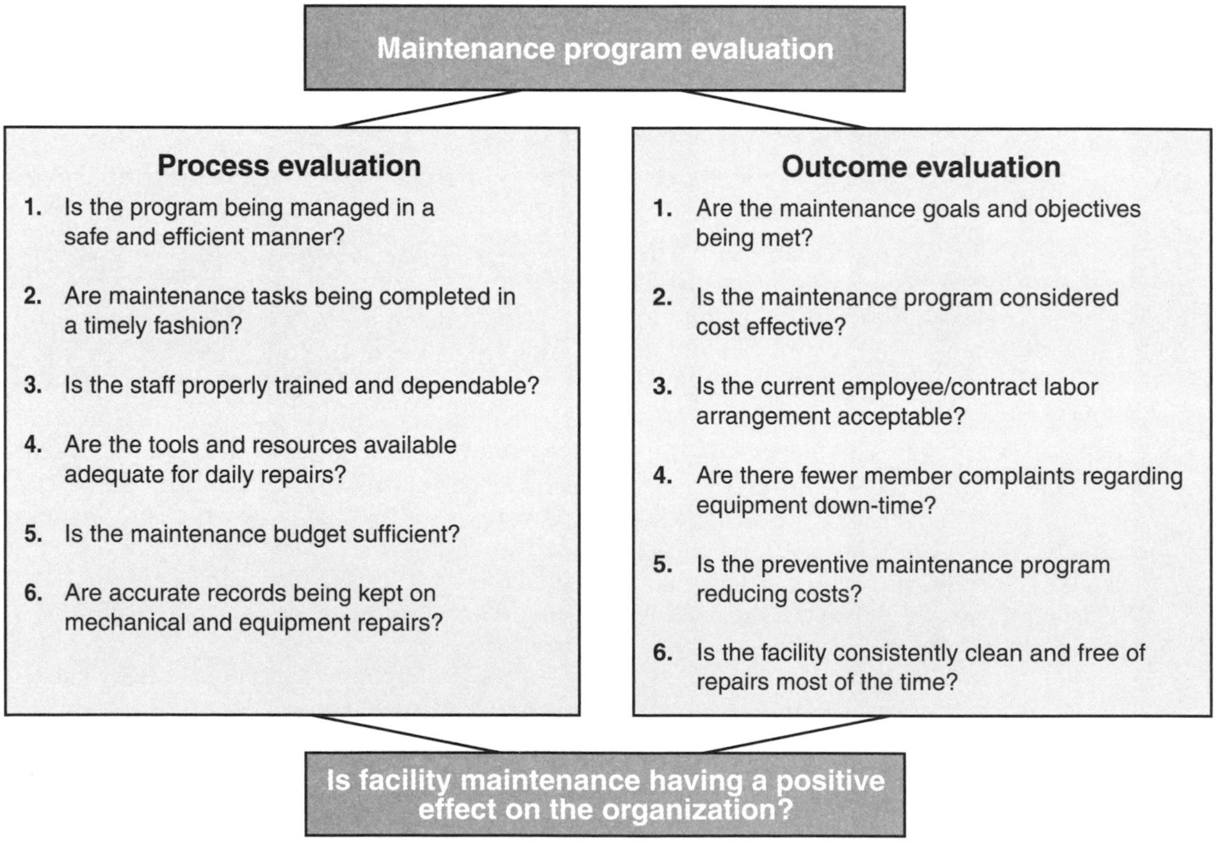

Maintenance program evaluation

Process evaluation

1. Is the program being managed in a safe and efficient manner?

2. Are maintenance tasks being completed in a timely fashion?

3. Is the staff properly trained and dependable?

4. Are the tools and resources available adequate for daily repairs?

5. Is the maintenance budget sufficient?

6. Are accurate records being kept on mechanical and equipment repairs?

Outcome evaluation

1. Are the maintenance goals and objectives being met?

2. Is the maintenance program considered cost effective?

3. Is the current employee/contract labor arrangement acceptable?

4. Are there fewer member complaints regarding equipment down-time?

5. Is the preventive maintenance program reducing costs?

6. Is the facility consistently clean and free of repairs most of the time?

Is facility maintenance having a positive effect on the organization?

Figure 14.6 Maintenance process and outcome techniques.

facility against an existing setting. Some areas to consider benchmarking might include the following:

- Estimated annual cleaning costs per square foot—annual cleaning budget divided by the square footage of the facility

- Wage rates—average hourly rates for shift supervisors, average cleaning worker, and starting cleaning worker

- Maintenance spending per facility—estimated costs for chemicals, paper products, powered cleaning equipment, nonpowered equipment (e.g., mops, brooms)

- Staff time allotment for common tasks—percent of total annual cleaning work hours spent by staff in such areas as floor care, vacuuming, locker-room care, trash collection, dusting, carpet cleaning (other than vacuuming), and other tasks

- Total annual cleaning budget—total cleaning budget compared with similar fitness settings of the same approximate size

THE BOTTOM LINE

Benchmarking assists managers and maintenance personnel in justifying and evaluating overall performance.

It is impossible to improve what you cannot measure. Measuring productivity does not always have to entail a sophisticated system. You can establish categories to provide baseline parameters that communicate the overall performance of the maintenance division. These categories could include weekly towel counts, numbers of work orders completed each week, and number of emergency response calls completed each week.

A system of this nature provides an objective means for determining maintenance effectiveness. In the past, many maintenance supervisors have used their sense of what was best. However, this method of evaluation is too subjective and does not always provide a definitive means for measuring performance.

Developing a Preventive Maintenance Program

Once the maintenance program is operating efficiently, organize and implement a preventive maintenance program. The amount of funds invested in mechanical, electrical, and exercise equipment certainly justifies the costs of maintaining the equip-

ment so it is safe and operational. In the health and fitness business, the cost of waiting until a system malfunctions is not worth the outcome.

The goal of any preventive maintenance program is to ensure the continuous operation of facility systems (HVAC, boilers, pool heaters, fire alarm, security systems) and equipment (cardiorespiratory equipment, strength equipment, computers). An organized preventive maintenance program facilitates continued operation either through completion of work that keeps equipment operating or through identification of substandard performance, faulty parts, or equipment failure. Table 14.1 provides a preventive maintenance schedule for a StairMaster Crossrobics machine.

You can categorize each preventive maintenance action according to how it reduces or avoids costs to the facility operation. These categories are described here.

- *Maintain operations.* The most obvious justification for preventive maintenance is to maintain facility operations. The continued operation of a facility directly relates to the preventive maintenance tasks performed to ensure equipment reliability. However, the functioning of some systems has a higher priority than others. For example, failure of a club water heater could disable operations, whereas failure of a pool or spa water heater may not completely impede usage but might result in disgruntled member feedback.

- *Lengthen service life.* Many preventive maintenance procedures are designed to ensure that a piece of equipment will not fail prematurely. Most equipment is designed for a specific service life. The duration of operation depends on timely servicing throughout use of the equipment.

- *Identify worn-out equipment.* Because exercise equipment does not always perform like new, you should implement a system to monitor its gradual deterioration. Planning specific preventive maintenance tasks to detect any subtle changes and to alert maintenance personnel to major changes in equipment performance is highly recommended. Regular preventive maintenance will reduce overall costs if you catch mechanical problems early enough to detect signs of premature equipment failure.

- *Prevent loss.* Certain installed systems exist to protect members and personnel within the facility. For example, a malfunctioning fire alarm system has no effect on the facility operation until there is a fire. Preventive maintenance performed on this equipment is justified because it prevents losses involving members, employees, and the facility.

Table 14.1 Preventive Maintenance Schedule for the StairMaster Crossrobics 1650 LE

Part	Recommended action	Frequency	Cleaner	Lubricant
Plastic side cover (exterior only)	Clean	Daily	Soap and water or diluted cleaner	N/A
Seat	Clean	Daily	Same as above	N/A
Console	Clean	Daily	Water	N/A
Weight stack belt and connectors	Inspect	Weekly or every 70 hours	N/A	N/A
Pedal arm return springs	Inspect, clean, and relube	Weekly or every 70 hours	Degreaser	Oil-dampened rag
Alternator and drive belts	Check tension and inspect for wear	Weekly or every 70 hours	Degreaser	30W motor oil
	Remove, clean, and lubricate	Every 3 months or 900 hours	Degreaser	30W motor oil
Guide rods	Clean and lubricate	Weekly or every 70 hours	Window cleaner	Silicone spray
Drive shaft and hub assembly	Grease	Every 3 months or 900 hours	N/A	Heavy multipurpose grease
Bottom stop sprint	Wipe clean and grease	Every 3 months or 900 hours	N/A	Heavy multipurpose grease

• *Ensure personal safety.* Regularly maintain any system or piece of equipment within a club that is installed to prevent bodily injury or possible death to members. Protective systems such as exit signs, fire alarms, and emergency lighting are required by local building codes or city standards. The costs of preventive maintenance for these systems are unavoidable.

• *Protect facility.* Some systems are installed to protect physical property. Sprinkler systems and burglar alarms reduce the risk of property loss and reduce insurance premiums. For these reasons, perform maintenance even if the insurance policy doesn't require proof of maintenance for these systems.

• *Comply with government standards.* Numerous aspects of a facility must comply with local, state, and federal standards. For example, swimming pool water must meet local health department regulations. Steam-room boilers must meet emission control standards to satisfy insurance companies. Paint or possible explosive materials cannot be stored next to electrical panels according to OSHA requirements. In each case, the existing equipment must be maintained to perform at the levels required. Failure to comply with these organizations will result in discipline that could range from verbal warnings to closing the facility.

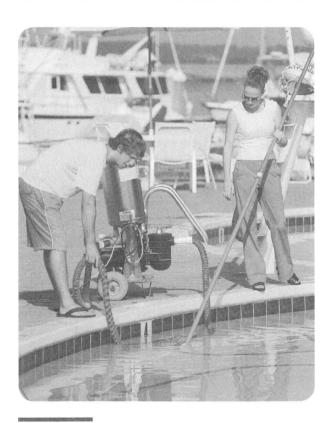

Regular swimming pool maintenance ensures the continuous operation of the pool and also enables the facility to comply with health regulations related to swimming pool water.

THE BOTTOM LINE

Preventive maintenance tasks are performed whenever the financial impact of failure to perform the activity exceeds the cost of its performance. For example, the cost of maintaining an air-conditioning system often outweighs the cost of periodically replacing condensers or complete systems.

Initiating a preventive maintenance program begins with identifying those areas that have the greatest impact on the facility if not maintained. Examine and classify each system and piece of equipment as to its level of importance in facility operations. Those items that are critical to safe and continued operation of the facility receive high priority.

A primary source for identifying preventive maintenance tasks is procedures recommended by manufacturers. Companies that produce cardio-respiratory or strength equipment provide a user's manual specifying recommended service frequency and procedures. Any warranties provided with such equipment usually depend on completion of recommended preventive maintenance.

Once you determine the need for preventive maintenance for a system or piece of equipment, establish the procedures to provide that preventive maintenance task. Develop a **preventive maintenance order (PMO),** a form that acts as more than just a how-to guide. Figure 14.7 shows a competed PMO. Properly prepared, it describes the physical actions of performing the maintenance. The PMO is a planning document and a safety document. It provides assistance in ordering parts, and you can

Preventive Maintenance Order

Equipment name *Concept II Rower*	Model no. *None*	Manufacturer *Concept II, Inc.*
Frequency: daily weekly monthly quarterly annual		
Location *cardio room*	Other location information *Unit next to window*	
Tools required	*wrench* *screwdriver* *pliers*	
Materials required	*1 – lubricant tube* *1 – nonabrasive scouring pad*	*1 set – footstraps*
Safety procedures	*watch tension on chain after cleaning*	
Maintenance procedures	*Clean monorail with nonabrasive scouring pad—daily* *Clean and lubricate chain—weekly* *Check cord tension—weekly* *Check chain for stiff links—monthly* *Check tightness of all nuts and bolts—monthly*	
Date completed	Completed by	Time to complete
Remarks		

Figure 14.7 Completed PMO form.

use it as an inspection and feedback tool. Although PMO forms have never been standardized and many variations exist, basic components of the form should include equipment data information, location, tools and materials required, safety procedures, maintenance procedures, and work completion data.

Each time preventive maintenance is to be performed on a system or piece of equipment, staff should prepare a PMO and forward it to the person administering the job. Once the work is completed, return the PMO to either the club operator or the maintenance supervisor. Pay close attention to any comments the worker makes that might initiate further investigation. File the completed order and establish a date for the next PMO for that piece of equipment. Record the date either manually or in a computer database for the next scheduled preventive maintenance.

Periodically evaluate the preventive maintenance program to determine its effectiveness. Measure the effectiveness by the performance of the facility and equipment and by the cost of the program. Address the following questions:

- Is the program running efficiently, or is preventive maintenance being forgotten or ignored?

- Has the number of maintenance request orders been reduced on those items receiving preventive maintenance?

- Have parts and equipment supply costs been reduced?

- Have there been fewer calls for outside repair workers?

- Have any equipment failures been the result of inadequate preventive maintenance?

KEY TERMS

benchmarking

contract labor

contract maintenance

heating, ventilation, and air-conditioning (HVAC)

iterative process

needs assessment

preventive maintenance

preventive maintenance order (PMO)

purchase order system

strategic plan

REFERENCES AND RECOMMENDED READINGS

Feldman, E. 1991. *How to save time and money in facilities maintenance management.* Latham, NY: Cleaning Management Institute.

Fried, G. 2005. *Managing sport facilities.* Champaign, IL: Human Kinetics.

Grantham, W.C., R.W. Patton, T.D. York, and M. Winick. 1998. *Health fitness management.* 1st ed. Champaign, IL: Human Kinetics.

Greenwood, M. 2000. Facility layout and scheduling. In *Essentials of strength training and conditioning,* eds. T.R. Baechle and R. Earle, 549-565. Champaign, IL: Human Kinetics.

———. 2004. Facility and equipment layout and maintenance. In *Essentials of personal training,* eds. T.R. Baechle and R. Earle, 587-601. Champaign, IL: Human Kinetics.

Greenwood, M., and L. Greenwood. 2000. Facility maintenance and risk management. In *Essentials of strength training and conditioning,* eds. T.R. Baechle and R. Earle, 587-601. Champaign, IL: Human Kinetics.

Hoke, J.R. 1975. *Designer's guide to OSHA.* New York: McGraw-Hill.

International Health, Racquet, and Sportsclub Association (IHRSA). 2006. *Global report: State of the health club industry.* Boston: IHRSA.

International Health, Racquet, and Sportsclub Association (IHRSA). 2004. *Profiles of success.* Boston: IHRSA.

Magee, G. 1988. *Facility maintenance management.* Kingston, MA: Means.

Patton, R.W., J.M. Corry, L.R. Gettman, and J.S. Graf. 1986. *Implementing health fitness programs.* Champaign, IL: Human Kinetics.

Patton, R.W., W.C. Grantham, R.F. Gerson, and L.R. Gettman. 1989. *Developing and managing health fitness facilities.* Champaign, IL: Human Kinetics.

Publishers Survey. 1995. 1995 in-house survey. *Cleaning and Maintenance Management* 32(12):2-8.

Ray, R. 2000. *Management strategies in athletic training.* 2nd ed. Champaign, IL: Human Kinetics.

Rice, R. 1995. Housekeeping benchmarks. *Cleaning and Maintenance Management* 32(3):62-65.

Tatum, R. 1995. How technology is reshaping facility management. *Building Operating Management* 42(1):24-30.

Tharrett, S.J., McInnis, K.J., and Peterson, J.A. 2007. *ACSM's health/fitness facility standards and guidelines.* 3rd ed. Champaign, IL: Human Kinetics.

Williams, T. 1994. How top managers evaluate their facilities. *Cleaning Maintenance Management* 31(9):40-42.

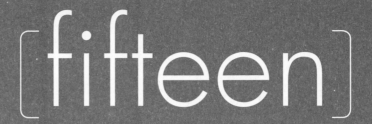

Choosing the Right Equipment

Mike Bates

LEARNING OBJECTIVES

After studying this chapter, the reader will be able to

- develop questions that should be asked when selecting exercise equipment,
- identify the expenses involved in purchasing and maintaining exercise equipment,
- recognize the safety concerns associated with exercise equipment layout and usage, and
- understand the criteria used when selecting other equipment.

Tales From the Trenches

Jake's 5-year-old fitness center was ready for an upgrade in equipment. His membership base had grown to more than 1,500 members and what was working for him a couple of years ago was no longer keeping his members happy.

Since he knew that he had many equipment options to choose from, he first gathered information from staff and members on what types of equipment people were looking for. With this information in hand and some of his own preferences in mind, Jake scheduled a trip to an industry conference where he would have the opportunity to talk with the major equipment suppliers. At the conference Jake made personal contacts with the sales reps for his area and had the opportunity to try out the equipment and collect marketing information. He found out about new industry trends and even learned about new equipment that would be available in time for his scheduled expansion.

When Jake arrived home from the conference, he narrowed his selections to three equipment suppliers. In talking with people at the conference, he learned that he might get a better price if he went with one company for all his needs. In the past he had used multiple companies for his equipment and even though this seemed to have worked out well, he was open to trying out one supplier for his next big purchase.

Jake sent the following list off to the three suppliers and asked for a quote:

- 6 treadmills
- 4 elliptical trainers
- 4 group cycling bikes
- 6 recumbent bikes
- 2 rowing machines

Within a week, each of the companies got back to Jake with a quote. Jake compared warranties, reputation, and the specific features on each machine to ensure the companies were quoting similar products. He also checked with the local equipment repair company to see what their experiences had been. He then asked the company about their lease rates. Each supplier sent him forms to fill out related to his current financial situation. In another week the leasing companies of each equipment supplier responded to Jake with an offer.

With all of this information, he then made a list of preferences and asked each company if these were the best prices he could get. Two companies were able to discount their pricing further, but the third did not change the quote. Jake made his decision and informed each company with a personal phone call. The winning bidder told him that his equipment would arrive in about 8 weeks.

As the date drew closer, the equipment company gave Jake a definite date and time for delivery. After the equipment arrived, Jake organized a membership party to celebrate the new equipment. Members and staff were happy with the equipment and were glad that Jake had asked for their input.

In the months that followed, any minor repairs were covered under warranties and were able to be fixed quickly since Jake had taken the equipment company's advice and had spare parts on hand at the club. This saved the time of ordering and delivering parts from the manufacturer. Jake's staff followed a scheduled maintenance program on all of the equipment, and personnel came in to regularly service the equipment that the club staff were not able to take care of.

Jake's experience with his new purchases was a smooth one because he took the time to research and plan for all the needs of the facility. Choosing the proper equipment and getting good prices for that equipment can have a major impact on the success of any fitness club.

The selection, purchase, maintenance, and operation of exercise equipment are an important process in the health and fitness industry. Each represents a significant investment of time and money, and any poor decisions made during the process can haunt you later. A wide selection of products in varied price ranges is available to choose from. In this chapter, we provide criteria for selecting equipment, as well as some ideas about purchasing, maintaining, and operating it. In addition, we offer insight into other equipment considerations. Many facilities have laundry equipment as well as water treatment systems for aquatics and supportive equipment for racket sports, so we offer guidelines for these areas as well.

Selecting Health and Fitness Equipment

Selecting equipment is a baffling process for the average buyer because of the many vendors and types of products on the market. Canvassing classified advertisements in trade journals and visiting exhibits at trade shows can certainly confuse all but a few professionals who spend most of their time dealing with such matters. We present the following information on selecting equipment without regard to priorities because each buyer has different priorities.

Function

A piece of exercise equipment is normally designed for a particular function or purpose. For example, a bicycle ergometer is designed to function as an exercise station for developing cardiorespiratory endurance; free-weight bars and the attached plates are designed primarily to develop muscle strength and endurance. However, you can use most equipment to accomplish secondary functions. For instance, you can use free-weight equipment with low resistance to accommodate a high number of exercise repetitions for achieving a moderate cardiorespiratory endurance. Thus, determining which functions a piece of equipment will serve is one of the first decisions you must make. When determining what kind of programming spaces a facility requires, you have to make arbitrary decisions about the need for strength training equipment, cardiorespiratory training equipment, and diagnostic and testing equipment, as well as support equipment such as laundry, computers, and office equipment. The focus of this chapter is exercise equipment.

The equipment you choose should match the marketing image you want to project. The hard-core power studio is probably dominated by free-weight equipment, whereas the executive fitness center probably has more selectorized, weight-stacked equipment. Thus, the questions to ask in the early stages of decision making include the following:

- What kind of image do you want to project?
- Who will be using the equipment?
- What is the basic purpose of the equipment?
- Will there be an emphasis on strength or endurance equipment?

Cost

The price of a single piece of exercise equipment can range from a few dollars to several thousand dollars. For example, you can use a dumbbell to assess or develop forearm strength and endurance at a cost of only a few dollars, and you can accomplish the same tasks using a high-tech computer product line for several thousand dollars. The difference, of course, is the degree of sophistication involved in the equipment. Most sophisticated equipment interfaces with a computer system for analysis, logging, or tracking purposes. There is a similar cost contrast among bicycle ergometers and treadmills in the cardiorespiratory area.

Exercise caution when selecting equipment. There is often a point of diminishing returns when upgrading older equipment lines for newer products, and the cost of equipment can easily place a program in financial difficulty. Moreover, expensive equipment can place such a burden on the budget that other important areas of the program, such as personnel, might suffer. Still, equipment is a highly visible marketing tool, especially in the early stages of program development. Personnel, on the other hand, become critical in member adherence and renewals. A balance of expenditures is essential.

Industry experts agree that the total cost of purchasing equipment consists of the following factors:

- Initial purchase price
- Sum of maintenance
- Power requirements
- Repair and downtime

Paying for exercise equipment is usually required before or at the time of delivery. Although delivery dates frequently extend to 8 weeks or longer, large expenditures of money over short periods can be burdensome. Consider alternatives to purchasing new equipment outright if you are already under the pressure of heavy expenditures.

A lease or a lease-purchase arrangement is the route most fitness clubs use to purchase their equipment. The benefits of leasing include the small outlay of cash and the ability to expense lease payments on the income statement. There are no

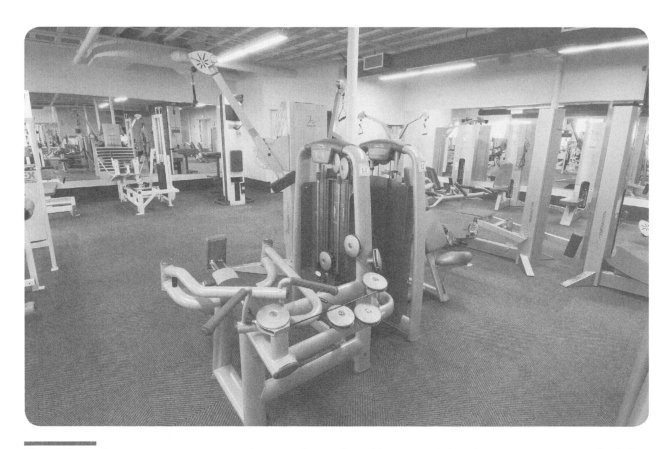

The selection of equipment requires consideration of a number of factors, including function, cost, space, durability, safety, versatility, and user appeal.
© Will & Lisa Funk/Alpine Aperture

industry standards for leasing equipment, but most clubs can expect to get lease terms of 36 to 48 months, with a small buy-back option at the end of the lease term. Interest rates on leased equipment will vary based on the leasing company and the financial situation of the club. Most leasing companies will expect you to place a deposit on any lease agreements before the start of the regular monthly lease payments. A general starting point is 10% down in addition to the lease payments of the first and last months. Everything is negotiable when leasing equipment, so make sure to get multiple quotes to ensure you are getting the best possible terms.

One alternative to purchasing new exercise equipment is to buy used equipment. A series of phone calls to equipment manufacturers may provide you with contacts for trade-in equipment. Many vendors are a good source for used equipment because they frequently have trade-in agreements with their customers. The secondhand market is becoming an affordable option for equipment. Many of these vendors refurbish the equipment to nearly new condition before resale. You may also

choose to recondition your own used equipment. Various companies now can restore your old equipment to a nearly new condition and save you about 30% of the cost of new equipment.

A combination of used and new equipment is also an option during the start-up period. If the new equipment is made more visible to the members, the general impression will be that you have purchased all new equipment for the facility. Although this arrangement is less than ideal, it can frequently be a necessary compromise when investors are seeking an early break-even period and a quick return on their investment.

Several companies are emerging as vendors of used and rental exercise equipment. You can obtain contact information for these companies through trade journals or even local classified advertisements. There are also leasing companies that advertise repossessed equipment with lease-purchase contracts. The purchase price on this equipment is discounted to as little as 10% of the original price. Several other businesses offer similar services and products to the resourceful consumer.

THE BOTTOM LINE

Expect to receive about 35% to 65% of the original purchase price when trading in used exercise equipment.

Depreciation and salvage value of exercise equipment after its usable life are other cost considerations. From an accounting perspective, the usable life of most exercise equipment is about 5 years; however, the life expectancy and salvage value of some equipment are better than others. Generally, brand-name equipment is superior in this regard, offsetting some of the extra expense during the initial purchase.

Finally, consider the operational expense of equipment. Electronic equipment, for example, is more expensive to operate than mechanical equipment. Electronic part replacements and ongoing electricity costs can become a major expense. For this reason, many clubs choose to lease their cardiorespiratory equipment, which is run electronically.

Space

The amount of space available often determines the type or amount of equipment selected in a health and fitness facility. This accounts for circulation of participants and the average space needed for larger items such as treadmills and smaller items such as bicycle ergometers, as well as large free-weight racks and single-station **selectorized equipment.** If your facility is planned for nothing but multistation selectorized equipment, then these assumptions are invalid and you should consult the vendor. Note that most equipment manufacturers offer space-planning services that are invaluable, especially if you are planning to use only one brand of equipment. Figures 15.1 and 15.2 illustrate two typical equipment layouts.

THE BOTTOM LINE

A rule of thumb for designing exercise spaces is that one station or footprint of exercise equipment occupies approximately 46 square feet (4 square meters) of floor space.

To optimize the use of space, plan for as many exercise patterns in one space as possible. For example, arrange a circuit on selectorized weight equipment around a group of ergometers to accommodate a super circuit if a member wants to cross-train for strength and endurance during the same workout.

Durability

Durability is an important consideration when selecting exercise equipment. There is no ironclad way to calculate the life expectancy of exercise equipment. Equipment of a particular type enjoys more use in some settings than it does in others. Also, users are fickle; they may drift from one type of exercise equipment to another in search of one that yields large gains with the least pain. Trendy equipment will experience intense periods of heavy use for short times, followed by periods of little or no use. Here we offer some guidelines for determining the probable durability of a given type of equipment.

- *Joints.* Welds should be sturdy, and the best equipment will have the welds ground smooth. Bolted joints are useful where equipment must be disassembled to move or to remove or replace connecting parts.

- *Chassis.* Moving parts should be enclosed to reduce cleaning and maintenance.

- *Padding.* Double stitching should be standard on the front and back of pads. No staples are used on quality pads. Closed-cell foam should be used in areas of heavy wear; softer material is used in support areas.

- *Bearings.* Bearings should be suited to their use: Delrin or nylon on weight stacks, self-lubricating brass bushings on pivots, and roller or pillow-block bearings on linear movements.

- *Chains, cables, and belts.* Chains, aircraft cables, and belts are usual choices for connecting to weight stacks. Cables and belts are quieter, and belts are thought to be more durable than cables.

- *Electronics.* Electrical components and moisture are not well suited for one another. Take care to avoid sweating onto display boards and to secure bottle holders on equipment at a level well below any circuitry.

The warranty on equipment serves as a rough indicator of its life expectancy. For example, manufacturers of selectorized strength equipment frequently warranty the structural frame for life, the moving parts for a year, and the upholstery for 90 days because each material has a different projected life span. Read the small print in a warranty that promises a lifetime guarantee; little in this world

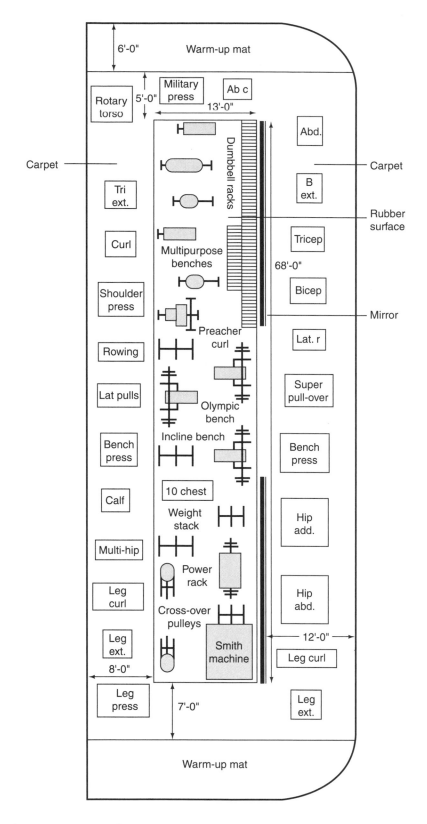

Figure 15.1 Weight-room equipment layout.

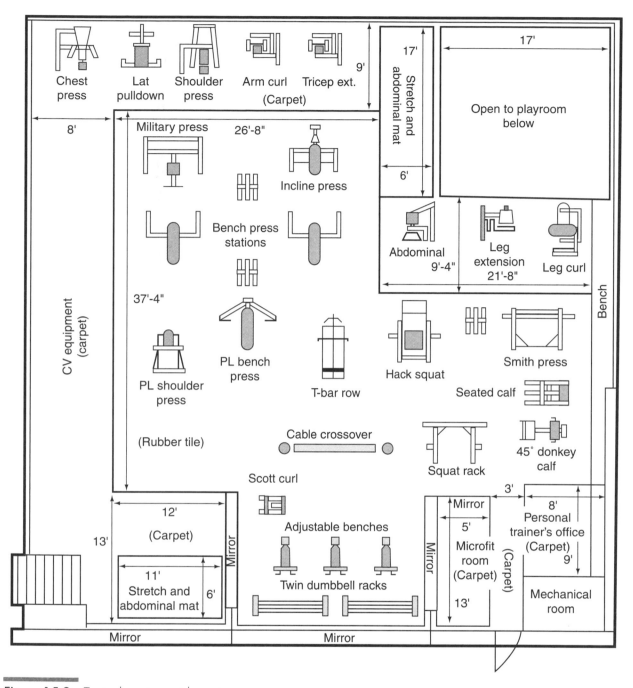

Figure 15.2 Typical equipment layout.

is guaranteed for life, especially in the realm of exercise equipment. Manufacturers are careful to extend a warranty that requires low repair activity at their expense. Therefore, assume that expected deterioration rates of equipment under normal conditions will exceed the warranty period advertised by the manufacturer.

Another indicator of durability is competitors' experiences with the equipment. A canvassing of other programs in your area that are similar in size and

clientele can give you a good idea about the durability of a type of equipment. This evaluation, coupled with trade journal commentary, will assist you in making the right decision about equipment durability.

Safety

The safety of intended users should be your first consideration when making decisions about exercise equipment. Formal law and legal precedent dictate that agencies and administrators of health and fitness programs have a responsibility to provide a reasonably hazard-free environment for exercise experiences. **Safe place statutes,** which entitle the users to safe environments, place an extra burden of care on activity providers. In any event, it is important that the equipment be as safe as possible for the intended users. Use the following suggestions to avoid trouble spots for exercise equipment and consult the other chapters in this book that discuss safety and maintenance concerns.

Weight Machines

- Cable systems should have plastic-coated cables, which are less likely to fray.
- Movable attachments should not have soft metal pulleys.
- Movable parts should be easily lubricated.
- Frames should have the capacity to be anchored to the floor or wall.
- Frames should have several welding marks at junctions.
- Equipment should be coated with corrosion-resistant paint.
- Safety stops in selectorized machines should be aligned.
- Cotter pins should not be difficult to place in stacks.
- Nonslip surfaces should surround lifting areas.
- Lifting areas should be free of clutter.
- Floor surfaces should be of high-density, shock-absorbing material.
- Plates, bars, and collars should be stored after each use.
- Appropriate fasteners of free weights should be available.
- Sleeves for bars should not be bent or frayed at the ends.
- Preset barbells and dumbbells should be welded in place.
- Benches should be sturdy enough to support anticipated loads.
- Bench bolts and nuts should be welded in place.
- Bench surfaces should be padded to avoid splinters and the like.
- Selectorized stacks should be shrouded with protective covering.

- Safety stops for preventing a crushing injury should be designed into equipment.

Cardiorespiratory Equipment

- Electrical plugs should be grounded. Ground fault interrupters should be on the power source.
- Treadmills should have an emergency stop button on the handrail.
- Spotter's platform should be available on treadmills that elevate.
- Cycles and rowers with turbines should have protective guards.
- Countdown timers should automatically stop equipment.
- Treadmills should have guardrails on three sides.
- Instructions for safe use should be permanently mounted on units.
- Preventive maintenance should be easily accomplished (e.g., lubrication).
- Climbing walls should have belaying systems.

THE BOTTOM LINE

Always assign a staff member to monitor areas where exercise equipment is available to members.

Versatility

Look for versatility when purchasing equipment. Each piece must be able to perform more than one function. For example, the equipment should be capable of diagnosing ability, rehabilitating injury, and training injury-free members. In addition, it should be reliable so that you obtain the same information on the same subject in repeated tests. It should also be accurate in that it truly measures what you intended in the test (e.g., treadmills may best measure running ability). Finally, the equipment should provide objectivity—the same results should be achieved when two different people test a member.

THE BOTTOM LINE

A major consideration for any equipment purchase is the ability to modify the equipment for different populations.

Can children, women, and large men use the same piece of equipment effectively? If not, then you might want to seek alternative product lines. Some vendors offer products that can accommodate a wide range of body sizes and types. Unfortunately, many manufacturers have developed their equipment for the standard man or woman. Such equipment cannot comfortably accommodate different populations with unusual sizes and shapes without using pads, pillows, and other devices to adjust the equipment. The versatility of product design should weigh heavily in your decision making. One way to assess the versatility of a piece of equipment is to ensure that it can adjust to members between 5 feet, 2 inches (158 centimeters) and 6 feet, 6 inches (198 centimeters).

User Appeal

The intended user must find the equipment appealing if it is to be successful in the club setting. Several factors are involved in making equipment appealing. For instance, name recognition is one important appeal factor. Precor, Star Trac, Cybex, Hammer Strength, Nautilus, and Life Fitness equipment, for example, have instant credibility and appeal among many users.

Free weights have recently enjoyed a groundswell of support. Although no particular product line has emerged as a consumer leader, sturdy and massive-looking equipment is desired by many devotees of powerlifting. This appeal is consistent with the concern for function over appearance. Most free-weight users are more concerned with results than with the convenience and appearance of the equipment. Harried club members, in contrast, may be concerned with getting a quick but effective workout by using the selectorized equipment that doesn't require a spotter and that they can use with minimal time and fuss. They will be concerned about efficiency as much as powerlifters are concerned about the effectiveness of the equipment. Be sure to deal with all these considerations when selecting exercise equipment.

Maintenance Contracts

Some manufacturers offer service contracts at the time of purchase. This is an important consideration for buyers who don't have access to maintenance and repair personnel. Typically, the maintenance contract dovetails with the warranty, and the fees are associated with the amount of equipment to be serviced. An average facility with a full complement of resistive and cardiorespiratory equipment should plan on spending anywhere from $300 to $800 per month for external maintenance contracts. Although this removes many headaches for the club, it places an extra burden on the budget. If the buyer has access to good maintenance personnel, the maintenance contract will not be a significant consideration in the decision-making process. This is especially true if a large inventory of spare parts is possible. We strongly recommend that you investigate the availability of parts and service before purchasing any equipment. A regional service center located nearby should place a vendor at an advantage over competing product lines that are of equal price and quality but farther from the club.

Warranties and Extended Warranties

As you can see, there are many things to consider before making an equipment purchase. **Warranties** and **extended warranties** are the final factor to consider when making an equipment purchase.

Although most equipment purchases come with some form of warranty, the reality is that these warranties are short lived and may be limited in their scope. The majority of equipment warranties only last for 2 to 3 years and only cover basic repairs. Beyond this, clubs have the option of purchasing an extended warranty.

According to Kurt Broadhag (2006), there are four things to look at when considering an extended warranty:

1. *Warranty coverage.* Both basic and extended warranties vary among manufacturers, especially involving wear and tear. Extended warranties that cover these items will protect you from paying out of pocket for repairs during the life of the warranty.

2. *Type of equipment.* Equipment with a high probability of costly repairs benefits more from an extended warranty. Treadmills have the most costly repairs due to the large forces created from usage and their many moving parts. Given the basic wear and tear of the deck and belt system and the manufacturers' recommendations of replacement once a year, it is easy to see how a $300 repair, not including labor, will be recuperated within the first 2 years based on the price of the extended warranty.

3. *Length of time equipment is in service.* The amount of time you plan to keep the equipment in service is another factor to consider. If you plan on selling or upgrading the equipment around the time the warranty expires, there is no need for an extended warranty.

4. *Preventive maintenance.* A proper preventive maintenance program is crucial to prolong the life of equipment and keep it repair free. Facilities that do not have an extensive preventive maintenance program in place should definitely consider the extended warranties on all their cardiorespiratory equipment given the greater risk of repair from neglect.

Purchasing Exercise Equipment

Purchasing equipment is a complex process influenced greatly by the setting. The procedures you employ to secure the equipment you need vary depending on whether the facility is corporate, community, clinical, or commercial. Government agencies, for example, may have a purchasing department governed by federal or regional laws. Hospitals may have corporate purchasing guidelines if they are members of a large group of hospitals, whereas community hospitals may have more latitude in the purchasing process. Commercial fitness centers may be similar to hospitals in that chain centers often have centralized purchasing to enjoy the economics of scale in large-volume buying. Smaller, sole proprietorships may have greater latitude in decision-making and procedural processes regarding equipment purchases.

Thus, it is difficult to generalize about purchasing procedures. This difficulty is compounded when we consider the geographic setting (concentration of indoor versus outdoor equipment), the intended users (upscale, single-station units versus downscale, multistation units), the desired image (lavish versus Spartan), and other factors that influence the decision-making processes. Notwithstanding these limitations, let's examine some broad concerns that most programs will need to address when purchasing equipment. Figure 15.3 outlines member participation levels for specific types of equipment.

Activity participation (millions)

Activity	Male	Female
Resistance machines	6.1	6.6
Treadmills	4.4	6.1
Free weights	4.8	4.1
Stationary bikes (net)	3.1	4.1
Elliptical trainers	2.7	4.4
Abdominal machines	2.4	3.7
Stair-climbers	1.9	2.9
Recumbent cycling	1.2	1.7
Swimming (laps)	1.0	1.5
Rowing machines	1.2	1.3
Aerobics (step)	0.3	1.9
Stationary cycling	1.0	0.8
Aerobics (low-impact)		1.5
Racquetball	1.0	0.5
Yoga/Tai chi	0.4	1.0
Aquatic exercise	0.3	1.1
Pilates training	0.2	1.0
Cardio kick boxing	0.3	0.8
Nordic ski machine	0.4	0.5
Aerobics (high-impact)		0.9
Tennis	0.2	0.1

Figure 15.3 Club members' use of equipment and participation in activities in 2005. Numbers are by the millions.

Reprinted, by permission, from IHRSA, 2006, *Profiles of success* (Boston: IHRSA), 17.

Taking Inventory

Unless you are opening a new facility and purchasing new equipment, it is important to begin the purchasing process with an **inventory** of current equipment. It is equally important to determine the condition of each inventory item. A complete list of equipment and its condition tells you not only what you need at the moment but also what you will need later. It is important to plan ahead when purchasing equipment for many reasons, including member needs, tax planning, program planning, and budget planning. Table 15.1 illustrates a sample format for taking inventory of equipment.

Consider replacing an item in the *poor* category of the equipment inventory when planning next year's budget. Flag the *average* category for ordering replacement parts to repair pads, cables, motors,

Table 15.1　**Sample Equipment Inventory**

Equipment	Good	Average	Poor
Treadmill 1	X		
Treadmill 2	X		
Treadmill 3			X
Cycle ergometer 1		X	
Cycle ergometer 2		X	
Cycle ergometer 3			X
Rower	X		
Mini trampoline		X	
Stair climber		X	
Ski trainer, downhill		X	
Ski trainer, cross-country	X		
Recumbent trainer		X	
Quadrupedal climber			X

Adapted, by permission, from R.W. Patton, et al., 1989, *Developing and managing health/fitness facilities* (Champaign, IL: Human Kinetics), 229.

and other equipment prone to breaking down. This inventory keeps track of equipment condition, ensures quality control of equipment condition, and permits a good system for budget planning.

Reviewing the Equipment Market

Taking stock of the available equipment on the market is no small task. It seems as if half the products at trade shows are computerized with a myriad of bells and whistles. One approach to avoiding purchasing errors in such a high-tech field is to hire an equipment consultant. A 1-hour consultation fee is money well spent to avoid costly mistakes, such as buying inappropriate, obsolete, or high-maintenance equipment. You can find consultants in the professional journals that advertise products, services, and consultants. Networking with colleagues in similar settings is usually a good referral source for consultants as well.

A second approach is to contact vendors who represent several product lines and who can offer opinions about available equipment. It is wise, however, to get a second vendor's opinion to account for the potential bias created by different profit-margin agreements between manufacturers and vendors. A third approach is to study the equipment on the market by spending time at trade shows and reading

the journals in which the equipment is advertised. Many facility managers and owners take pride in their expertise regarding exercise equipment. A better approach for internal surveillance of equipment on the market might be to assign staff members various areas of responsibility and get input from them before you make equipment purchases. A final approach is the trial method—vendors are frequently willing to place a piece of their equipment in your facility for a short trial period.

Writing Specifications

Once you have determined what kind of equipment you want in your facility, it is necessary to write down clear **specifications** to ensure that you get exactly what you want. Equally important, you want to get the equipment for the least amount of capital expenditure. If you use a bidding system to purchase equipment items, then precise specifications are essential. Poor specifications are often the greatest source of purchasing mistakes; avoid these mistakes by following the suggestions described here.

The first step in writing specifications is to get as much information about the desired equipment as possible. This can be your best defense against demanding club members, owners, and purchasing

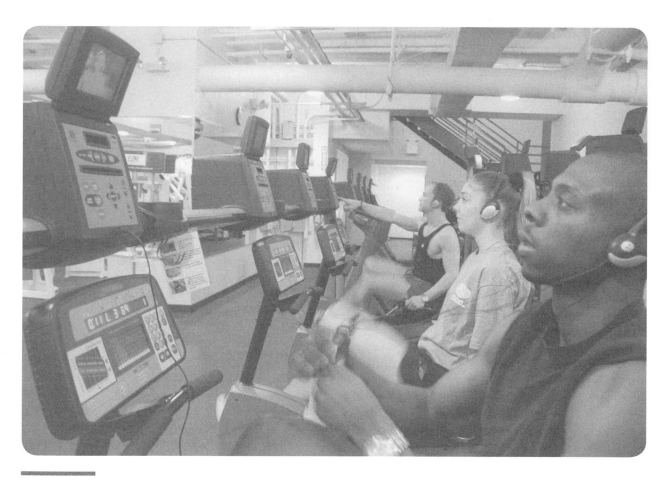

The purchase of high-tech exercise equipment with a lot of computerized features might warrant the hiring of an equipment consultant.
© Frances M. Roberts

agents. Armed with the details of the equipment features and construction, you can write lockout specifications for the equipment type and model you want to purchase. Lockout specifications are prepared in such a way that you are assured of getting a bid only on the product that you have decided is best for your needs. It is not sufficient to state merely that you want brand X, model B, or equivalent. Substitutions are commonplace among purchasing agents trying to save money. You may also be deceived by a lower bid and buy what turns out to be an undesirable piece of equipment.

Be specific! State the previous information, but be careful to add the size, color, materials, design, and performance characteristics that are necessary. In addition, it is helpful to contact the manufacturers of the equipment, because they can help you prepare the specifications. This lessens your chance of disappointment but does not always guarantee satisfaction. To guarantee satisfaction, provide all necessary information and indicate that no substitutions are acceptable. Unfortunately, this is not permissible in many purchasing environments unless the equipment is an accessory to a previously purchased item that needs an attachment.

There is a trend toward listing not only the brand, model, and detailed characteristics of a piece of equipment but also two or three acceptable brand names and models that meet the specifications. For example, you may list Nautilus single-station leg extension equipment in the description but include Body Masters and Cybex as acceptable alternatives that meet the specifications. This gives the bidder the flexibility to offer competitive **bids** on acceptable equipment.

The detailed specification of equipment can also intimidate potential bidders, however. If you write absolute lockout specifications without providing alternative brands and models, there will be little variability and competitiveness in the bid returns. Indeed, such tight specifications deny you the opportunity to learn of legitimate alternatives to the product. One approach to take when an acceptable alternative item comes in well under

Equipment Trends in the Fitness Industry

The following is a list of the most popular trends and things to consider when purchasing fitness equipment.

- Prospects and members don't want to work out in a fitness club that just has four walls and some equipment. Fitness clubs are selling a total experience, so the equipment needs to match the ambience and aesthetics of that club and its overall experience.
- Choose equipment that will help you sell your club. The equipment you choose has the potential to differentiate you from your competitors. Equipment should be nice to look at, nonthreatening, and easy to use.
- Your space should be used wisely. Choose equipment that meets your needs and uses up the least possible amount of space.
- Choose equipment that will be easy for members to get in and out of or on and off of.
- Consider adding equipment that matches the way your members move. This equipment is referred to as **user-defined equipment,** as opposed to **machine-defined equipment.**
- Any equipment that focuses on the mind–body connection (e.g., pieces related to yoga, Pilates, or tai chi) should be seriously considered due to the rapid increase in participation in these areas.
- User-defined or functional training equipment is a great way to add something new to your programs while also giving a more complete workout.
- Equipment companies are building machines with every piece of feedback imaginable. Make sure the feedback matches your membership base. For example, most users are not likely to use more than two or three programs, so having programs like a fitness test and a fitness challenge may not be necessary for the majority of clients.
- Technology constantly influences the fitness industry. Make sure you choose equipment with a proven track record and with technology that won't be out of date tomorrow.

In terms of programming, consider the following areas when making equipment purchases:

- Personal trainers offer a different level of service to your members. Specialized equipment for this area can also help your trainers sell their services.
- Group strength training is a popular form of group training that requires specialized equipment.
- Pilates and yoga continue to be major areas of growth. Consider adding specialized equipment in these areas.
- Wellness and rehabilitation continue to play an increasingly important role with fitness club members. This area, like the others, requires specialized equipment.

the price of the originally identified item is to ask for a nonreturnable sample that the staff and club members can field test before the final decision for equipment purchase is made. Many manufacturers will accommodate serious requests for field testing a new product or product line. Strategically placed products in prestigious facilities are frequently viewed by vendors and manufacturers as inexpensive advertising.

Here are some other things to consider while writing specifications:

- What type of equipment does your competition have? Will the equipment you choose act as differentiator or a competitive advantage? Will this equipment match the mission and overall atmosphere of the club?
- The type of equipment you choose will affect the type of clientele you attract. It is critical to take this into consideration before specifications are finalized. Will you be attempting to attract athletes, seniors, people with

disabilities, people focused on weight loss, or all of these?

- Though it can prolong the process, it is always a good idea to get feedback from staff and members on any equipment purchases.

The following is a list of general prices from the major commercial equipment suppliers as of 2007:

- Bikes (upright): $1,500 to $2,500
- Bikes (recumbent): $2,000 to $3,000
- Treadmills: $4,000 to $6,500
- Elliptical machines: $3,500 to $5,500
- Leg extension machines: $2,600
- Seated chest press machines: $2,800
- Shoulder press machines: $2,800
- Functional training system with dual adjustable cables: $3,600

Getting Bids

Getting bids is not a simple process. It is important to issue bids far enough in advance to attract responsible bidders. Cut-rate vendors, who may submit alternative and frequently unacceptable equipment bids, can often respond on a moment's notice.

THE BOTTOM LINE

The responsible bidder requires enough time to adequately evaluate the specifications, service, and warranty requirements of the bid, so be sure to develop a bidder list and get bids far enough in advance.

The bidder list is important to the purchasing process. It defines the competition you want in providing the needed equipment and sometimes the follow-up service of warranty performances. The list of criteria for suitable bidders should include history of delivery and service, dependability, size of inventory, financial stability, and promptness in financial matters. The bidder list is further reduced if you insist that the bidder provide installation, on-site repair, backup parts in stock, and a 2-year warranty. All these requirements add to the cost of the equipment; therefore, you should not impose them in the specifications unless they are necessary to the operation of your program. It is handy to put the bidder lists in a database management system that can update your list with minimum

effort. You may wish to notify the bidders on your list that you are accepting bids by using a form similar to the Notice to Bidders on page 328.

In some situations, there is a distinction between informal and formal bidding processes. Informal bidding frequently involves several phone calls to vendors on the bidder list, and this process can come down to repeated calls to negotiate the final price. Such arbitration is effective in many situations, if permitted. The sole proprietorship uses this process to the maximum since large-volume purchasing is not possible. The formal approach necessitates that a bid sheet be developed and distributed to a number of the vendors on the bidder list. Many large programs and institutional settings require that you ensure competitive bidding by having a minimum of three bidders. Even in a formal bidding process, it is customary to use informal communication at the end to maximize the competition between close bids. This ensures that you receive the lowest bid.

The lowest bidder usually gets the contract to supply the equipment. After all, the competitive process was established to get the lowest price for tightly specified equipment. Often the lowest bidders will have cut their profit margin to get your bid, and thus they will be less likely to overwhelm you with follow-up service calls if there is little profit in the offing. This is one reason why service is frequently built into the bidding process.

Another factor that influences bid selection is the proximity and history of the bidders. A local bidder with whom you have had a good relationship over the years might be selected over an outsider with whom you have never done business. However, exceptions to accepting anything but low bids are rare, and you should apprise your local vendor of being underbid. If you ever get in the habit of buying from one vendor, you can forget competitive bidding. Temper your decisions about going with the low bidder only with good judgment. If everything is equal, stay with a standardized equipment line. The more equipment you have from a single manufacturer or vendor, the better. Some other factors to consider in choosing a vendor are as follows:

- Your relationship with the vendor
- Vendor's years in business
- References from other installations
- Sales rep's service
- Training after sales (on-site training, audiovisual tools, use and maintenance)

Notice to Bidders

The Board of Education of _____ School District

No. _____ of the town(s) of _____ popularly

known as_____ , (in accordance with Section 103 of

Article 5-A of the General Municipal Law) hereby invites the submission of sealed bids on

_____ for use in the schools of the district. Bids will be

received until _____ on the _____ day of _____ , _____ ,
                 (hour)   (date)   (month)   (year)

at _____ at which time and place all bids will be

publicly opened. Specifications and bid form may be obtained at the same office. The Board of Education

reserves the right to reject all bids. Any bid submitted will be binding for _____ days

subsequent to the date of bid opening.

Board of Education _____ School District No. _____

of the Town(s) of _____ County(ies) of _____

By _____ _____
                (Purchasing agent)   (Date)

From M. Bates, 2008, *Health Fitness Management*, 2nd ed. (Champaign, IL: Human Kinetics).

As a rule of thumb, it is always in your best interest to get at least three bids for any major equipment purchases. Rushing to buy something you need because of an unexpected situation is likely to cost more money in the long run.

Purchasing the Equipment

For institutions that must adhere to legal procedures and policies, the process becomes more complicated than a simple phone call from the sole proprietor of a local fitness center. In any event, the purchasing process should begin well in advance of the need for equipment, and it should follow a consistent order of procedures. The following procedures are tailored to a medium-size institutional setting, but they are applicable to all settings:

1. *Initiation.* A request is made to the manager to fulfill, augment, supplement, or improve the program.

2. *Request review.* Approve or reject the request after careful consideration of needs and budget.

3. *Budget review.* Review the request and, if approved, assign a code number to the equipment item in the identified budget category.

4. *Specifications prepared.* Prepare detailed specifications and make them available to vendors.

5. *Bid evaluation.* Evaluate bids to ensure quality requirements and examine the lower bids to make recommendations for purchase.

6. *Development of purchase order.* Develop **purchase orders** and send them to the vendor.

7. *Payment.* Cut the check and mail it on delivery and performance of contract.

8. *Payment schedule.* The general rule is 50% down and 50% on receipt of equipment.

Sometimes you can arrange cash on delivery (COD). Plan on freight, installation, and taxes being added to the cost. Withhold 10% of the payment for 30 days to encourage prompt, effective installation.

Maintaining Exercise Equipment

Once you have purchased the equipment, the endless process of maintenance begins. The stress of 500 to 1,000 users per day on the equipment in a facility is considerable. The life span of equipment parts and materials can be short if you do not employ proper maintenance procedures.

Internal Maintenance

The day-to-day maintenance of equipment is considered internal maintenance. Establish external maintenance through contractual agreements with vendors and professional service companies that maintain exercise equipment in a given service area. The internal maintenance of equipment is critical because it limits the amount of external service needed and preempts or delays costly breakdowns. Moreover, many internal maintenance procedures are also considered cleaning procedures. Cleanliness is imperative in the health and fitness business and cannot be overemphasized. Therefore, internal maintenance must be a highly organized and ongoing process. Checklist for Internal Maintenance of Exercise Programs on page 330 gives equipment maintenance guidelines to follow for internally maintaining equipment. (See chapter 14 for more on maintenance.)

Note that some vendors assist buyers with maintenance of exercise equipment. For example, in-service training is available from many vendors to train staff in the care and service of their products. Some vendors provide national hotlines to address concerns about maintenance or emergency parts. A few vendors notify buyers when warranty periods are about to expire and offer extended maintenance contracts.

External Maintenance

Consider the first aspect of external maintenance before the purchase: Don't buy anything you can't get repaired. If the equipment is mechanical, anticipate problems in advance and plan on breakdowns. Pay attention to warranty conditions and durations and the location of the nearest service center. Warranty conditions are calculated from the average amount of maintenance-free service for a given product; therefore, expect service demands to increase when the warranty expires. Location of service centers in the immediate area is a favorable factor when buying a product.

Another external maintenance consideration is the service contract. In large metropolitan areas, companies are emerging to meet the equipment service needs of the health and fitness profession. You can contract any equipment services, including many internal maintenance procedures identified. The fees vary depending on the degree and amount of services required.

In most settings your staff will have some responsibilities in the areas of internal and external maintenance. These responsibilities could range from notifying the manager when a piece of equipment breaks down to having a daily cleaning schedule that all staff are responsible for. Regardless of your situation, it is critical to keep staff accountable in these areas just as you would keep staff accountable for meeting their job responsibilities in other areas of the club.

Maintaining Support Equipment

There are numerous other types of equipment that most health and fitness facilities must have to operate their programs—laundry equipment, office equipment, fitness testing equipment, health promotion items, and various sport and games apparatuses, to mention a few.

Laundry

Many fitness programs need equipment to launder uniforms and towels. Although some settings, such as hospital-based facilities, can farm out their laundry services to other departments within the organization, most health and fitness settings perform their laundry in-house. Larger operations are now using washer-extractors. These are heavy-duty units that take up to 125 pounds (56.5 kilograms) and are capable of almost completely drying the materials by spinning the loads at 300 g. Moreover, most newer units have advanced programmable microprocessors that simplify operations and expand their capabilities.

The net effect of this process is that large laundry loads can be handled efficiently, and the materials come out of the spin cycle damp but not wet. This reduces the amount of drying time and, consequently, the need for as many dryers. Although washer-extractors are more expensive than traditional washing

Checklist for Internal Maintenance of Exercise Programs

Equipment frames

_____Tighten all nuts and bolts.

_____Use chrome polish on chrome as glass cleaner shows fingerprints.

_____Use car polish on painted surfaces.

_____Use fine steel wool to remove rust; then use nonabrasive polish.

Upholstery

_____Clean daily with upholstery cleaner. Wipe frequently with warm water and mild soap.

_____Remove pad for repair at first sign of hairline crack.

_____Have backup pads available for high-use equipment.

_____Wax upholstery monthly with hard floor wax.

_____Rotate cushions if possible.

_____Remove chewing gum by carefully scraping and wiping with kerosene.

_____Remove ball point ink with rubbing alcohol. Remove shoe polish or paint with kerosene or turpentine and rinse.

Pulley systems

_____Inspect all parts and connections regularly.

_____Replace damaged pulleys and frayed cables immediately.

_____Adjust cables and chains regularly for proper tension.

_____Watch for and correct slack developing in pulley systems.

_____Wipe chains and cables regularly with oiled cloth.

_____Don't spray systems with oil as it will drip onto floor or soil clothes.

Treadmills

_____Adjust rear drums to ensure proper belt tracking.

_____Put dance wax between belt and platform bed periodically.

_____Lubricate all moving parts regularly, except sealed bearings.

_____Mount control panel away from moving parts if possible, as vibrations are a major cause of control panel repairs.

_____Clean treadmill belt regularly with mild soap and water.

_____Inspect electrical cords and plugs regularly; replace as needed.

_____Locate equipment near electrical outlets to avoid injury to members and damage to equipment.

Bicycle ergometers

_____Inspect electrical cords and plugs regularly; replace as needed.

_____Clean upholstery and frames daily with mild soap and water.

_____Wax upholstery periodically with a hard wax.

_____Polish painted surfaces periodically with car wax.

From M. Bates, 2008, *Health Fitness Management*, 2nd ed. (Champaign, IL: Human Kinetics).

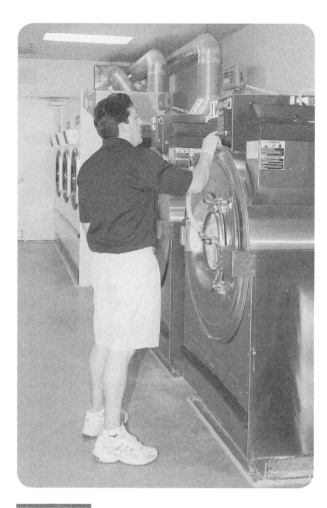

In addition to a club's exercise equipment, other types of equipment will have to be maintained. Most clubs have in-house laundry facilities for uniforms and towels.
© Will & Lisa Funk/Alpine Aperture

machines, they have been proven cost effective in that they are durable, require about half the total number of washers and dryers needed in a traditional laundry room, and conserve energy costs. The space recommendation of 150 to 300 square feet (14-28 square meters) when standard washers and dryers are used in the laundry area is reduced by more than half. Consequently, with building and maintenance costs rising, the trend is toward smaller, more compact laundry areas with more efficient and durable equipment.

Office Equipment

Most fitness clubs have business offices of varying sizes. Once again, corporate and clinical programs may defer some office functions to other places within their organization. Commercial programs dealing with most of the business concerns will normally require more office equipment than most other settings. Some equipment that supports office functions includes the following:

- Telephone systems
- Desks and chairs
- Computers
- Postage meters
- Fax modems
- Card readers
- Printers
- Pager systems
- Answering systems
- Lounge furniture
- Scanners
- Copiers

As business and communication technology inevitably expands, so will the need for increased office equipment.

Locker-Room Equipment

The locker room should provide approximately 15 to 25 square feet (1.4-2.3 square meters) of space for each person expected to use the locker room at any time. This range is due to the different locker configurations and equipment used in the environment. In most instances, no more than 10% to 15% of members will be occupying the locker room at any one time; therefore, there should be enough lockers to accommodate this load. If the facility provides permanent rental lockers, there should be enough lockers to handle 70% to 85% of the users, with some additional daily-use lockers for other members and guests.

Facilities should have an adequate number of showers in the locker room to handle expected usage; a shower total of approximately 1% of the total membership is usually adequate (e.g., for 2,000 members there should be a total of 20 showers), although different regions will have specific standards. An architect or club designer will be able to give you specific information on your area. Most facilities have abandoned gang shower arrangements for single-stall setups. Other equipment, such as hair dryers and grooming accessories, are frequently provided in locker rooms as well.

Space for Fitness Testing, Health Promotion, and Wellness

For certain programs, the availability of space can be classified as an equipment consideration. Allocate enough space and equipment for the fitness testing, health promotion, and wellness areas to perform their expected functions. Table 15.2 gives some guidelines about the type and amount of space as well as the equipment requirements for fitness testing, health promotion, and wellness programs.

Gymnasium

A gymnasium is frequently provided in health and fitness facilities. The minimum space needed for a gymnasium is a full-size basketball court of 50 by 84 feet (15 by 25.5 meters) with at least 5 feet (1.5 meters) of unobstructed area around the court. Consider overlapping markings for basketball, volleyball, and badminton along with appropriate equipment for each sport. Also consider wall clocks and scoreboards. Ceiling heights of at least 22 feet (7 meters) are the minimum in these spaces. If you provide spectator seating, you need 3 square feet (.3 square meter) per spectator; portable bleachers can be a solution to spectator seating. You also need a variety of equipment to accommodate the activities in this area.

There are a host of other equipment concerns that we could address for health and fitness programs. We address some of these equipment needs elsewhere in the book, including equipment in areas such as spas, child care, and aquatics, but for now you have an idea of the overall considerations involved in choosing equipment.

Table 15.2 Space and Equipment Needs for Fitness Testing, Health Promotion, and Wellness Programs

Type of space	Amount of space	Equipment needed
Fitness testing	120-180 ft² (11-17 m²)	Bicycle ergometer or treadmill, skinfold caliper, anthropometric tapes, sit-and-reach bench or goniometers, tensiometers or strength equipment, BP equipment, scales
Counseling room	90-120 ft² (8-11 m²)	Office furniture
Seminar room	20 ft² (2 m²) per person	Audiovisual equipment, tables, chairs

KEY TERMS

bids

extended warranties

inventory

machine-defined equipment

purchase orders

safe place statutes

selectorized equipment

specifications

user-defined equipment

warranties

REFERENCES AND RECOMMENDED READINGS

American College of Sports Medicine (ACSM). 2006. *ACSM's health/fitness facility standards and guidelines.* Champaign, IL: Human Kinetics.

Broadhag, K. 2006. Extended warranty protection? *Fitness Management,* Feb. 2006.

International Health, Racquet, and Sportsclub Association (IHRSA). 2006. *Profiles of success: Industry data survey of the health and fitness club industry.* Boston: IHRSA.

———. 1997. *Health club trend report.* Boston: IHRSA.

[sixteen]

Understanding Legal and Insurance Issues

John Wolohan

LEARNING OBJECTIVES

After studying this chapter, the reader will be able to

- identify the legal duty that health and fitness providers owe their clients,
- discuss the tort of negligence and its defenses,
- recognize potential danger areas in health and fitness clubs,
- explain the importance of contract law to health and fitness providers,
- understand the importance of employment law in managing employees, and
- discuss the importance of insurance to clubs.

Nicole Wolf, a 43-year-old school teacher, came to a fitness center to use the lap pool as part of a physical therapy and rehabilitation program. Upon entering the facility, Wolf was assisted at the front desk by an employee and informed that because she was not a member of the center, she was required to fill out a guest registration card and pay a fee before swimming. Figure 16.1 shows the guest registration card.

Soon after Wolf began swimming, a club employee who was walking into the pool area spotted her lying motionless underwater near the bottom of the pool. The employee yelled to the lifeguard on duty, who pulled her from the pool and administered CPR. Wolf died the next day and drowning was listed as the official cause of death on the coroner's report.

Her only child has just filed a wrongful death action against the fitness center, claiming that the center was negligent in the operation of the pool facility and that the negligence of its employees caused Wolf's death. Consider these questions:

- Were the actions of the fitness center employees negligent?
- Are there any defenses?
- Is the waiver valid?
- If so, what effect does it have on the case?
- If not, what can be done to correct the waiver?

Guest Registration

Name _____

Address _____

City _____   State _____

Zip code _____   Home phone _____

Reason for visit _____

How did you hear of the fitness center? _____

I would like membership information (circle one):
Yes   No

Waiver Release Statement
I agree to assume all liability for myself without regard to fault while at the fitness center. I further agree to hold harmless the fitness center or any of its employees for any conditions or injury that may result to myself while at the fitness center. I have read the foregoing and understand its contents.

Signed _____

Date _____

From M. Bates, 2008, *Health Fitness Management*, 2nd ed. (Champaign, IL: Human Kinetics).

Figure 16.1 Guest registration card that includes a waiver release statement. Is this particular waiver valid?

As this scenario demonstrates, it is essential that health and fitness managers have at least a basic understanding of certain legal principles. The purpose of this chapter is to provide managers with a basic understanding of the law as it relates to managing and operating a facility.

After reading this chapter, managers should be able to identify and evaluate the risks involved in operating a health and fitness facility and determine when to obtain formal legal advice from competent counsel. In order to assist in identifying potential liability, a Legal Liability Checklist is included below. Please note that the checklist is not intended to cover every legal area but to provide a framework for identifying major areas of risk.

Although the purpose of this chapter is to provide health and fitness managers with a basic understanding of the law, it is not meant to take the place of an attorney. Managers must seek competent legal counsel for periodic review of any documents or contracts used by the organization and for help with any legal questions that may arise.

Civil Versus Criminal Liability

The difference between **civil liability** and **criminal liability** lies in the interests affected and in the remedy afforded (Keeton et al. 1984). In criminal law, a crime has been committed against society, and the state, as the protector of society, is responsible for bringing any criminal prosecution. The purpose of criminal law, therefore, is to protect society by punishing antisocial behavior. Civil cases, however, are filed by the injured party with the primary purpose of recovering money damages against the person who caused the injury. The purpose of civil cases, therefore, is to compensate the injured party by the payment of money. Even though the same action can give rise to both criminal and civil liabilities, a tort or civil wrong is legally not a crime.

For example, if during a basketball game, one of the players intentionally punched another player and caused physical injury, the injured party could file a civil lawsuit (tort of battery) to recover any damages, such as medical costs, pain and suffering, and lost wages. In addition, the state could also file a separate criminal complaint resulting in jail or probation.

Legal Liability Checklist

- Do professional staff have appropriate credentials?
- Are all staff CPR certified?
- Are adequate staff available in the exercise and activity areas?
- Do all new members go through a thorough orientation program?
- Are safety notices clearly posted on or near all equipment?
- Are all public areas regularly inspected for unsafe conditions?
- Is all equipment inspected regularly?
- Is a standard procedure in place to respond to discovery of unsafe equipment or dangerous conditions?
- Are safety inspection records documented and kept current?
- Has equipment layout been evaluated to determine safety concerns related to location and arrangement?
- Are internal and external lighting adequate to enhance safety?
- Is a standard health and fitness screening protocol used to check for unsafe medical conditions?
- Does the facility have a written emergency plan available for review?
- Does the facility have adequate first aid supplies that are checked and refreshed regularly?
- Are all activity areas free from environmental hazards?
- Does the organization have written personnel policies that are available to all employees?
- Has the organization provided training for all staff in the areas of discrimination and harassment?
- Does management have clear procedures for responding to and documenting violations of personnel policy?
- Do all staff participate in safety training and review sessions for emergency procedures?
- Is a formal policy in place for making statements on behalf of the organization?

Tort Law

Generally, a **tort** is a private or civil wrong or injury, other than a breach of contract, committed upon a person or property as the result of another person's conduct. The three main areas of tort law that health and fitness managers need to be aware of are negligence, intentional torts, and reckless misconduct.

Negligence

The most common tort in the health and fitness industry is the **negligence tort.** Negligence is an unintentional tort that is based on the legal theory that people are required to act in a way that avoids creating an unreasonable risk to others (Schubert, Smith, and Trentadue 1986). Therefore, any conduct or action that falls below this standard and creates an unreasonable risk is considered negligence. In determining whether the conduct was reasonable, the courts use what is known as a *reasonable person test.* The reasonable person test examines whether a reasonable, prudent person in the same circumstances would have acted in the same manner.

In order to establish a claim of negligence, a person must establish all four of the following elements:

- Duty of care
- Breach of duty
- Causation
- Damages

Duty of care refers to the standard of care the law has established for the protection of others (Schubert et al. 1986). In determining whether one person owes another a duty of care, there needs to be a special relationship between the parties. Some examples of relationships in a health and fitness setting that create a legal duty of care include employer to employee; employer or employee to guest or member; and teacher, coach, or trainer to student.

The law of negligence does not require that you ensure the safety of every person using the facility from every conceivable injury; it merely requires that you do not create an unreasonable risk and that you protect people from risks that are foreseeable. If the risk is not foreseeable, there is no liability. People breach their duty of care when they create an unreasonable risk of injury. Therefore, if someone acts in a way that a reasonable, prudent person under the same circumstances would not, that person has breached the duty of care.

The standard of care is based on the qualifications or certification of a prudent professional in that industry, not on the individual's professional experience. Everyone, no matter how experienced or inexperienced, must meet the same standard of care. In determining the appropriate standard of care for the health and fitness industry, it is important to look at the guidelines developed and published by the AHA, ACSM, American Medical Association (AMA), and American Physical Therapy Association (APTA). Where appropriate, these standards should be incorporated into the written policies of the organization, including employee manuals, job descriptions, and training procedures.

Once injured parties are able to establish that the defendant breached their duty of care, they still must show that the conduct actually caused the injury. Causation is established when there is a causal connection between the negligent conduct and the injury.

The final element of any negligence claim is damages—the person must also suffer some form of injury or damages. In awarding damages, the court will look at lost wages, pain and suffering, and medical expenses. In extreme cases, the court can also award punitive damages, which are designed to punish the party that caused the injury. If there is no injury, there is no liability.

THE BOTTOM LINE

Negligence, the most common tort in the health and fitness industry, is based on the legal theory that people are required to avoid creating an unreasonable risk to others.

Legal Status of Guests, Members, and Program Participants

To determine the duty of care that health and fitness facilities owe people using the facility, the courts examine the relationship between the user and the facility. These relationships can be divided into four groups: invitee, licensee, trespasser, and recreational user (van der Smissen 2004).

Invitees An **invitee** is any person whose presence produces a direct or indirect economic gain for the facility operator (Keeton et al. 1984). Members and guests of health and fitness facilities are generally classified as invitees. As a result, club operators have a legal duty or obligation to exercise reasonable care to keep members or guests safe, to protect them from unreasonable risk, and to avoid acts that can create risks. To meet the duty of care, the owner or occupier

1. must warn of any known defects on the premises,
2. is responsible for any unknown defects that could reasonably be discovered, and
3. must make the premises safe and free from such defects or dangers.

The theory behind this rule is that the owner or occupier of the facility is in the best position to discover and control any risks or hazards. It is essential, therefore, that health and fitness managers conduct frequent facility and equipment inspections.

Licensee A licensee is any person who has the permission or consent of the operator to use the facility but provides no real or expected benefit to the facility owner. Unlike with an invitee, the facility owner has no duty or obligation to inspect the premises to discover dangers or to give any warnings of obvious dangers (Keeton et al. 1984).

Trespasser A trespasser is any person who enters the facility without the permission of the operator. Generally, since no consent has been given to use the facility, the only obligation of the facility owner or operator is to refrain from any intentional conduct that would cause injury to the trespasser (Keeton et al. 1984).

Recreational User A **recreational user** is any person who is on the premise specifically for recreational purposes. Generally, the owner's only obligation is to provide a warning of any known concealed danger that would not be apparent to the recreational user. The owner has no duty to warn of open and obvious hazards or of conditions that are unknown to the owner (Wolohan 2004). (For more information on recreational users, see Immunity on page 339.)

THE BOTTOM LINE

The relationship between the user and the facility determines the duty of care that health and fitness facilities owe to people using the facility.

Potential Danger Areas

Since providing a safe facility is the responsibility of the possessor or occupier of the property, health and fitness managers must take reasonable steps to protect members from any potential dangers. The follow are just some of the potential danger areas.

Floor Surfaces, Preparations, and Coverings As stated, since people using a club are invitees, health and fitness managers have an obligation to exercise reasonable care to keep them safe and to protect them from unreasonable risks. As a result of this duty, managers need to provide proper floor surfaces throughout the facility to avoid what are commonly called *slip-and-fall situations*. All slippery, oily, overwaxed, wet, dusty, or damaged floors must be cleaned or repaired before they cause serious falls, collisions, or other related injuries.

Ignorance of the defect is no defense, either. Since managers have a duty to inspect for dangerous conditions, it is essential that, upon discovering a dangerous situation, the club immediately either correct the condition or limit access to the location until correcting the problem.

Equipment Health and fitness managers also have a legal duty to ensure that the equipment used in the facility is safe for its intended purpose. Therefore, it is critical that someone at the facility visually

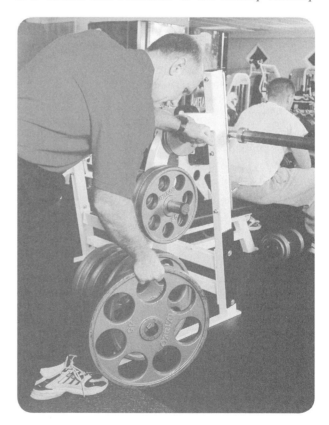

Returning weight plates to weight trees after use is one way to reduce physical hazards in health and fitness clubs.

inspect the equipment on a daily basis and replace or remove any equipment that is in disrepair or defective.

Besides inspecting the equipment, employees must teach members or anyone else using the equipment how to use it. This should be done as part of a new-member orientation, at the conclusion of which new members should sign an acknowledgment that they were provided proper instructions and warnings, and facilities should also post the instructions. By posting instructions that are clear, concise, and easily understood in an area that is visible to all users, managers ensure consistent and accurate communication of not only the instructions but also adequate warnings of reasonably foreseeable and known risks.

Equipment Design or Manufacturing Defects   Since most, if not all, of the equipment used in a facility is not designed, manufactured, or built by program personnel, liability for injuries due to defective equipment will usually rest with the equipment manufacturers under the theory of product liability. However, even though product liability claims are usually against the manufacturers or sellers of the equipment, heath and fitness organizations are not excused from inspecting the equipment, testing it for defects, and replacing any defective parts.

Fitness Activities   In addition to providing proper instructions on how to use equipment, facilities also have an obligation to provide adequate supervision during fitness activities and to warn people of any risks associated with an activity. In assessing the type of warnings necessary for a particular activity, managers must assess the nature of the activity and the skills and abilities needed in order to successfully and safely participate in the activity. For example, if the activity is difficult or potentially dangerous, direct supervision by experienced professionals is required. If, on the other hand, the activity is simple and safe, less direct supervision is required. It is the duty of the person supervising the activity to identify the inherent risks of the activity and warn the participant of these risks.

Emergency Medical Care   Another potential problem area is medical care. Generally, health and fitness clubs have a duty to provide timely and reasonable medical assistance. Additionally, they have a duty to refrain from taking any actions that could aggravate the injury. This means that the operator has to be able to recognize when serious injury has occurred (Wong 2002).

Just as in supervision, the definition of reasonable medical care depends on the type of activity

being performed. In addition, the duty to provide emergency care not only includes caring for injuries once they occur but also preparing for emergency care before the activity. For example, although a club does not need to have an ambulance in the parking lot, it does need to be able to contact one quickly in an emergency situation.

Legal Documents   One of the best ways to protect your organization in the event of an injury is to keep detailed, written records on everything from facility and equipment repairs and maintenance to injury and treatment reports. In the case of a lawsuit, these records can be vital in demonstrating that the organization acted reasonably.

Vicarious Liability   The owners and managers of health and fitness facilities need to be aware that under the theory of **vicarious liability,** they can be held accountable for the negligent actions of their employees.

There are three main exceptions to this rule.

1. Employers are generally not liable for the negligence of independent contractors, unless they closely supervise the contractor's activities.
2. Employers are generally not liable for any intentional torts committed by employees.
3. Employers are generally not liable for employee conduct that is outside the scope of employment.

Defenses of Negligence

Even if someone is injured, a number of defenses are available to clubs. Following are five of the most common defenses:

1. Assumption of risk
2. Agreements to participate
3. Waivers
4. Immunity
5. Contributory negligence

Assumption of Risk   Under the theory of **assumption of risk,** health and fitness managers are not liable for injuries resulting from risks that are inherent to the activity. In order for assumption of risk to apply, a person must voluntarily participate in an activity, knowing the inherent risks involved in an activity or event.

As a general rule, the assumption of risk defenses do not apply to minors (children under the age of 18). Therefore, although there are limited exceptions to this rule, such as if a minor is highly experienced in an activity, managers should not depend on assumption of risk when working with minors.

Agreements to Participate   One way to strengthen the assumption of risk defense is through the use of an agreement to participate. The **agreement to participate**, which is different from a waiver, is a document that helps managers inform participants of the nature of the activity, the risks involved in the activity, and the behaviors expected of the participant (Cotten and Cotten 2004).

Waivers   A **waiver** is a written contract between the facility or service provider and a club member or guest in which the person using the facility or services agrees to relinquish the right to pursue legal action in the event of an injury caused by the negligence of the provider.

Though waivers are not valid in Louisiana, New Mexico, Montana, and Virginia, in all other states a well-written, properly administered waiver voluntarily signed by an adult is an effective tool in protecting health and fitness facilities and providers from liability for ordinary negligence (Wolohan 2005).

The laws in each state are different; however, the following 12 guidelines should be used when developing a waiver (Cotten and Cotten 2004).

1. The document should be titled properly: "Waiver" or "Waiver of Liability."

2. The font size should be at least 10 point.

3. The language should be clear and unambiguous.

4. The waiver should be one page.

5. The waiver should stand alone and not be part of another document.

6. Since the waiver is designed to excuse negligence, the word *negligence* should be used in the document.

7. The waiver should not contain any fraudulent statements.

8. Since a waiver is a contract, it should state something like, "In consideration for waiving the right to sue for negligence, the signer is given the right to use the facility and equipment."

9. The waiver should specify the parties covered under the waiver.

10. The waiver should contain information covering the inherent risks of activity.

11. The waiver should include a statement that the signer understands the risks and assumes responsibility for the risks.

12. The waiver should include a statement indicating that the signer read the document.

Just as with assumption of risk, as a general rule waivers are not enforceable against minors. Due to the value of waivers in showing that the parties were aware of the risks associated with the activity, even if you live in a state where waivers are unenforceable due to public policy or other reasons, you should still require minors and their parents to sign waivers when they participate in potentially dangerous activities.

Immunity   Traditionally, there were two types of immunity: sovereign immunity, which prevents an injured party from suing the government or its political subdivisions without consent, and charitable immunity, which prevents an injured party from suing charitable organizations. Due to the hardship the immunities caused to the injured people, most states have modified or abolished the two traditional immunities.

While most states have modified or abolished the two traditional immunities, every state has created another immunity in an effort to open up more land for recreational use. The immunity, also called a recreational user statute, is designed to encourage landowners to open their property to the public for recreational use by giving them immunity from liability if someone is injured while on the property for recreation.

Each state has its own variation of recreational user statute, but most statutes have four common characteristics (Wolohan 2004):

1. *Type of property.* Originally, immunity was designed to protect private landowners only. In some states, however, the owners of public lands (i.e., local, state, and federal government agencies) are also afforded immunity.

2. *Free use of property.* Landowners cannot charge a fee for people to use the premises.

3. *Condition of property.* The land must be unimproved or undeveloped rural land retained in its natural condition.

4. *Obligations of the landowner.* The owner's only obligation is to provide a warning for any known concealed danger that would not be apparent to the recreational user.

In addition to recreational user statutes, most states have also enacted volunteer immunity statutes with the goal of protecting people who volunteer with nonprofit organizations from liability for negligence.

Contributory Negligence Under contributory negligence, if the injured person's conduct contributed in any way to the injury, no matter how small, the person is barred from recovering any damages. Due to the injustices caused by the rule, most states replaced it with comparative negligence. Under comparative negligence, damages are awarded according the person's degree of negligence or fault. For example, if a person was 5% at fault in the injury, the courts will reduce the amount received in damages by 5%.

Only four states (Alabama, Maryland, North Carolina, and Virginia) plus the District of Columbia still use contributory negligence as a valid defense. The rest of the states have adopted a form of comparative negligence either by statute or judicial decisions (Robertson, Powers, Anderson, and Wellborn 2004).

Intentional Torts

Intentional torts, as the name implies, arise out of an intentional or willful action. For example, if a club member violently and intentionally strikes another member during an argument, the violent member has committed the intentional tort of battery. The legal remedy is to force the violent member to pay for any damage caused and possibly impose punitive damages to deter the activity from being repeated. Other intentional torts include assault (an apprehension of immediate harm), slander (false and defamatory verbal statements), libel (false and defamatory written statements), fraud (intentionally misleading someone to cause a financial loss), false imprisonment (wrongful detention), trespass (unlawful use or injury of property), and conversion (unlawful taking and keeping of property).

Reckless Misconduct

Although not as common as negligence or intentional torts, the tort of **reckless misconduct** can be important when someone is injured while participating in group activities. For example, if a softball player intentionally slides into another player in an attempt to break up the play even though sliding is not permitted, the person who slid is said to have acted with reckless disregard for the safety of the other person. The key to any reckless misconduct is that the intentional action, especially if it is in violation of an established and known safety rule, must be done in a reckless, willful, or wanton manner. The conduct is not an intentional tort, however, since it is usually performed with no intent to harm or touch.

Contracts

Health and fitness managers use **contracts** on almost a daily basis. An exhaustive discussion of contract law is well beyond the scope of this brief chapter; the following section simply outlines certain essential concepts of contract law.

Contract Essentials

A contract is "a promise, or set of promises, for breach of which the law gives a remedy, or the performance of which the law in some way recognizes as a duty" (Restatement of Contracts 1979). However, since not all promises are contracts, it is important to understand how a promise is transformed into a legally binding contract. In order for a promise to become a valid contract, it must contain the following five elements:

1. Offer
2. Acceptance
3. Consideration
4. Intent
5. Legality

An offer is a conditional promise made by one party, the offeror, to another party, the offeree, to do or refrain from doing something in the future (Calamari and Perillo 1998). To be valid, an offer usually must contain the parties involved, the subject matter, the time and place for performance, and the price or consideration to be paid.

In order for the offer to be binding, the offeree must accept the offer. Acceptance must be made in some positive form, whether in words or by conduct, and can only be made by the party to whom the offer was made. If an offer has been made and the offeree proposes to change one of the terms, such a counteroffer is considered a rejection of the original offer. In addition, an offer may no longer be accepted by the offeree in circumstances where the offer has lapsed due to time or has been revoked by the offeror, or when either of the parties dies or loses mental capacity before acceptance (Calamari and Perillo 1998).

The next element of a valid contract is consideration. Consideration is the mutual exchange of value that induces a party to enter into a contract and may include money, services, goods, or any other thing of value. Therefore, although the parties may exchange promises, any agreement that does not contain a mutual exchange of value is void for lack of consideration. The final two elements require that all the parties have a genuine intent to create an enforceable contract and that the performance involved in the contract is for legal activity or does not violate public policy.

Although technically not a required element for a valid contract, the legal capacity of a person can also affect the enforceability of a contract. For example, the law seeks to protect people who lack the capacity to understand the essential terms of the contract by making such contracts, except for necessaries, voidable at the individuals' option but enforceable by them against the other contracting party.

The courts generally consider that minors and other people with diminished mental capacity lack the ability, competence, or capacity to enter into contracts. As a result, minors may often disregard their promises with impunity, as, for example, when a minor signs a waiver agreeing to relinquish the right to pursue legal action against a service provider. As discussed previously, in most circumstances, the waiver will be ineffective in shielding the provider from suit by the minor.

Finally, most contracts do not need to be in writing to be legally enforceable, but the law does require that certain contracts must always be in writing. The three areas most relevant to health and fitness managers include

1. contracts involving the sale, mortgage, or lease of an interest in land (e.g., facility lease agreements, land purchases);
2. contracts that cannot be performed within 1 year from the date of their making (e.g., long-term vendor or employment contracts); and
3. contracts for the sale of goods for $500 or more.

As a matter of good business practice, managers should put all contracts in writing in order to reduce future problems and misunderstandings over the actual terms of the contract.

THE BOTTOM LINE

A contract is a promise that the law recognizes as a duty. However, not all promises are contracts, so it is important to understand what turns a promise into a legally binding contract.

Types of Contracts

Some of the most common contracts found in the health and fitness industry include membership,

independent contractor, vendor, and employment contracts.

Membership Agreements

All relationships between a health and fitness organization and its members are based on contracts. This is true whether a written, signed agreement exists or members are merely paying a daily entry fee each time they visit the facility.

Because of the wide range of health and fitness settings, it is difficult to generalize about membership contract requirements. Some states have passed specific laws requiring fitness clubs to include certain contract terms related to duration of the contract, cancellation of the contract, refund of deposits, automatic billing to checking accounts and credit cards, and transferability of the contract. Because these laws are enacted at the state level, managers must obtain copies of their state's laws and regulations related to spas, fitness centers, and health clubs.

In general, it is to the mutual benefit of the health and fitness organization and the member to have a clearly worded, complete written agreement that identifies the obligations of the organization and the member. See the membership agreement on pages 342-344 for a sample agreement. Examples of issues that a membership contract should address include the following:

- Names and addresses of the parties
- Duration of the contract with clearly stated starting and ending dates
- Signatures and dates
- Location of the facilities; specific facility access concerns such as time of day, days of the week; facility use limitations (i.e., tennis only, cardiorespiratory areas only, classes only)
- Membership fees and terms of payment
- Rights, penalties, and fees associated with cancellation or transferability
- Renewal options
- Direct billing terms for checking accounts or credit cards

In addition, the agreement should contain the following obligations of members:

- Pay amounts due in a timely manner.
- Abide by all rules and regulations.
- Operate equipment safely and cautiously.

Membership # _____

Membership Agreement Part I

_____ / _____ / _____ / _____ / _____
Name   Birth Date   Marital Status   Spouse's Name   Birth Date

_____ / _____ / _____ / _____
Address   Home Phone   Teen 1 Name   Birth Date

_____ / _____ / _____ / _____ / _____
City   State   Zip   Business Phone   Teen 2 Name   Birth Date

_____ / _____
Occupation/Employer   E-mail

_____
How did you hear about us?

_____ / _____
Emergency Contact   Emergency Phone Number

Buyer's Right to Cancel

If you wish to cancel your membership, you may cancel by delivering in person or via certified mail, return receipt requested, written notice to the Club. The notice must say that you do not wish to be bound by the Membership Agreement and must be delivered or mailed before 12-midnight of the third business day after opening or if opened, by the 3rd business day after you sign and receive a copy of the Agreement. The notice must be delivered or mailed to the Club. In some cases, as described in the Agreement, you may also cancel your membership if you sign the Agreement before the Club was completed, if the Club moves or goes out of business, if you become permanently disabled, or if you move from within a 30-mile radius. If you cancel, the Club may be entitled to retain a certain portion of the money you have paid. If the Club goes out of business or refuses to give you a refund, there may be a bond or letter of credit under which you are entitled to collect. For details, read the Agreement carefully. If you feel your rights have been violated, you may contact the Consumer Frauds and Protection Bureau of the state Attorney General's office.

Notice

Any holder of this contract is subject to all claims and defenses which the debtor could assert against the seller of goods or services obtained persuant hereto or with the proceeds hereof. Recovery hereunder by the debtor shall not exceed amounts paid by the debtor hereunder.

Conditions

Please see membership agreement Part II for all terms and conditions of this agreement.

I have read and fully understand all the terms and conditions of this agreement.

Member's signature: _____ Date: _____

Club representative: _____ Date: _____

From M. Bates, 2008, *Health Fitness Management*, 2nd ed. (Champaign, IL: Human Kinetics). Reprinted, by permission, from Island Health & Fitness, Ithaca, New York.

Membership Agreement Part II

1. **Terms.** The membership period is _____ months / month-to-month, beginning _____. A member may resign from the Club prior to the end of the agreement if they meet any of the criteria outlined in the Membership Agreement "Buyer's Right to Cancel." A member may resign from the Club after the initial _____ month term by providing a written notice to the Club. A Club member's resignation becomes effective on the first day of the month following the expiration of the notice period. Notices must be received before the end of business hours on the 10th of the month in order to terminate the following month. If notice is received after the 10th of the month, termination will occur the 1st of the month after the following month. Prior to the effective date of termination, the member shall be responsible for the payment of all fees, dues, and other charges due the Club.

2. **Buyer's Right to Cancel/Terminate.** A Member has the right to cancel this contract under certain circumstances:

   (A) Move. The Member may cancel the contract if the Member provides written verification of having moved to a new permanent residence beyond a thirty (30) mile radius from the Club, in which event the Club may make a prorated refund of prepaid dues if appropriate.

   (B) Disability or Death. You may also cancel if you become disabled, and your estate may cancel in the event of your death. The Club will make a prorated dues refund within 30 days of the written notice of this cancellation.

   (C) End of Term. After the expiration of the initial _____ month term, the Member may terminate this agreement by written notice as indicated in "TERMS" above. Such notice must be delivered in person or by certified mail and will be effective on the first of the month as described above.

3. **Member Obligation.** Failure to use the facilities will not relieve the Member of the obligation to pay the monthly dues during the initial _____ month term or any monthly renewal term of the contract. If for any reason, my bank or credit card does not honor any membership draft, I understand that I am responsible for said payment plus a penalty fee payable to the Club (currently $25.00). This will be in addition to any bank service charge fee(s).

My signature below indicates that I have read and fully understand the
above (3) points relating to payment for membership.

Enrollment Fee and Prorated Dues Payment

Primary Member _____   Enrollment Fee $ _____

Associate Member _____   Prorated Dues $ _____

Teen Member(s) _____   Total Fees Paid $ _____

Fees paid by CHECK (or CASH):   ### Fees paid by CREDIT Card

Financial Institution _____ Card type: MC   VISA   AMEX   DISC

Check # _____   Credit card # _____

Payment amount _____   Credit card expiration date: _____

Monthly Dues Draft Information   ### Fees paid by CREDIT Card

Monthly dues (and other fees, as applicable)   Bank Debit   Credit Card   Payroll Deduction
(attach voided check)

Check or savings acct # _____ Card type: MC   VISA   AMEX   DISC

Check # _____   Credit card # _____

Routing # _____   Credit card expiration date: _____

I have read and fully understand the contents of this document. I verify that the above financial information is accurate and understand that my monthly dues (and other fees as applicable) will be drafted each month following the terms and conditions of my membership agreement.

Member signature_____ Date _____ Staff initials _____

From M. Bates, 2008, *Health Fitness Management*, 2nd ed. (Champaign, IL: Human Kinetics). Reprinted, by permission, from Island Health & Fitness, Ithaca, New York.

Terms and Conditions

1. The club maintains a variety of services including strength training, cardiovascular fitness, pools, and aerobic studios. From time to time mechanical problems, maintenance, or other issues may arise that cause these areas to be out of service. Should any of these major areas of the Club be unavailable to members for more than 90 consecutive days, an adjustment in monthly membership rates may be made.

2. The Club retains the right to suspend or cancel this membership and/or impose fines of $25.00 plus costs on any member for violation of the following rules:

   a. Theft, damage, or destruction of Club property or the property of other members.

   b. Failure to pay dues or charges when due, or returned check or credit card payments.

   c. Fighting with or harassing other members or guests.

   d. Conduct of behavior found to be offensive or unacceptable.

   e. Any other violation of the rules of conduct as described in the Membership Handbook and any subsequent policies that the Club issues.

3. Members are responsible for the conduct, damages, and charges of their guests.

4. The Club reserves the right to amend its rules and regulations at any time. Changes will be posted on the Club bulletin board or communicated through other appropriate means.

5. The member acknowledges and accepts the risk inherent in the use of Club services and facilities. By using the club the member hereby assumes the risk of injury, accident, death, disability, loss cost, or damage to his or her person or property that may arise from use of the Club's services or facilities. The member, his or her heirs, executors, representatives of assigns hereby release the Club from all claims or liabilities for personal injury or loss of or damage to property of any kind sustained by the member while on the premises of the Club except where this is the direct result of negligence or willful misconduct by the Club.

6. The member certifies that he or she is in good physical health and is able to undertake and engage in the physical activities, exercise, or sports activities in which he or she has chosen to participate.

7. Members shall dress in an appropriate manner while in all public areas.

8. By signing the Agreement, the member agrees to adhere to and be bound by the Club's rules, to pay all fines levied for misconduct and to forfeit membership without refund of dues or initiation/assessment fees if terminated by the Club for cause.

9. The member agrees to pay, when due, all initiation/assessment fees, charges and guest charges in accordance with this Agreement and in accordance with the rules and regulations of the Club. If a member should fail to pay when due, any amounts payable to the Club, then the unpaid balance will be assessed an interest charge at the rate of 1.50% per month until paid plus any penalty the Club imposes for nonpayment. Should collection efforts be required, the member shall be fully responsible for payment of all costs of collection, including reasonable attorney fees.

10. MEMBERSHIP FREEZE. Members may freeze their membership only for specific reasons and only by submitting their request in writing. For a Primary Member, freezes will only be allowed for medical reasons or temporary relocation in conjunction with their employment OR VACATION, more than 30 miles from their home. A doctor's letter or a letter from an employer is required to freeze a Primary Member. When a Primary Member freezes, all remaining family members are automatically frozen as well, and are unable to use the club. The EXCEPTION is when associate or teen members take over the responsibility of the Primary Member's dues. A minimum of one full calendar month notice is required to freeze a membership. The freeze shall be effective on the 1st of the month following the expiration of the previous calendar month. Associate and Teen members may freeze their membership without providing a reason. The length of freeze for Primary Members may not exceed 5 months. A service charge of $25.00 for Primary and Associate, $10 for Associates or Teens, is required at the time of freeze. If primary and associate freeze together, the charge is $25. Freezes by telephone or fax are not permitted. Any freeze must be in person or sent via certified mail, return receipt requested. The Club reserves the right to change this or any other policy at its discretion. For more information on this or any other Club policy, consult the Member Handbook. If you have signed for a 3, 6, or 12 month period, the frozen months are added at the end.

TERMINATION POLICY. Except for a doctor's official note contraindicating exercise, after you have completed your _____ contract a minimum of Twenty days (if received by the 10th of the month) notice is required to terminate a membership.

Initial and Date

Member   Member

From M. Bates, 2008, *Health Fitness Management*, 2nd ed. (Champaign, IL: Human Kinetics). Reprinted, by permission, from Island Health & Fitness, Ithaca, New York.

- Notify health and fitness management immediately about any observed unsafe condition, equipment, or practice.
- Notify the health and fitness management of any personal health or fitness conditions that affect the member's ability to participate in health or fitness activities, programs, or use of equipment.

Waivers and Releases

As part of the membership contract, but on a separate, stand-alone form, health and fitness clubs should also require each member, or anyone just using the facility for the day, to sign a waiver. The purpose of the waiver is to expressly waive the member's right to sue the organization for any injury, damage, or loss suffered while on the premises as a result of negligence by the organization or its employees. (See Defenses of Negligence on page 338)

Independent Contractors

In order to keep costs low while at the same time providing a wide variety of services, it is essential to use the services of **independent contractors.** In addition to keeping employee costs down, using independent contractors can also cut down on liability. For example, as long as the organization uses reasonable care in selecting a qualified and competent independent contractor, the legal liability for any injuries that are caused by the independent contractor's ordinary negligence generally shifts from the organization to the independent contractor (van der Smissen 1990).

Besides shifting liability, in the United States the health and fitness organization is not required to pay FICA (Federal Insurance Contributions Act, or Social Security), FUTA (Federal Unemployment Tax Act), or state unemployment taxes on independent contractors. Plus, employers do not pay independent contractors' health care benefits, retirement benefits, vacation pay, sick-leave pay, or any other employee benefits.

To prevent organizations from classifying everyone as independent contractors and to ensure that employers are paying the appropriate unemployment and social security taxes, the IRS has developed guidelines to help identify who is an employee and who is an independent contractor. As a general rule, however, an individual is an independent contractor if the person for whom the work is being performed has the right to control or direct only the result of the work, and not what will be done and how it will be done or the method of accomplishing

the result. If an organization improperly designates an employee as an independent contractor, it is subject to back taxes, interests, and penalties. For more information, see the IRS Web site at www.irs.gov/charities/article/0,,id=128602,00.html.

Vendor Contracts

In order to provide a wide range of services, health and fitness organizations are also required to enter into contracts for various services and products. To protect the organization, it is essential that these agreements be in writing. Although most of the agreements will be standard form contracts, managers should feel free to negotiate any of the terms found in the contract. Critical terms in vendor agreements include the right to terminate the agreement without cause, return unused goods without charge, maintain a nonexclusive relationship that allows the organization to use other products or services, and be indemnified by the vendor for any loss or damage caused by the vendor's services or products.

In some cases, the organization may select a vendor to subcontract operation of one or more membership or operational services. Examples of operations frequently contracted out to vendors include pro shops, food and beverages, vending machines, specialty health services (e.g., massage therapy, health and beauty services, sports medicine services), facility maintenance (e.g., night janitorial services), and towel laundry service. Whenever subcontracting with a vendor, establish written contracts that outline the relationship of the parties.

Employment Contracts

In most cases, the employer–employee relationship is based on contract law. Whenever one person agrees to work for another person or legal entity in exchange for wages and other benefits, an employment contract is in place. The rights and obligations of the employer and employee are governed by a combination of general contract law and state and federal regulations and statutes. In many states, unless a written employment contract is signed, employment is considered to be **employment at will.** Employment at will means that, absent a discriminatory motive, an employer may terminate an employee at will and without cause. Likewise, the employee is not required to give notice or reasons for quitting and may do so at any time without liability.

Since most employees in the health and fitness industry do not have employment contracts, employee manuals and handbooks take on an added importance as the most effective method of defining the employer–employee relationship. Many organizations require that all new employees sign a document stipulating that they have read or been provided with a copy of the employee handbook. Because of the importance of these issues in determining employer liability, the last section of this chapter reviews the subject matter that an employee handbook should include.

Employment Law

There are two distinct areas of employment law (van der Smissen 2004):

1. Employment process
2. Workplace environment

Employment Process

The employment process is concerned with fundamental concepts related to the recruitment, selection, and hiring process. Two of the most important items in the employment process are the employee handbook and the personnel policy manual.

Employee handbooks are addressed to employees and generally communicate in clear, direct terms the more important policies that govern employment, such as employment benefits, vacation, sick leave, holidays, and grievance and discipline procedures. In addition, handbooks should also include guidelines defining inappropriate conduct that may result in disciplinary action and list the circumstances under which the company will consider an employee to have voluntarily terminated employment.

The main benefit of an employee handbook is that it informs employees what they may expect of their employer and what the organization expects of them. In the absence of any written guidelines, an employer is more likely to encounter problems arising from ignorance of its policies, inconsistent application, and confusion about what is expected. An employee handbook can help avoid some of these problems.

Personnel policy manuals, by comparison, are addressed to managers and personnel professionals who must administer the employer's policies. The manuals not only describe the policies but also designate administration procedures. Personnel policy manuals, therefore, are more comprehensive. They address a larger number of policies, such as background and criminal checks for employees and volunteers, and address each in greater detail.

Personnel policy manuals can be accessed by all employees, but they usually are not distributed to each employee.

Developing a personnel policy manual is a detailed and extensive process. Large organizations consider policy manuals necessary to maintain consistency and to ensure compliance. For all employers, personnel policy manuals are a two-edged sword. To the extent that the manual defines standards and procedures for discipline, performance evaluations, and payment of wages and to the extent that these policies and procedures are followed, it can help avoid legal problems. However, if the personnel policy manual is overly complex, not properly distributed, or not enforced, different legal issues and liabilities may arise.

A checklist of items that should be included in an employee handbook or personnel policy manual is included on page 347.

Workplace Environment

In addition to making sure that the environment is safe for club members and guests, health and fitness managers also need to ensure that they do not violate any laws governing the workplace environment. The following are some of the most common laws governing the workplace environment:

- Title VII of the Civil Rights Act of 1964
- Americans with Disabilities Act of 1990
- Age Discrimination in Employment Act of 1967
- Sexual harassment policy (Title VII of the Civil Rights Act)
- Occupational Safety & Health Administration (OSHA)

Title VII of the Civil Rights Act of 1964

Title VII of the Civil Rights Act of 1964, which applies to organizations with 15 or more employees who are employed for at least 20 weeks a year, prohibits discrimination in employment by making it illegal for an employer "to fail to hire or to discharge an individual, or otherwise discriminate against any individual with respect to compensation, terms, conditions, or privileges of employment, because of such individual's race, color, religion, sex or national origin" (Title VII 2003).

If people believe that they were discriminated against under Title VII, they must file a claim with the EEOC. The EEOC will investigate all charges and attempt to resolve any disputes. If the discrimination continues and the organization will not remedy

Policies to Include in an Employee Handbook

- Introduction to the manual
- Equal employment opportunity
- Employment at will
- Orientation and probationary period
- Hours of work, overtime, and payday
- Vacation
- Holidays
- Sick leave
- Other leaves of absence, including disability and family and medical leave
- Internal complaint review procedure
- Termination, discipline, and rules of conduct
- Employee classifications
- Performance and pay review
- Personnel records

- Dress and grooming standards
- Smoking
- Recruitment and selection, employment of relatives, and rehires
- Safety program
- Security and confidential information
- Bloodborne and airborne pathogens in the workplace
- Employee benefits
- Nonfraternization
- Conflicts of interest
- Proof of right to work
- Medical examinations
- Inspections for prohibited materials or substances, including concealed weapons
- Drug-free workplace
- Harassment
- Employee assistance program

it, the EEOC has the power to file suit in federal court (Masteralexis 2004).

Americans with Disabilities Act of 1990

The **Americans with Disabilities Act of 1990 (ADA)** is divided into five sections covering the rights of people with disabilities in the areas of employment, public services, transportation, and telecommunications. Title I of the ADA, which covers employment, provides that "no covered entity shall discriminate against a qualified individual with a disability because of the disability of such individual in regard to job application procedures, the hiring, advancement, or discharge of employees, employee compensation, job training, and other terms, conditions, and privileges of employment" (Age Discrimination in Employment Act [ADA] 2003).

Title I covers any organization with 15 or more employees who work for 20 or more calendar weeks in the current or preceding calendar year. If covered under the ADA, an organization must make reasonable accommodations for any qualified person with a disability. However, employers only need to do so if providing the reasonable accommodation

does not result in undue hardship. Examples of reasonable accommodation include the following (Hums 2004):

- Making existing facilities reasonably accessible to and usable by people with disabilities
- Job restructuring; part-time or modified work schedules; reassignment to a vacant position; acquisition or modification of equipment or devices; appropriate adjustment or modifications of examinations, training materials, or policies; the provision of qualified readers or interpreters; and other similar accommodations

When an employee's excessive absenteeism or tardiness is related to a disability, the organization may be required to make reasonable accommodations in the form of leave or a modified work schedule. Although *reasonable accommodation* is a term defined by courts, many courts have held that if regular attendance is an essential job component, an organization is not required to accommodate a disabled employee's high rate of unpredictable absences if it would result in an undue hardship.

Organizations facing these issues would be well served to consult with legal counsel before disciplining a possibly disabled employee for absenteeism or tardiness.

In addition to employment, people with disabilities have also used the ADA with varying degrees of success to force health and fitness facilities to accommodate their disabilities when providing recreational activities. As a general rule, if accommodating a person with a disability does not pose a direct threat to the safety of the other participants or require a fundamental modification of the activity, the organization must accommodate the individual.

For more information on the ADA, see the **U.S. Department of Justice** Web site at www.usdoj.gov/crt/ada/adahom1.htm.

Age Discrimination in Employment Act of 1967

Based on Title VII of the Civil Rights Act of 1964, the **Age Discrimination in Employment Act of 1967 (ADEA)** makes it unlawful "to fail to hire or to discharge an individual, or otherwise discriminate against any individual with respect to compensation, terms, conditions, or privileges of employment, because of such individual's age" (Age Discrimination in Employment Act [ADEA] 2003).

As baby boomers age, ADEA, which covers all employees or potential employees over the age of 40 in the United States, has the potential to become extremely important to health and fitness professionals. However, like Title VII, ADEA applies only to those organizations with 20 or more employees who are employed for at least 20 weeks a year.

For more information on age harassment, see the EEOC Web site at www.eeoc.gov/policy/adea.html.

Sexual Harassment

Sexual harassment is a form of sex discrimination under Title VII of the Civil Rights Act of 1964, which prohibits any unwelcome sexual advances, requests for sexual favors, or other verbal or physical conduct of a sexual nature imposed on the basis of sex.

There are two theories of sexual harassment: quid pro quo and hostile environment. **Quid pro quo sexual harassment** occurs when a manager grants or withholds employment opportunities or benefits as a result of another person's willingness or refusal to submit to the manager's sexual

demands. Because the pressure may be either an explicit or implicit term or condition of the person's employment, the critical point is not whether the victim submits voluntarily but whether the conduct is unwanted.

Hostile environment sexual harassment exists when a manager or coworker's conduct has the purpose or effect of unreasonably interfering with an employee's work performance or creates an intimidating, hostile, or offensive work environment. Some examples of hostile environment sexual harassment would be unwelcome verbal expressions of a sexual nature, including graphic sexual commentaries about a person's body or dress and the use of sexually degrading language or jokes or sexually suggestive objects, pictures, videotapes, audio recordings, or literature in the work area, that may embarrass or offend an individual (Wolohan 1995).

Sexual harassment does not require the people involved to be of different sex. The U.S. Supreme Court has recognized that individuals of the same sex can create a hostile environment of sexual harassment with each other, as long as the harassment is motivated by the victim's sex (Wolohan 1995).

To discourage such behavior and to protect the organization from costly lawsuits, all health and fitness organizations should proactively take the following steps:

1. Include a sexual harassment policy in all employee handbooks and make sure that the policy clearly communicates to employees that sexual harassment will not be tolerated and that no retaliation will be permitted against employees who file a complaint.

2. Provide all employees with sexual harassment training.

3. Establish an effective complaint or grievance process that encourages all employees to report any incident to an appropriate manager. To be safe, and to ensure that the person doing the harassing is not the person who receives the complaint, employees should be offered two different sources for reporting sexual harassment complaints.

4. Immediately review and investigate all complaints as thoroughly and confidentially as possible. If the facts are discovered to be true, the employee's relationship with the organization should be terminated.

For more information on sexual harassment, see the EEOC Web site at www.eeoc.gov/types/sexual_harassment.html.

Employee Safety

The health and safety of all employees is regulated by OSHA. Some of the areas affected by OSHA regulations include injury and illness records, employee safety posters, posting of signs, bloodborne pathogens, written plans and training, personal protective equipment, safety equipment, electrical safety, toilet facilities, regular inspections, housekeeping, safety conditions, emergency evacuation, machine guarding, hazard communication, and chemicals (van der Smissen 2004).

For more information, see www.osha.gov/pls/publications/pubindex.list.

THE BOTTOM LINE

Health and fitness clubs must not only ensure a safe environment for club members and guests, they also must ensure that they do not violate any laws governing the workplace environment.

Insurance Considerations

A health and fitness facility can present a number of potentially dangerous conditions for members, guests, and personnel. An environment with cardiorespiratory machines, resistive weight training equipment, locker rooms with wet areas (i.e., showers, saunas, whirlpools, and steam rooms), and a pool all possess the possibility for accidents and injuries. Combine these facilities with a membership comprising men and women of every age range, fitness level, and health status, and the potential for injury seems almost endless.

The easiest way to protect yourself and your organization from the legal liability and financial loss associated with these risks is through insurance. Insurance allows the facility to transfer the potentially devastating financial risk of a future loss for the cost certainty of a monthly or yearly payment (premium).

Determining Insurance Needs

Since insurance is a vital part of any risk management plan, it is essential that the facility take the time to determine its specific insurance needs. The first step in determining insurance needs is iden-tifying the potential risks within the facility. For example, if the facility has a pool, the potential risks involve someone drowning or slipping and falling. Once the risks are identified, the next step involves analyzing the potential risks and weighing them against any potential financial loss. Once again using the pool example, since both types of incidents could result in lawsuits and potentially substantial financial losses, it would be in the best interest of the club to obtain insurance, thereby transferring the risk of such losses to the insurance company.

In examining your insurance needs, it is important to not only identify potential problem areas in the facility but also evaluate all the programs, activities, and equipment used in the facility. Identifying and evaluating everything will ensure that proper coverage is given to the entire facility and help guard against possible gaps in the policy.

In addition, insurance policies should be tailored for each individual club since every club is different. Therefore, it is important to study each policy before signing it in order to determine the areas specifically covered by the policy and, more importantly, to identify areas not covered by the policy. Finally, although entering into an initial insurance contract or renewing a policy may represent the final stage of the process, it is necessary to take time during the year to evaluate the coverage and make changes or additions as needed.

THE BOTTOM LINE

Insurance is the easiest way to protect a health and fitness center from legal liability and financial loss.

Types of Insurance

Purchasing adequate and affordable insurance can be a frustrating task for health and fitness professionals. However, two types of insurance every facility should have are property insurance and general liability insurance. The following section examines some of the most common types of insurance in the health and fitness industry.

Property Insurance

Property insurance is the primary means of protecting the facility from accidental losses resulting from damage or destruction. The two primary areas covered by property insurance are (1) the buildings and (2) business and equipment contents contained within the designated buildings.

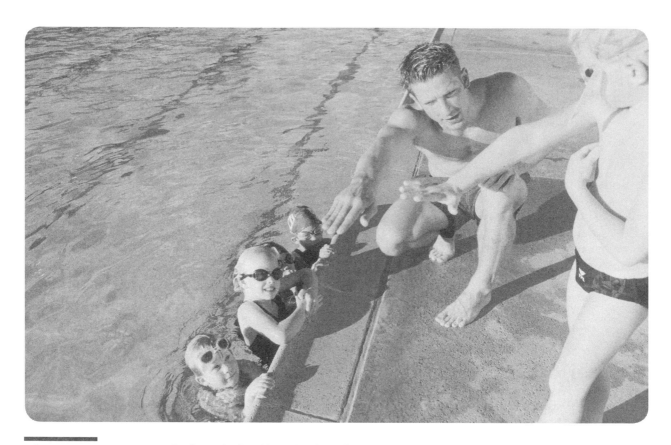

All wet areas pose potential risks to the health and safety of members and guests. Accidents could result in lawsuits and financial loss, and it's in the best interest of the club to obtain insurance.
© Getty Images/Rob Gage

There are three levels of property insurance: basic, extended coverage, and special form, also sometimes referred to as *open perils* (Cotten 2007). The basic coverage protects against a limited number of hazards, such as fire, weather-related damage, and vandalism. Extended coverage not only includes the same protections as in the basic coverage but additional hazards, such as ice, water, and smoke damage. Special form coverage is designed to protect against any losses except those specifically excluded from coverage (Cotten 2007).

Even with special form coverage, there will be some property risks that are not covered under the policy. If the facility believes that more coverage is needed, it can purchase additional endorsements. An example of one such endorsement is **business interruption,** or loss of earnings coverage for disasters that temporarily affect the daily operations of a facility. This can be significant if, for example, an organization is damaged by a fire and must wait 9 to 12 days to reopen. The damage is not just the cost of renovation; it also involves lost revenue and expenses that are ongoing even when the club is not operational (i.e., debt service, real estate taxes, insurance, the demand portion of utilities). In addi-

tion, in some situations, key employees will need to be retained during the reconstruction phase and a temporary office and furniture may be required.

General Liability Insurance

General liability insurance is designed to protect businesses from any financial losses due to the negligence of the owner and employees. General liability insurance is often referred to as *third-party insurance* because if a business is sued, the insurance company protects the owner against suit by a third party. A general liability insurance policy generally provides for investigating and negotiating private settlements. In addition, it covers the defense of lawsuits brought against the owner and the payment of judgments up to the limit of the policy, usually $500,000 to $1 million.

Umbrella Liability Insurance

Although general liability insurance will cover most risks associated with running a health and fitness facility, the policies are subject to financial limits that ordinarily do not exceed $500,000 to $1 million. Therefore, in order to protect businesses from a catastrophic loss where liability may exceed the limits of the general liability insurance, the business must have an **umbrella liability** policy.

In addition to general liability claims, an umbrella liability policy can allow a business to greatly increase its coverage in other key areas, such as auto liability, workers' compensation, and employer liability. Umbrella liability policies also usually provide broader coverage than most underlying policies, thus providing primary coverage for certain occurrences that would not be covered by an existing policy.

Event Liability Coverage

When planning a special event or trip, it is essential that managers contact their insurance agents to determine if the event is covered under the existing general liability policy. If not, the business should purchase additional event liability coverage. If a business offers off-site trips, it should ask the coordinating outside party to provide the necessary insurance. This applies to ski tours, white-water rafting companies, and even the charter bus company that transports members to an event. Generally, such companies do not have to pay anything extra to name the club on their insurance coverage for an outing or event. However, if the outside party chooses not to provide insurance coverage, it is the responsibility of the club to obtain an insurance rider on its liability policy to cover the event.

Automobile Insurance

A significant liability exposure facing virtually all businesses comes from operating automobiles. In the United States, automobile accidents produce the greatest number of liability claims and account for most of the liability awards higher than $1 million. Even businesses not owning a vehicle can be held liable for the operation of a vehicle by others. For example, an employee could take the day's cash deposit to the bank and have an accident on the way. If the employee is at fault, the business can be held responsible because the employee was acting on behalf of the business.

In addition to liability and physical damage coverage, several other endorsements are available that you can add to a standard commercial auto policy, such as protecting employee-owned cars and rental vehicles while on company business. It is recommended that a club representative discuss all the vehicle-related situations that may exist in the daily operation of the club with the insurance agent to ensure that proper coverage is obtained at the best rate.

Workers' Compensation

Most work-related accidents, diseases, and disabilities are subject to state **workers' compensation** statutes, which require employers to provide compensation for covered injuries without regard to fault. The scope of coverage varies in each state with respect to benefits payable in the case of early death, total disability, and partial disability due to specific injuries.

Every state has its own workers' compensation laws, but there are two requirements that injured employees must satisfy before they can recover workers' compensation benefits (Wolohan 2007):

1. They must show that they were an employee of the organization.
2. The injury must have occurred in the course of employment.

The benefits paid in the event of a valid workers' compensation claim include medical expenses, disability income or death benefits to replace lost wages, and rehabilitation services to assist the employee in getting back to work.

Although the U.S. government and every state have enacted workers' compensation laws, recent changes in some state statutes no longer require workers' compensation to be mandatory. Instead, these states have made workers' compensation elective; that is, the employer may elect to be governed by the provisions of the act. An employer electing not to be governed cannot use as a defense employees' negligence as a contributing factor, or that the accident was due to the actions of a coworker, or that the accident was a normal risk of the business.

Independent Contractor Liability

General liability insurance will usually protect employers from liability due to the negligent acts of their employees, but such policies do not currently cover independent contractors (i.e., aerobics instructors, sport instructors, personal trainers) while working on the premises of a club. Consequently, club managers must require self-employed contractors to obtain their own coverage.

Typically, the insurance agent requests copies of independent contractors' insurance certificates before underwriting their liability insurance. Because the liability associated with being an independent contractor varies from the standard commercial liability policy, insurance companies have established different policies for specific groups. For example, companies specializing in health and fitness insurance offer a separate personal trainer insurance program.

KEY TERMS

Age Discrimination in Employment Act of 1967 (ADEA)

agreement to participate

Americans with Disabilities Act of 1990 (ADA)

assumption of risk

business interruption

civil liability

contract

criminal liability

duty of care

employee handbook

employment at will

general liability insurance

hostile environment sexual harassment

independent contractor

intentional tort

invitee

negligence tort

personnel policy manual

quid pro quo sexual harassment

reckless misconduct

recreational user

sexual harassment

Title VII of the Civil Rights Act of 1964

tort

umbrella liability

vicarious liability

waiver

workers' compensation

U.S. Department of Justice

REFERENCES AND RECOMMENDED READINGS

Age Discrimination in Employment Act, 42 U.S.C. §623 (4) (2003).

Americans with Disabilities Act, 42 U.S.C. § 12112 (2003).

Calamari, J., and J. Perillo. 1998. *The law of contracts.* 4th ed. St. Paul: West.

Cotten, D.J. 2007. Managing risk through insurance. In *Law for recreation and sport managers,* 4th ed., eds. D.J. Cotten and J.T. Wolohan. Dubuque, IA: Kendall/Hunt.

Cotten, D.J., and M.B. Cotten. 2004. *Waivers and releases of liability.* 4th ed. Statesboro, GA: Sport Risk Consulting.

Hums, M.A. 2004. Title I of the Americans with Disabilities Act. In *Law for recreation and sport managers,* 3rd ed., eds. D.J. Cotten and J.T. Wolohan. Dubuque, IA: Kendall/Hunt.

Keeton, W., et al. 1984. *Prosser and Keeton on the law of torts.* 5th ed. St. Paul: West.

Masteralexis, L. 2004. Title VII of the Civil Rights Act of 1964. In *Law for recreation and sport managers,* 3rd ed., eds. D.J. Cotten and J.T. Wolohan. Dubuque, IA: Kendall/Hunt.

Restatement (second) of Contracts §1 (1979).

Robertson, D., W. Powers, D. Anderson, and O. Wellborn. 2004. *Cases and materials on torts.* 3rd ed. St. Paul: West.

Schubert, G.W., R.K. Smith, and J.C. Trentadue. 1986. *Sports law.* St. Paul: West.

Title VII of the Civil Rights Act of 1964, 42 U.S.C. §§ 2000e *et seq.* (2003).

van der Smissen, B. 1990. *Legal liability and risk management for public and private entities.* Cincinnati: Anderson.

———. 2004. Human resources law. In *Law for recreation and sport managers,* 3rd ed., eds. D.J. Cotten and J.T. Wolohan. Dubuque, IA: Kendall/Hunt.

Wolohan, J.T. 1995. Sexual harassment of student athletes and the law. *Seton Hall Journal of Sport Law* 5:339-357.

———. 2004. Land reform: Recreational-use statutes are expanding to include public fields, playgrounds and pools. *Athletic Business* 28:22-26.

———. 2005. Faulty waivers: A drowning death leaves all exculpatory agreements in state of Wisconsin under water. *Athletic Business* 29:20-26.

———. 2007. Workers' compensation. In *Law for recreation and sport managers,* 4th ed., eds. D.J. Cotten and J.T. Wolohan. Dubuque, IA: Kendall/Hunt.

Wong, G.M. 2002. *Essentials of sports law.* 3rd ed. Westport, CT: Preager.

seventeen

Evaluating Your Operation

Dave Hardy

After studying this chapter, the reader will be able to

- identify evaluation goals and processes to determine program efficiency,
- understand the importance of and implement evaluation processes related to additional profit centers,
- acknowledge that what is measured is easily managed, and
- determine the best evaluation method for a fitness facility.

As the owner of ABC Fitness for 5 years, Paula had seen ups and downs, but the past 2 years had been very smooth with steady growth—up until the last 3 months. During this time a new competitor had come into the market and began offering programs that Paula's club was not, and she had lost many members to the competitor. Although the new programs of the competitor were a factor, there were also other reasons why her members were leaving.

In order to get to the bottom of this decline, Paula personally called many of the members who had left, something the club had never done in the past. The information she gathered opened her eyes to things that she was not aware of. Some of the comments included the following:

- "The change rooms were getting dingy and needed some upgrades."
- "I've asked about Pilates and yoga classes for the past 2 years and no one has ever given me a good reason why this club won't offer them."
- "The new club has personal trainers."

These were just a few of the comments she received. She was shocked because had she known about these concerns previously, she could have easily addressed them. Her club actually had personal trainers but apparently most members didn't know how to approach them and what they had to offer. Paula was not even aware that members were interested in Pilates or yoga, and she thought members would prefer to see more treadmills as opposed to upgraded locker rooms.

These comments made Paula aware of the fact that she needed to spend more time working on her business as opposed to working within her business. If she had been paying better attention to the needs of her members, she could have dealt with many of these concerns. A formal member feedback program and more informal contact with members would have easily revealed that these problems existed.

Paula also realized that there were probably other problems in her business that she was not aware of. With this mind, she met with her key staff and decided to conduct a full evaluation of the entire business. This was a time-consuming endeavor, but the end result was a much more effective and efficient fitness facility. Paula planned to implement formal and informal methods for evaluating the entire operation throughout the year. She realized that one big evaluation each year was simply too much work and also did not meet club needs throughout the year.

The evaluation tools discussed in this chapter provide a generic approach to outcome-oriented management practices. This permits a snapshot view of the performance of an organization that may be useful to club operators in planning for the future.

Within the fitness industry, there is a growing awareness of the need to develop meaningful standards and quality controls to measure the extent to which a program has achieved its stated objectives. Because the industry has evolved significantly over the last 40 years, the evaluation process is becoming increasingly important in terms of documenting the outcomes and processes involved in health and fitness services.

Evaluation Defined

Evaluation is the process of determining the extent to which an organization has achieved its stated objectives. It measures the efficacy of programs as well as the overall performance of an organization based on industry standards. If evaluation is performed honestly, it may yield negative rather than positive findings and may ultimately result in program downsizing or elimination.

Goals of Evaluation

Clearly defined goals and objectives are essential components of evaluation. You must measure each one to determine program effectiveness. Program participation rates, attrition, postprogram behavior changes (e.g., weight loss, fitness improvements, stress reduction), and staff satisfaction are examples of areas that must be measured in determining program success. Evaluation is part of the control function of club operations.

The overall goals of evaluation in the fitness industry are as follows:

1. To determine how effective a program is in meeting predetermined goals and objectives

2. To provide comprehensive information about the full range of program achievements as well as possible weaknesses

3. To measure the quality of a program based on accepted standards and criteria

4. To appraise the quality of organizational management, such as the performance of staff or the effectiveness of policies and procedures

5. To provide feedback for improving programs and recommending a direction for future reference

6. To provide information for internal and external marketing of program achievements

Models of Evaluation

The following section will compare various evaluation methods necessary in determining whether the goals and objectives of a fitness facility are being met.

Summative and Formative Models

In the past, evaluation was primarily thought of as summative. **Summative evaluation** provides information on efficacy—that is, the ability of a program to do what it was designed to do. Summative evaluation is carried out at the end of a program to measure its success or failure and make recommendations for the future.

Today, however, much of the evaluation process is formative, providing continual monitoring of a program while it is being planned and implemented. **Formative evaluation** is a method of judging the worth of a program while the program activities are forming or occurring. This type of evaluation establishes whether goals and objectives are being met, modifying them as necessary throughout the process.

In order to maintain their competitive edge, managers should routinely conduct evaluations on all aspects of the business and regularly adjust the mode of operation to fit the needs of the consumer.

Process and Preordinate Models

Process evaluation models delineate a set of steps and procedures to use in conducting an evaluation without identifying the judgment criteria, whereas **preordinate evaluation models** provide a process and specify the criteria necessary in determining the worth of a program. Preordinate models begin with determining exactly how an evalua-

tion should be carried out, the type of information that will be required, and the best way to gather it. Member participation, interest, feedback, and instructor evaluation are examples of preordinate evaluation.

No single approach is correct in all situations. A combination is often used in evaluating fitness facilities and the operations.

Health and Fitness Evaluation Model

Maintaining a competitive edge over similar facilities is a matter of survival. The quest for excellence separates the marginal operator from the successful operator. Whether a facility is small, medium, or large, striving to be the best should be the goal.

Elements of quality may be measured in various ways. Regardless of the measuring system used, the end result should be to identify those areas that meet or surpass acceptable industry standards and pinpoint areas that need further investigation and improvement. As an example, one of the most widely used systems for measuring quality in the fitness industry is **total quality management (TQM).** TQM involves observing and measuring everything occurring within an organization so you can identify weaknesses and improve operations. Operational procedures and policies must be reviewed and revised to examine how and by whom decisions are made and carried out within the organization. TQM may improve worker performance, productivity, customer service, and profitability.

The purpose of an evaluation model is to develop an awareness of the management policies and procedures used in various health and fitness settings, provide a means to measure the quality of those policies and procedures against proven methods, and point out the need to assess, improve, and change any areas deemed deficient. Use evaluation as a vehicle for improvement and as an indicator of where to concentrate efforts within the business.

Within most health and fitness settings there are various levels of communication that are important to the success of the business. When conducting a facility evaluation, the groups involved in the evaluation process generally include management, an evaluation coordinator or consultant, an evaluation committee, and staff. Figure 17.1 illustrates how the flow of information obtained from a facility evaluation reaches the appropriate people.

• *Management.* It is the responsibility of management to take the data obtained from the evaluation

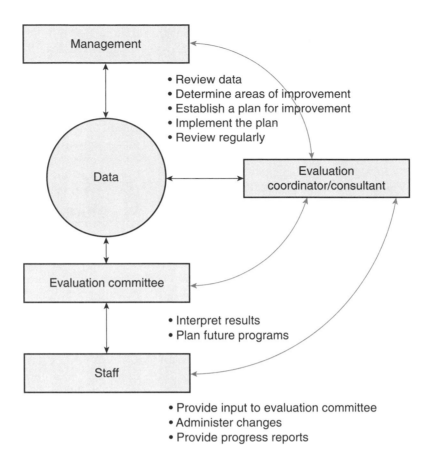

Figure 17.1 Communication network for evaluation.

Adapted, by permission, from Association for Fitness in Business, 1992, *Guidelines for employee health promotion programs* (Champaign, IL: Human Kinetics), 83.

and use it to monitor established goals. Managers should look for areas considered deficient, establish a plan for improvement, implement the plan with the assistance of personnel, and regularly review the results. Having the support of management for short- and long-term planning is essential; consequently, a strong line of communication is needed between managers and other members of the evaluation group. You can obtain this interaction through regular presentations and reports that focus on significant findings and recommendations for improvement.

• *Evaluation coordinator or consultant.* The role of the evaluation coordinator is to be the intermediary between management and staff. This task is often performed by an independent, impartial consultant who has no ties to the organization. If you use an in-house employee, we recommend that both management and staff approve the selection. The person chosen to manage this process will be responsible for analyzing data, reviewing results, comparing data with industry benchmarks, and determining pertinent conclusions.

• *Evaluation committee.* The evaluation committee usually consists of supervisors or personnel who have a vested interest in the evaluation process. They are responsible for developing and administering the evaluation, reviewing the results with the evaluation coordinator, and providing recommendations for improvement. The committee performs these tasks through regular meetings and brainstorming sessions for solving problems associated with the evaluation process. Committee members obtain input from other staff to incorporate their ideas and to make them feel a part of the operation.

• *Staff.* Staff members assist the evaluation committee in planning and conducting the evaluation, but more importantly, they are responsible for administering the changes approved by management. We cannot overstate their involvement in the evaluation process. Providing a sense of ownership during the evaluation phase helps ensure that staff members implement planned program, facility, or operational changes in a positive manner. Staff members are also responsible for providing regular feedback on these changes so the organization can make refinements as needed.

Evaluation findings may be used as an external marketing tool. Promotional and advertising vehicles, such as newsletters and direct or private mailings, may be implemented to communicate evaluation results to members.

As shown in figure 17.2, an ongoing cycle for evaluation implementation will help define new goals and objectives, establish strategic planning, and follow up on plan implementation. This cycle allows for the continual evaluation of the business to ensure proper managerial techniques are incorporated.

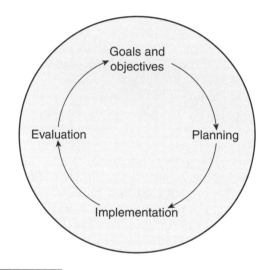

Figure 17.2 Implementation cycle of evaluation.

Location Analysis

Many club operators believe a facility either makes or loses money the day the lease for the location is signed. As in most retail operations, the three most important factors of success are location, location, location.

Four primary factors affect demand in the health and fitness industry:

1. Population density
2. Travel time to the health club
3. Household income
4. Educational attainment

In terms of population density, sophisticated club operators generally operate in markets where at least 50,000 people or more are within close proximity. Concerning travel time, the primary trading area should extend no more than 12 minutes from

the point of departure. The **primary trading area** is the area closest to the club location, possesses the highest density of clientele, and extends no more than 10 to 12 minutes travel time from the location. Demographic studies have shown that 85% of club members come from within 12 minutes of travel time, equivalent to approximately 4 to 5 miles (6-8 kilometers) by car (McCarthy 2002).

Household income is a key determinant of member penetration rates and club pricing. There is a strong correlation between household income and club memberships. One out of eight members of the general population is a health club member; however, member penetration rates among high-income segments approach nearly 30% (McCarthy 2002). Educational attainment also dictates demand for memberships. In general, the higher the education attainment of the people in the primary trading area, the higher the membership penetration rates among that community.

The ultimate goal of location evaluation is to determine if there is an available market to support the new facility, and, for budgeting purposes, to estimate the number of monthly memberships the facility would likely sell. Both quantitative and qualitative approaches must be used in evaluating a location for a new fitness facility. **Quantitative research** refers to the collection of statistical data, whereas **qualitative research** refers to information based on opinions and values.

Quantitative Methodology for Evaluating Locations

In evaluating a location, the following information should be researched:

- *Population density within the primary target trading area.* For example, if a facility is seeking to target 18- to 55-year-olds, population density should be determined for everyone in this age range within the primary trading area. As mentioned, this is generally within 12-minute travel time; however, it must be determined location by location.

- *Education attainment and average income.* This information helps determine if the area will have a higher- or lower-than-average market penetration. Another influential factor is market positioning of the facility (for example, low-cost facilities would be more appealing to lower-income participants).

- *Traffic flow.* This should also be researched since there is generally a positive correlation between traffic flow and the number of guests willing to drop in to the facility.

Once secondary data are collected, it is necessary to collect primary data on the existing market area in terms of over- or underfilled demand. **Secondary data** come from the collection, analysis, and interpretation of sources of primary data, whereas **primary data** are collected firsthand, including original materials, surveys, experiences, and so on.

To accomplish this, all potential competitors within the primary trading area should be plotted on a map. The following information should also be collected:

- A map of competitors' primary trading areas
- An estimate of competitors' current membership
- The number of current competitor members who are inside the proposed trading area of the new facility

Then, using the abovementioned secondary demographic information of the population within the target market of the new facility, determine how many members would potentially purchase memberships at a fitness facility. A reasonable estimate must be made based on the available secondary data.

Finally, a calculation of the total potential market within the trading area less existing competition must be completed to determine whether the market has excess capacity for a new facility or whether excess supply already exists. See figure 17.3 for an example. A location analysis examines averages relevant to the primary trading area; most licensed real estate leasing agents are able to provide these averages based on a mapped primary trading area as laid out by the facility operator. Averages are dependent on the facility size, operating costs, and overall operating budget, and they determine whether the facility will be profitable as indicated by a mean average of attending members. This mean average does not take into account members who change facilities based on differences in services offered.

Qualitative Methodology for Evaluating Locations

Real estate evaluation must also consider qualitative factors to determine the percentage of the market that the proposed facility will access. Some qualitative factors include the following:

- *Brand awareness.* **Brand awareness** is a measure of how readily members of a target audience remember a product, service, company, or commercial brand and what the brand is about, as well as the consumer's level of trust in the brand.

- *Product offering.* This includes facility size and amenities as compared with existing competition, such as the amount of equipment, type of equipment, and other amenities (e.g., pool, racket sports, ingress and egress into the location, ease of parking).

Qualitative factors will vary significantly by market area.

Industry Evolution and Differentiation

With the evolution of the fitness industry has come increased sophistication in operators and business practices. In the early days of the fitness industry, operators were typically focused on leasing space or providing equipment to members for an annual or monthly fee. The evolution of the fitness industry has seen significant increases in consumer expectations.

From a competitive perspective, the number of clubs has increased at a significant pace. Based on information released by IHRSA, the number of adult commercial fitness clubs has increased significantly over the past 10 years, as shown in figure 17.4 (International Health, Racquet, and Sportsclub Association [IHRSA] 2006). In addition, there has been a significant increase in the not-for-profit and government sectors, including YMCAs, hospital-based facilities, and government-operated facilities.

The commercial fitness industry originated in the United States in the 1950s and 1960s, with industry growth strongest over the last 25 years. There have been significant changes in the competitive landscape during this time. In previous years, competition was limited to other commercial entities. However, today in Canada, for example, the largest competitors of the adult commercial fitness industry come from the government and the not-for-profit sector.

Increases in competition have forced operators to focus on differentiation. Many operators differentiate their business by creating additional **profit centers** within their facilities (see chapter 11 for more details). These centers include the following:

- Juice bars
- Group exercise
- Personal training

	Target Location	Municipality Averages
	-----	13
	-----	-----
	-----	19,705
	-----	5.00%
Total population	114,080	666,104
20-59 years old	44,532	394,295
20-34 years old	25,443	160,545
35-54 years old	39,003	204,565
55-59 years old	5,102	29,185
Completed university	12.6%	19.2%
Attending/attended university	8.8%	8.0%
Completed college	15.8%	17.0%
Attending/attended 2-year college	7.5%	7.4%
Trades certificate or diploma	14.8% 59.5%	12.5% 64.1%
Completed high school	12.5%	10.8%
Attending/attended high school	24.5%	18.7%
Completed less than grade 9	9.4%	6.5%
Average household income	$52,816	$57,418

Target Market Penetration Rates

Penetration rate, 20-34 years old	20%	5,089
Penetration rate, 35-54 years old	15%	5,850
Penetration rate, 55-59 years old	10%	510
Total potential members in market area		**11,449**

Total Estimated Members at Competitors' Locations

Competitor club A	4,000
Competitor club B	3,500
Competitor club C	2,500
Competitor club D	500

Percentage That Infringe on Market Area of Proposed Facility

Competitor club A	75%
Competitor club B	85%
Competitor club C	85%
Competitor club D	25%

Number of Members Already Serviced in Market Area

Competitor club A	3,000
Competitor club B	2,975
Competitor club C	2,125
Competitor club D	125
	8,225

Available/Oversold Market	**3,224**

Figure 17.3 Sample location analysis.

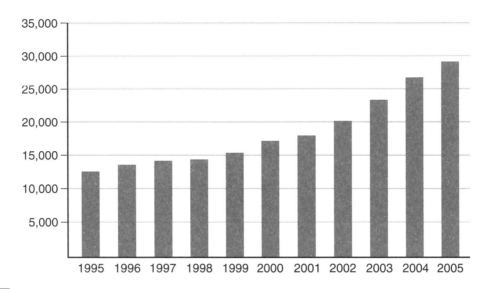

Figure 17.4 The number of successful operating fitness facilities in the United States has grown consistently between 1995 and 2005.

Adapted, by permission, from IHRSA, *Profiles of success* (Boston: IHRSA).

- Nutrition
- Apparel sales
- Special paid programming
- Massage services
- Kids' clubs (child minding)
- Tanning

Some areas of differentiation may not be profit centers, but they are almost all cost centers that require an increased level of evaluation to ensure they are operating in the most efficient manner possible. As such, fitness operators today may operate 5 to 10 different cost or profit centers within their facilities, each requiring a different level of expertise.

Management of Multiple Profit Centers

The management of multiple profit centers within a fitness facility requires an operator to use consistent terminology and identify fixed and variable costs. Before evaluation can occur, subjective evaluations must be determined for the fixed and variable costs associated with that profit center. Management capital may be attributed to operating a profit center. This section will evaluate the different types of profit centers, focusing on both possible financial returns and management costs.

Juice Bars

The incorporation of a juice bar or other food and beverage component into the operation of a fitness center followed a trend explosion in the 1980s alongside the growth of the fast-food industry across North America. Consumers would often request that fitness operators provide beverages or other nutritional products, which eventually led to the evolution of the juice bar. In addition to juice, sandwiches, and other such products, fitness operators would also often provide nutritional or supplement products.

Juice bars became a point of differentiation and a selling feature used by fitness facilities to attract new members. This evolution continued as operators looked for branded offerings, including franchises. These franchise offerings often resulted in a significant increase in sales per square foot because of members' acceptance of the brand and interest in the products.

Many fitness operators complain that a food service operation is one of the most difficult to operate within a fitness facility. It is not uncommon for such operations to require hundreds of stock-keeping units (SKUs) for selling food and beverages. In addition to the large inventory that is required, staffing is also usually difficult to manage. Regulations for the operation of food services also place further restrictions on the operator of the fitness facility to ensure the proper and profitable operation of the profit center.

The primary evaluation reports used in profit and loss statements on a gross margin and net income basis, including a provision for rent, are as follows:

- Weekly or monthly food costs
- Weekly or monthly labor costs

A trend appears to be growing in the fitness industry whereby operators are outsourcing the operation of their food and beverage services to third-party operators. In many cases, the third-party operators are coordinated through franchise companies who are able to offer a branded product and, as a result of doing higher sales, are able to pay a higher rent to the operator. Thus, many operators are finding they are able to generate more income with fewer requirements for capital.

Group Exercise

Group exercise is generally offered in fitness clubs as an included service. Some classes are often on a drop-in or fee-for-service basis. As such, this section will provide comments on both.

Although many fitness facilities offer some or all group exercise classes as included in the membership fee, the vast majority of facilities do not evaluate them based on performance or on return on investment. As a cost center, a free group exercise program may cost an operator 5% to 10% of the overall operating costs of the facility. These costs should be controlled and funds should be expended in such a way as to generate the highest return on investment for the operator. Although returns may not be quantified in terms of profit, the more people who take advantage of the service, the more likely those people are to maintain their membership and refer others, all of which will increase memberships and reduce attrition.

In the last 10 years, there has been a movement to adopt prechoreographed group exercise programs. These programs provide choreographed classes, including music, which allows operators to outsource the development and management of programs. The classes are generally developed to appeal to a wider range of participants, thus increasing interest in the programs. However, training instructors is often a challenge for fitness operators given labor shortages in these areas.

The primary selling feature of group exercise programs is the increased number of participants who attend group fitness classes, thus generating a greater return on investment. Evaluation techniques include the following reports:

1. Cost per participant. This calculation takes into consideration the cost of providing the class divided by the number of participants in each class. Operators are encouraged to track the number of participants in each class and then use this information to track and trend classes in order to eliminate nonperforming classes and reward instructors who have high-performing classes.
2. Average number of participants per class.
3. Average number of participants per instructor.

Both the second and third evaluation methods encourage the operator to focus on which classes are successful and which classes need to be revamped based on instructor or class. These results will skew based on time of day, club location, and so on; as such, they should not be the definitive method used to evaluate classes.

Case Studies

This section explores case studies of programs offered within existing fitness facilities and how the programs can be evaluated to determine efficacy and membership retention. By collecting pertinent information, management can apply this data to improve program implementation and create innovative ways to stimulate business growth.

Case Study: Group Exercise Evaluation   The membership of a specific fitness facility will determine the number and type of group exercise classes offered. It is important to take into consideration the average age of the membership for that specific location, patterns in traffic, and past participation rates.

In evaluating group exercise programs, it is essential to track the total number of classes taught per week, the total number of participants per club, and the percentage of participation based on class **capacity.** By tracking this information, the cost per participant can be determined. In tracking the average cost, you may determine the minimum cost per participant if and when the class is at 100% capacity. Capacity is based on room size and amount of equipment available. Figure 17.5 outlines three different measurement devices used for evaluating the success of a group exercise program.

Case Study: Personal Training Evaluation   In evaluating the effectiveness of a personal training program, it is necessary to compare the return on investment with the intrinsic value of the program. Fitness

	January	February	March
1. How much does the class cost per person?			
Total participants	5,993	5,460	6,001
Total program costs	$15,270.50	$14,537.00	$15,626.00
Cost per participant	$2.55	$2.66	$2.60
2. How full is the class?			
Maximum capacity	30	30	30
Average class attendance	17.7	16.8	17.4
Percent of maximum class participation	59%	56%	58%
3. What is the participation?			
Total number of visits that participated in a group exercise class each month	5,993	5,452	6,001
Total club attendance (the total visits for each month)	82,817	78,602	89,840
Group exercise participation as a % of total attendance (participation divided by total attendance)	7.2%	6.9%	6.6%

Figure 17.5 Three measurement devices that evaluate the success of a group exercise program.

facilities will often offer a personal training program on a break-even basis or at the risk of losing revenue simply because the intrinsic value of the program contributes to overall membership retention.

When evaluating the return on investment for a personal training program, the accrued gross margin should maintain at least a 30% contribution rate for the program to provide any return to the company. Depending on how the program is offered

(for example, whether training sessions are offered on a pay-per-service delivery or pay-per-session basis), **bad debt,** or outstanding fees collected on a monthly or per session basis, must also be taken into account before calculating the gross margin contribution rate. See figure 17.6 for a personal training accrual statement.

A personal training program must be evaluated by considering a number of **key performance**

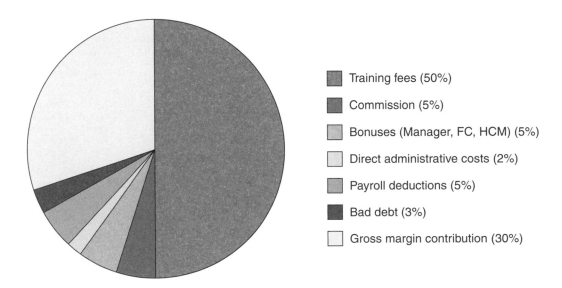

- Training fees (50%)
- Commission (5%)
- Bonuses (Manager, FC, HCM) (5%)
- Direct administrative costs (2%)
- Payroll deductions (5%)
- Bad debt (3%)
- Gross margin contribution (30%)

Figure 17.6 Sample business model for personal training.

indicators (KPIs). For instance, has the trainer maintained an average minimum number of hours of training per day? Has the trainer renewed a certain percentage of clients? Has the trainer recruited a certain number of new clients? Individual evaluation indicates consistency of service across the personal training program as a whole and ensures success of the program through maintenance of quality of service. See Key Performance Indicators for Personal Trainers for a sample form.

Personal training is one of the best ways to retain membership while providing clients with results-based training. A trainer's service allows for the success of members and is more likely to lengthen the life span of a membership. Having trainers on the facility floor also improves the overall optics of the facility—trainers are more apt to keep the gym floor in order and operative, and they are able to maintain the value of the overall facility by providing staff presence.

Advent of Technology

The sophistication of the fitness industry has increased significantly with the advent of various new technologies. As more facilities add computer

---

Key Performance Indicators for Personal Trainers

Personal trainer: _____

Month: _____

	Yes	No
1. Trainer has performed 5 hours minimum (on average) of training per day.	❑	❑
2. Trainer has attended and was on time for all appointments and staff meetings and the monthly review meeting.	❑	❑
3. Trainer has thoroughly completed all paperwork and tracking forms this month and submitted them on time.	❑	❑
4. For every day that the trainer hasn't had at least 7 appointments, the trainer has done the required member assistance and passed the names of the members on to the club manager.	❑	❑
5. Trainer has had 10% or less of their scheduled appointments not show this month. If there were more no-shows than this, trainer has called appointments.	❑	❑
6. Trainer renewed a minimum of 70% of clients who came up for renewal this month. If not, trainer placed follow-up calls with these clients to check progress, encourage renewals, and get referrals.	❑	❑
7. Trainer has received and closed at least 2 referrals from existing clients.	❑	❑
8. Trainer has worn the complete club uniform every day worked this month.	❑	❑
9. If the trainer is not completely full, has sold packages to 20% of training demos.	❑	❑
10. Trainer has recruited a minimum of 2 clients off the floor.	❑	❑
11. Trainer has handed out client satisfaction survey to at least 80% of active clients (and manager has received these from the clients).	❑	❑
12. Trainer has worked a minimum of 40 hours per week (in appointments, doing member assistance, doing follow-up calls—not working out).	❑	❑
13. Manager has not received any complaints about the trainer from members.	❑	❑

Trainer will receive 10 points for each indicator to which yes has been answered. Trainer is expected to receive a minimum score of 80% on the KPIs.

Personal trainer (signature): _____

Personal trainer coordinator (signature): _____

Date: _____

From M. Bates, 2008, *Health Fitness Management*, 2nd ed. (Champaign, IL: Human Kinetics).

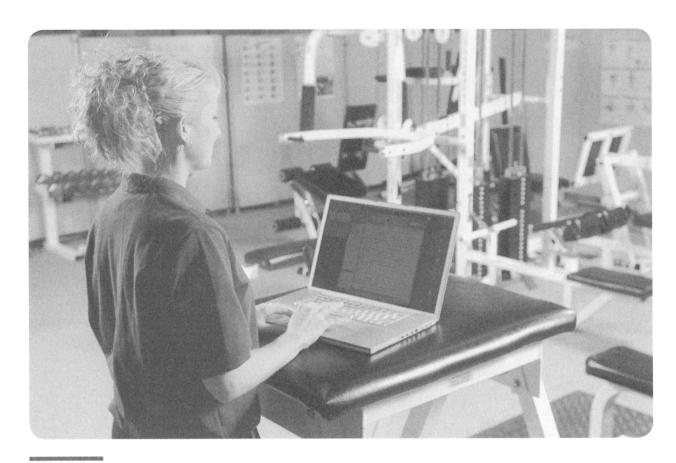

Evaluating your facility will be made easier by using a computer system to track member activity and services.

systems that allow tracking of member activity and services, managers are able to use this information to evaluate trends and anticipate opportunities.

There are a number of fully integrated software programs that allow operators to track almost every area of their business. Functionality among software products varies; however, management services typically include the following abilities, which all have advanced evaluation or reporting standards:

- Membership management and tracking
- Prospect management tracking and scheduling
- Sales-lead tracking and custom contracts
- Front-desk and check-in solutions
- Workout manager for member fitness tracking
- Data entry for information management
- Performance reporting for club management
- Health club business modeling with artificial intelligence

- Billing and accounting system
- Cash or financial accrual reporting
- Payroll and commission modeling
- Collections solution for overdue payments

Increased Activity by Private Investors and Public Markets

The final aspect of the fitness industry evolution is the increased activity by private investment groups and the public markets in this sector. Listed in "What a Year!" are a number of significant transactions that have occurred between 2003 and 2005 that show the increased interest of the public market and the banking sectors.

With billions of dollars being attracted to this industry, club sophistication is increasing to keep pace with the demands of the investment community. Investors are looking for more sophisticated operators and as such are putting pressure on the entire industry to squeeze more juice out of the orange, so to speak.

What a Year!

John McCarthy, executive director of IHRSA in 2005, summarized the record-breaking sales, brand expansions, and impressive metrics that made 2005 memorable.

- The sale of 24 Hour Fitness Worldwide, Inc., to Forstmann Little for $1.6 billion, approximately 9 times EBITDA (earnings before interest, taxes, depreciation, and amortization).
- The sale of Fitness First to BC Partners, Ltd., for $1.5 billion (approximately 8.5 times EBITDA).
- The sale of LA Fitness, the U.K.-based chain, to Mid Ocean Partners for $158 million (approximately 6.9 times EBITDA).
- The sale, by Bally Total Fitness (NYSE: BTF), of its Crunch brand to Sports and Fitness Ventures, LLC, for $45 million.
- The sale, by Bridgepoint Capital, of its 55% stake in Virgin Active, for $235.6 million to Sir Richard Branson, who plans to accelerate the chain's expansion in the Far East.
- The Sports Club Company (SCC) agrees to sell its East Coast operations to Millenium Partners.
- The launch of Town Sports International's (TSI's) initial public offering (IPO).
- Curves International surpasses 8,000 franchises.
- TRT Holdings moves to transform Gold's Gym International, Inc. (GGI), into a flagship franchise organization.
- Life Time Fitness, Inc. (NYSE: LTM), consistently trades at 30 times earnings, with a market cap of more than $1.2 billion.
- Marriott International teams up with Leisure Sports, Inc., to build 15 sports resorts.
- The industry is awash in new, fast-growing, fitness-franchise operations, such as Cuts, It Figures, Fitness 19, 1-2-3 Fit, Anytime Fitness, Planet Fitness, etc.
- Midsize companies—such as XSport, In-Shape, Spectrum Clubs, Lifestyle Family Fitness, and Gold's Utah, Gold's TKO, and Gold's Galiani Group—press the "pedal to the metal" and accelerate expansion.
- LA Fitness, the U.S.-based chain, tops 150 wholly owned sites and accelerates its growth in the northeast corridor.
- Bally updates its financial statements and refocuses on building its brand.
- The industry raises $1.2 million for the Muscular Dystrophy Association (MDA) in just three hours with "Augie's Quest," a charitable initiative created by Augie Nieto, the founder and past president and CEO of Life Fitness.
- Jerry Noyce's Health Fitness Corporation (OTC: HFIT) tops 400 units.
- David Patchell-Evans' Goodlife Group reaches 110 units in Canada.
- Tony de Leede masterminds Fitness First's impressive Australian rollout.
- Bally moves into China aggressively.
- The U.S. health club industry tops 28,500 commercial fitness centers.
- The U.S. health club industry tops 41.3 million members.
- The global health club industry tops 85 million members.

2005—what a year!

Reprinted, by permission, from IHRSA, 2005, "What a year!" *Club Business International*, Dec. 2005: 100.

KEY TERMS

bad debt

brand awareness

capacity

formative evaluation

key performance indicator (KPI)

preordinate evaluation models

primary data

primary trading area

process evaluation models

profit centers

quantitative research

qualitative research

secondary data

summative evaluation

total quality management (TQM)

REFERENCES AND RECOMMENDED READINGS

Association for Fitness in Business. 1992. *Guidelines for employee health promotion programs.* Champaign, IL: Human Kinetics.

International Health, Racquet, and Sportsclub Association (IHRSA). 2006. *U.S. health club facility growth 1995-2005.* Boston: IHRSA.

McCarthy, J. 2002. *Evaluating a loan or investment proposal.* Boston: IHRSA.

Looking Toward the Future

Each year numerous industry publications and experts weigh in on where they feel the fitness industry is going. Although there are many different approaches to this, most experts agree on a core group of trends that will affect the industry. As you prepare for your career in the fitness industry, it is critical that you are not only aware of what is happening now but that you are also aware of what is going to happen in the future. The trends we will identify here are not listed in any particular order.

• *Continued popularity of group fitness.* Group training has been popular for many years, and we see no reason why this will change. Group fitness has changed over the years in terms of what is offered in various facilities, but the underlying group dynamics have not. Groups meet the social demands of many members and have been shown to have higher retention rates than activities where the individual is the focus.

One of the major changes that has occurred in the group fitness studio is a move toward a student-centered experience as opposed to one that is teacher centered. In a student-centered environment, the teacher's focus is on all of the participants and what the teacher can do to help each participant have the best experience possible. In the past, on the other hand, the focus may have been on the instructor getting a workout or competing with participants in the front row, while the first-time exerciser was lost in the back of the room and most likely did not return.

Group training can be applied to just about any activity within a health and fitness setting. The list of potential group activities is endless and is entirely up to your imagination and discretion. A few examples are as follows:

- Group exercise classes (e.g., Pilates, yoga, step, kickboxing, stretching)
- Group personal training
- Specialized programming (e.g., running clubs, Women on Weights)
- Nutritional groups
- New-member orientation groups
- Weight-loss groups

• *Expansion of mind–body programming.* This is another area that has been popular for quite a few years now, and we see no reason why it will slow down. Mind–body programming can be described as "activities that offer an inward, meditative state as one of their activities" (Brehm 2006).Yoga and Pilates are the most popular forms of mind–body programming, but this approach can be included as part of most exercise programs. That is, the entire session doesn't have to focus on this one area. A traditional group aerobics class can incorporate mind–body principles when the instructor focuses the participants on breathing and asks them to relax and become aware of their bodies. Some of the reasons why these types of classes are so important are as follows:

- There is a connection between the mind and the body, and including a holistic point of view shows that we are aware of the mental and physical sides of exercise.
- The spiritual component is attractive for many people. This is evident in activities like yoga and tai chi. Although these disciplines do not ask people to follow a specific religion, they do have certain moral values like integrity and respect for others.

- A strong therapeutic value is associated with many of these activities. Some of these benefits include reduced stress, improved posture, and overall body mechanics. Health benefits are similar to those of regular exercise.
- The perceived calmness of the exercises may be attractive because the activities are seen as less stressful than lifting weights or jogging on a treadmill.

• *Increased emphasis on management expertise.* As you have seen throughout this text, running a fitness club is like running any other business. It requires all the management and business expertise that any other business requires. The difference is that now the fitness industry understands this. Clubs that do not have this type of expertise will need to get trained in the area or hire people who can come in and contribute right away. As more clubs open and others expand, the most successful clubs will be the ones with strong management personnel who not only have a passion for fitness but also understand financial, human resources, sales, marketing, and operational concerns. The days of fitness enthusiasts running clubs and getting by simply on their passion for the field are long gone. Passion is still a key criterion for success, but it is no longer the only one.

• *Shift in focus from gaining new members to retention.* The concept of member retention has been around for a while, and if you look at the topics at the various fitness conferences it is usually a common one. The reality is that as an industry we are still not very good at keeping the members we have. The greater focus is still placed on generating new memberships even though we all know that it is more expensive to get a new member than to keep one you already have. Unfortunately, there are not a lot of good data on this topic since few clubs are actually tracking this number. The clubs that do track this number are often the ones that excel at retention, and this artificially inflates the industrywide data.

Recent industry data from IHRSA show that there have been increases in this area, but as we have already stated, there is such a small number of respondents to these research questionnaires that it is not realistic to say that it represents the entire industry. These numbers should be used as benchmarks of the most successful clubs. Most large club chains will tell you that their retention levels have improved, but few of them will share specific numbers for competitive reasons. Our experience is that clubs do not consistently do enough in this area and they rarely have a specific game plan to address retention. The tracking of retention would be a great start for many clubs because it would open their eyes to the real numbers and the members they are losing.

• *Increased demand for personal training.* This continues to be one of the fastest-growing areas within the industry. As clubs struggle to find qualified personal trainers due to demand outpacing supply in most areas, the general public is becoming more aware of what personal trainers do and the benefits of these services. Postsecondary institutions continue to expand their curricula in these areas, and certification organizations continue to expand as more people look to get into the field.

• *Move toward niche marketing.* As larger clubs gain control in the market, the only way for smaller clubs to thrive is to fine-tune their operations and focus on specific parts of the marketplace. A few examples of niche clubs are those for

- baby boomers,
- sport conditioning,
- youth training,
- older adults,
- boutique-style clubs, and
- personal training–only studios.

• *Increased awareness of the sedentary audience.* The fitness industry will continue to attract this portion of the market. Few clubs have taken the necessary steps to attract this crowd, even though this is the largest portion of the marketplace. The traditional advertising, hiring, and training practices and programming options within most clubs do not meet the needs of this group, which makes up anywhere from 70% to 80% of the population depending on the study and parameter you are looking at.

• *Political lobbying.* The fitness industry in many countries is now organized on a national and international level. This level of organization allows the industry to be at the decision-making table when governments are making decisions about new laws and changes to existing laws. In the past, the fitness industry has reacted to changes in the laws that have affected them. Unfortunately, these reactions have come too late and have had little impact. The industry is now in a position to take a stance on certain topics, make proposals for changes, and actually be invited to the table when decisions are being made. One of the issues the industry is currently working on is the tax deductibility of fitness club memberships.

- *Health care costs and insurability.* As major U.S. corporations try to deal with the aging population and the effect this is having on their health care benefits, many businesses are looking to wellness programs as a proactive measure to decrease their costs. Progressive fitness companies are working with businesses and insurance providers to include fitness club memberships as part of a company's benefits package. There are also some insurance companies that offer discounted rates to people who exercise on a regular basis.

- *More functional training equipment.* You can't sit in a personal training session recently without hearing the term *functional training.* Essentially, these are exercises that mimic the activities a person does throughout the day. Functional exercises are about helping people maximize their body mechanics, as opposed to traditional fitness equipment, which is more focused on appearance. We refer to traditional equipment as *machine defined* and functional equipment as *user defined.* Cables are usually referred to as *user defined* when they are not guided entirely by the machine. That is, the person should be free to move the cable in various directions and not be restricted by the direction that the machine defines. We will see more user-defined or functional training equipment in the marketplace in the coming years. As consumers are educated on this type of equipment, they will expect their clubs to keep up with their needs.

In summary, the industry will continue to evolve as it has over the past few decades. Some trends will turn into fads and will quickly disappear, and others will be here to stay. As a successful manager, it is critical that you stay on top of industry trends so that you can meet the needs of your current and future members.

REFERENCES AND RECOMMENDED READING

Brehm, B. 2006. Why mind/body exercise? Retrieved May 3, 2007, from www.fitnessmanagement.com/FM/tmpl/genPage.asp?p=/information/articles/library/lab-notes/labnotes0806.html.

index

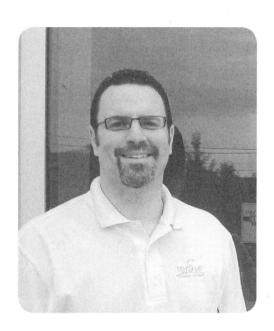

Mike Bates is the owner of Refine Fitness Studio located in Windsor, Ontario. Bates is also a lecturer at the University of Windsor, teaching courses in sport management, human resource management, and strength and conditioning. He coordinates and teaches personal training and sports conditioning certification courses and is a regular speaker at IHRSA, Can-Fit-Pro, and Club Industry. He was also the Managing Director of Human Kinetics Canada from 1999–2007. Bates holds a BHK and an MBA from the University of Windsor.

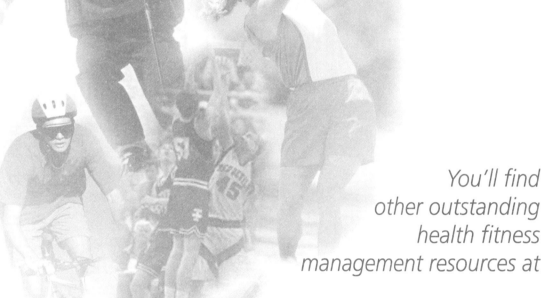

*You'll find
other outstanding
health fitness
management resources at*

www.HumanKinetics.com

In the U.S. call

1-800-747-4457

Australia...08 8372 0999
Canada 1-800-465-7301
Europe..+44 (0) 113 255 5665
New Zealand......................................0064 9 448 1207

HUMAN KINETICS
The Information Leader in Physical Activity
P.O. Box 5076 • Champaign, IL 61825-5076 USA